D1766030

Psychiatric Diagnosis
and Classification

Psychiatric Diagnosis and Classification

Edited by

Mario Maj
University of Naples, Italy

Wolfgang Gaebel
University of Düsseldorf, Germany

Juan José López-Ibor
Complutense University of Madrid, Spain

Norman Sartorius
University of Geneva, Switzerland

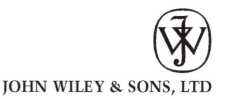

JOHN WILEY & SONS, LTD

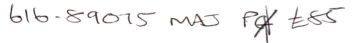

Other Wiley Editorial Offices

John Wiley & Sons, Inc., 605 Third Avenue,
New York, NY 10158-0012, USA

WILEY-VCH Verlag GmbH, Pappelallee 3,
D-69469 Weinheim, Germany

John Wiley & Sons Australia, Ltd., 33 Park Road, Milton,
Queensland 4064, Australia

John Wiley & Sons (Asia) Pte, Ltd., 2 Clementi Loop #02-01,
Jin Xing Distripark, Singapore 129809

John Wiley & Sons (Canada), Ltd., 22 Worcester Road,
Rexdale, Ontario M9W IL1, Canada

Library of Congress Cataloging-in-Publication Data

Psychiatric diagnosis and classification / edited by Mario Maj . . . [et al.].
    p. cm.
    ''Based in part on presentations delivered at the 11th World Congress of Psychiatry
    (Hamburg, Germany, August 6–11, 1999)''
    Includes bibliographical references and index.
    ISBN 0-471-49681-2 (cased)
    1. Mental illness—Diagnosis—Congresses. 2. Mental illness—Classification—Congresses.
    I. Maj, Mario, *1953*–II. World Congress of Psychiatry (11th: 1999: Hamburg, Germany)

    RC469. P762 2002
    616.89'075—dc21

                                                                        2001057370

British Library Cataloguing in Publication Data

A catalogue record for this book is available from the British Library

ISBN 0-471-49681-2

Typeset in 10/12pt Palatino by Kolam Information Services Private Ltd, Pondicherry, India
Printed and bound in Great Britain by TJ International Ltd, Padstow, Cornwall, UK
This book is printed on acid-free paper responsibly manufactured from sustainable forestry,
in which at least two trees are planted for each one used for paper production.

Contents

Contributors

Gavin Andrews *School of Psychiatry, University of New South Wales at St. Vincent's Hospital, 299 Forbes Street, Darlinghurst, NSW 2010, Australia*

Somnath Chatterji *Classification, Assessment, Surveys and Terminology, Department of Evidence for Health Policy, World Health Organization, Geneva, Switzerland*

C. Robert Cloninger *Department of Psychiatry, Washington University School of Medicine, Campus Box 8134, 660 S.Euclid, St. Louis, Missouri 63110–1093, USA*

Jean-Marc Cloos *Centre Hospitalier de Luxembourg, 4, rue Barblé, L-1210 Luxembourg*

Horacio Fabrega Jr. *Department of Psychiatry, University of Pittsburgh, 3811 O'Hara Street, Pittsburgh, PA 15213, USA*

Michael First *NYS Psychiatric Institute, 1051 Riverside Drive, New York, NY 10032, USA*

David Goldberg *Institute of Psychiatry, King's College, London, UK*

Assen Jablensky *University Department of Psychiatry and Behavioural Science, University of Western Australia, MRF Building, Level 3, 50 Murray Street, Perth, WA 6000, Australia*

Aleksandar Janca *Department of Psychiatry and Behavioural Science, University of Western Australia, Perth, Australia*

Marianne C. Kastrup *International Rehabilitation and Research Center for Torture Victims, Copenhagen, Denmark*

Robert E. Kendell *University Department of Psychiatry and Behavioural Science, University of Western Australia, MRF Building, Level 3, 50 Murray Street, Perth, WA 6000, Australia*

Tina Marshall *Division of Research, American Psychiatric Association, 1400 K Street N.W., Washington, DC 20005, USA*

Juan E. Mezzich *Division of Psychiatric Epidemiology and International Center for Mental Health, Mount Sinai School of Medicine of New York University, New York, USA*

R. Srinivasa Murthy *National Institute of Mental Health, Department of Psychiatry and Neuroscience, Post Bag 2900, Bangalore 56002-9, India*

William E. Narrow *Division of Research, American Psychiatric Association, 1400 K Street N.W., Washington, DC 20005, USA*

Josef Parnas *Department of Psychiatry, Hvidovre Hospital, Brondbyoestervej 160, 2650 Hvidovre, Denmark*

Charles B. Pull *Centre Hospitalier de Luxembourg, 4, rue Barblé, L-1210 Luxembourg*

Marie-Claire Pull-Erpelding *Centre OMS Francophone de Formation et de Référence, 4, rue Barblé, L-1210 Luxembourg*

Darrel A. Regier *American Psychiatric Institute for Research and Education, 1400 K Street N.W., Washington, DC 20005, USA*

Greg Simon *Center for Health Studies, Group Health Cooperative, 1730 Minor Ave. #1600, Seattle, WA 98101–1448, USA*

T. Bedirhan Üstün *Classification, Assessment, Surveys and Terminology, Department of Evidence for Health Policy, World Health Organization, Geneva, Switzerland*

Narendra N. Wig *Postgraduate Institute of Medical Education and Research, Chandigarh 160012, India*

Dan Zahavi *Danish Institute for Advanced Studies in the Humanities, Vimmelskaflet 41 A, DK-1161 Copenhagen K, Denmark*

Preface

The next editions of the two main systems for the diagnosis and classification of mental disorders, the ICD and the DSM, are not expected before the year 2010. The most frequently alleged reasons for this long interval are: (1) the satisfaction with the performance of the systems as they are now, since they are achieving their goals of improving communication among clinicians and ensuring comparability of research findings; (2) the concern that frequent revisions of diagnostic systems may undermine their assimilation by clinicians, damage the credibility of our discipline, and hamper the progress of research (by making the comparison between old and new data more difficult, impeding the collection of large patient samples, and requiring a ceaseless update of diagnostic interviews and algorithms); (3) the presentiment that we are on the eve of major research breakthroughs, which may have a significant impact on nosology. There is a further reason, however, for the current hesitation to produce a new edition of the above diagnostic systems, which is seldom made explicit, but is probably not the least important: i.e. the gradually spreading perception that there may have been something incorrect in the assumptions put forward by the neo-Kraepelinian movement at the beginning of the 1970s, which have guided the development of the modern generation of diagnostic systems.

That current diagnostic categories really correspond to discrete natural disease entities is appearing now more and more questionable. Psychiatric "comorbidity", i.e. the coexistence of two or more psychiatric diagnoses in the same individual, seems today the rule rather than the exception. Thirty years of biological research have not been able to identify a specific marker for any of the current diagnostic categories (and genetic research is now providing evidence for the possible existence of vulnerability loci which are common to schizophrenia and bipolar disorder). Also the therapeutic profile of newly developed psychotropic drugs clearly crosses old and new diagnostic boundaries (e.g. new generation antipsychotics appear to be as effective in schizophrenia and in bipolar disorder, and new generation antidepressants are effective in all the various disorders identified by current classification systems in the old realm of neuroses).

The fact that current diagnostic categories are unlikely to correspond to discrete natural disease entities has been taken as evidence that the neo-Kraepelinian (or neo-Pinelian) model was intrinsically faulty, i.e. that psychopathology does not consist of discrete disease entities. This has been recently maintained from several different perspectives, including the psychodynamic [1], the biological [2], the characterological [3], and the evolutionary [4] ones. Of note, Kraepelin himself, in his late years, questioned the validity of the "discrete disease" model, by stating that "Many manifestations of insanity are shaped decisively by man's preformed mechanisms of reaction" and that "The affective and schizophrenic forms of mental disorder do not represent the expression of particular pathological processes, but rather indicate the areas of our personality in which these processes unfold" [5].

A second possibility, however, is that psychopathology does consist of discrete disease entities, but that these entities are not reflected by current diagnostic categories. If this is the case, then current clinical research on "comorbidity" may be helpful in the search for "true" disease entities, leading in the long term to a rearrangement of present classifications, which may either involve a simplification (e.g. a single disease entity may underlie the apparent comorbidity of major depression, social phobia and panic disorder) or a further complication (e.g. different disease entities may correspond to major depression with panic disorder, major depression with obsessive-compulsive disorder, etc.) or possibly a simplification in some areas of classification and a further complication in other areas.

There is, nevertheless, a third possibility: that the nature of psychopathology is intrinsically heterogeneous, consisting in part of true disease entities and in part of reaction types or maladaptive response patterns. This is what Jaspers [6] actually suggested when he distinguished between "true diseases", like general paresis, which have clear boundaries among themselves and with normality; "circles", like manic-depressive insanity and schizophrenia, which have clear boundaries with normality but not among themselves; and "types", like neuroses and abnormal personalities, which do not have clear boundaries either among themselves or with normality. Recently, it has been pointed out [7] that throughout medicine there are diseases arising from a defect in the body's machinery and diseases arising from a dysregulation of defenses. If this is true also for mental disorders, i.e. if a condition like bipolar disorder is a disease arising from a defect in the brain machinery, whereas conditions like anxiety disorders, or part of them, arise from a dysregulation of defenses, then different classification strategies may be needed for the various areas of psychopathology.

The present volume reflects the above developments and uncertainties in the field of psychiatric diagnosis and classification. It provides a survey of the strengths and limitations of current diagnostic systems and an overview of various perspectives about how these systems can be improved in the future. It is hoped that, at least for the eight years to come, the book will be of some usefulness to the many clinicians and researchers around the

world who are interested in the future of psychiatric diagnosis and classification.

Mario Maj
Wolfgang Gaebel
Juan José López-Ibor
Norman Sartorius

REFERENCES

1. Cloninger C.R., Martin R.L., Guze S.B., Clayton P.J. (1990) The empirical structure of psychiatric comorbidity and its theoretical significance. In: *Comorbidity of
   Mood and Anxiety Disorders* (Eds J.D. Maser, C.R. Cloninger), pp. 439–498. American Psychiatric Press, Washington.
2. van Praag H.M. (1996) Functional psychopathology: an essential diagnostic step
   in biological psychiatric research. In: *Implications of Psychopharmacology to Psychiatry* (Eds M. Ackenheil, B. Bondy, R. Engel, M. Ermann, N. Nedopil), pp.
   79–88. Springer, Berlin.
3. Cloninger C.R. (1999) *Personality and Psychopathology*. American Psychiatric
   Press, Washington.
4. McGuire M., Troisi A. (1998) *Darwinian Psychiatry*. Oxford University Press, New
   York.
5. Kraepelin E. (1920) Die Erscheinungsformen des Irreseins. *Z. ges. Neurol. Psy-
   chiat.*, **62**: 1–29.
6. Jaspers K. (1959) *Allgemeine Psychopathologie*. Springer, Berlin.
7. Nesse R. M. (2000) Is depression an adaptation? *Arch. Gen. Psychiatry*, **57**: 14–20.

This volume is based in part on presentations delivered at the 11th World
Congress of Psychiatry (Hamburg, Germany, 6–11 August 1999)

1

Criteria for Assessing a Classification in Psychiatry

Assen Jablensky and Robert E. Kendell

Department of Psychiatry and Behavioural Science, University of Western Australia, Perth, Australia

INTRODUCTION

Three decades after the introduction of explicit diagnostic criteria and, subsequently, rule-based classifications such as DSM-III [1], DSM-III-R [2], ICD-10 [3] and DSM-IV [4], it should be possible to examine the impact of these tools on psychiatric nosology. The worldwide propagation of the new classification systems has resulted in profound changes affecting at least four domains of professional practice. First and foremost, a standard frame of reference has been made available to clinicians, enabling them to achieve better diagnostic agreement and improve communication, including the statistical reporting on psychiatric morbidity, services, treatments and outcomes. Secondly, more rigorous diagnostic standards and instruments have become the norm in psychiatric research. Although the majority of the research diagnostic criteria are still provisional, they can now be refined or rejected using empirical evidence. Thirdly, the teaching of psychiatry to medical students, trainee psychiatrists and other mental health workers is now based on an international reference system which, while reducing diversity due to local tradition, provides a much needed "common language" to the discipline worldwide. Fourthly, open access to the criteria used by mental health professionals in making a diagnosis has helped improve communication with the users of services, carers, and the public at large, by demystifying psychiatric diagnosis and making its logic transparent to non-professionals.

While acknowledging such gains, it is important to examine critically the current versions of standardized diagnostic criteria and rule-based classification systems in psychiatry for conceptual and methodological shortcomings. At present, the discipline of psychiatry is in a state of flux. Advances in

Psychiatric Diagnosis and Classification. Edited by Mario Maj, Wolfgang Gaebel, Juan José López-Ibor and Norman Sartorius. © 2002 John Wiley & Sons, Ltd.

neuroscience and genetics are setting new, interdisciplinary agendas for psychiatric research and the results to be expected within the next few decades are likely to affect profoundly the theoretical basis of psychiatry, in particular the understanding of the nature and causation of mental disorders. New treatments targeting specific functional systems in the brain will require more refined definitions of the clinical populations likely to benefit from them than is possible at present. Even more importantly, the realization that, in all societies, mental disorders contribute a much larger burden of disease than previously assumed [5] will raise critical questions about cost-benefit, equity, right to treatment, and feasibility of prevention.

The conjunction of these powerful factors is likely to have major implications for the future of psychiatric classification as a conceptual scaffold of the discipline. There is little doubt that the classification of mental disorders will undergo changes whose direction and extent are at present difficult to predict. Although the prevailing view is that an overhaul of the existing classification systems will only be warranted when an accumulated "critical mass" of new knowledge makes change imperative, processes aiming at revisions are already under way and the debates about the future shape of DSM and ICD are gathering momentum. In the light of this, a discussion of the basic principles and "rules of the game" should be timely. Of course, the complexity of the subject makes it unlikely that any sort of quality assessment checklist will soon emerge and become generally accepted in reviewing new proposals. Nevertheless, a step in that direction is needed if further progress in consolidating the scientific base of the discipline is to be achieved.

GENERAL FEATURES OF CLASSIFICATIONS

To clear the ground, we review briefly certain terms and concepts relevant to the subsequent discussion of specific aspects of classification in psychiatry.

Why Do We Wish To Classify? Purposes and Functions of Classifications

The term classification denotes "the activity of ordering or arrangement of objects into groups or sets on the basis of their relationships" [6]; in other words, it is the process of *synthesizing* categories out of the raw material of sensory data. Modern cognitive science is echoing Kant: "the spontaneity of our thought requires that what is manifold in the pure intuition should first be in a certain way examined, received and connected, in order to produce knowledge of it. This act I call synthesis" [7]. The recognition of similarities and the ordering of objects into sets on the basis of relationships is thus a fundamental cognitive activity underlying concept formation and naming. This activity is present at every level, ranging from the child's acquisition of cognitive maps of the surrounding world, through coping with everyday life, to the development of a scientific theory [8]. Research into the cognitive psychology of daily living has highlighted the computational intricacies of so-called natural, or "folk" categorization systems which people intuitively use to classify objects [9]. Such systems provide for economy of memory (or "reduction of the cognitive load"); enable the manipulation of objects by simplifying the relationships among them; and generate hypotheses and predictions.

Classification, Taxonomy, Nomenclature

Classification in science, including medicine, can be defined as the "procedure for constructing groups or categories and for assigning entities (disorders or persons) to these categories on the basis of their shared attributes or relations" [10]. The act of assigning a particular object to one of the categories is *identification* (in medical practice this is diagnostic identification). Diagnosis and classification are interrelated: choosing a diagnostic label usually presupposes some ordered system of possible labels, and a classification is the arrangement of such labels in accordance with certain specified principles and rules. The term *taxonomy*, often used as a synonym for classification, should refer properly to the metatheory of classification, including the systematic study of the various strategies of classifying. In medicine, the corresponding term *nosology* denotes the system of concepts and theories that supports the strategy of classifying symptoms, signs, syndromes and diseases, whereas *nosography* refers to the act of assigning names to diseases; the names jointly constitute the *nomenclature* within a particular field of medicine.

Taxonomic Philosophies and Strategies

The classical taxonomic strategy, exemplified by grand systems of classification in the natural sciences such as the Linnaean systematics of plants or the Darwinian evolutionary classification of species, assumes that *substances* (i.e. robust entities that remain the same in spite of change in their attributes) exist "out there" in nature. When properly identified by sifting out all accidental characteristics, some such substances reveal themselves as the *phyla* or *species* of living organisms underlying the manifold appearances of nature and thus provide a "natural" classification. In medicine, an essentialist view of diseases as independently existing agents causing illnesses in individuals was proposed by Sydenham in the eighteenth century [11]; its vestiges survive into the present in some interpretations of the notion of "disease entity".

A radically different philosophy of classification evolved more recently in biology as a way out of certain difficulties in applying the Darwinian phyletic principle to the systematics of bacteria and viruses. In contrast to the essentialist strategy, this approach, known as *numerical taxonomy*, shifts the emphasis to the systematic description of the *appearance* of objects (hence the approach is also called *phenetic*) and treats all characters and attributes as having equal weight [6]. Groups are then identified on the basis of the maximum number of shared characteristics using statistical algorithms. An approximation to such a strategy in medical classification would be the empirical grouping of symptoms and signs using cluster or factor analysis.

Another recent taxonomic strategy, based on the analysis of "folk" systems of categories referred to above, is the prototype-matching procedure [12, 13]. In this approach, a category is represented by its *prototype*, i.e. a fuzzy set comprising the most common features or properties displayed by "typical" members of the category. The features describing the prototype need be neither necessary nor sufficient, but they must provide a theoretical ideal against which real individuals or objects can be evaluated. Statistical procedures can be used to compute for any individual or object how closely they match the ideal type.

The taxonomic strategies described above employ different rules for identifying taxon membership. Thus, the classical phyletic strategy presupposes a *monothetic* assignment of membership in which the candidate must meet exactly the set of necessary and sufficient criteria that define a given class. In contrast, both numerical taxonomy and the prototype-matching approach are *polythetic*, in the sense that members of a class "share a large proportion of their properties but do not necessarily agree on the presence of any one property" [6]. The periodic table of the elements, where atomic weight and valence are the only characteristics that are both necessary and sufficient for the ordering of the entire chemical universe, is a pure example of a monothetic classification. DSM-IV and ICD-10 research criteria are examples of a polythetic classification where members of a given class share some, but not all, of its defining features.

THE NATURE OF PSYCHIATRIC CLASSIFICATION: CRITIQUE OF THE PRESENT STATE OF NOSOLOGY

No single type of classification fits all purposes. It is unlikely that the principles underlying the classification of chemical elements, or subatomic particles, would be of much help in classifying living organisms or mental illnesses since the objects to be classified in these domains differ in fundamental ways. Medical classifications are created with the primary purpose of meeting pragmatic needs related to diagnosing and treating people experiencing illnesses. Their secondary purpose is to assist in the generation of new knowledge relevant to those needs, though progress in medical research usually precedes, rather than follows, improvements in classification. According to Feinstein [14], medical classifications perform three principal functions: (a) denomination (assigning a common name to a group of phenomena); (b) qualification (enriching the information content of a category by adding relevant descriptive features such as typical symptoms, age at onset, or severity); and (c) prediction (a statement about the expected course and outcome, as well as the likely response to treatment).

As these are the purposes and functions of medical, including psychiatric, classifications, a critical question that is rarely asked is: what is the nature of the entities that are being classified? (Or what are the objects whose properties and relationships psychiatric classifications aim to arrange in a systematic order?)

Units of Classification: Diseases, Disorders or Syndromes?

Simply stating that medical classifications classify *diseases* (or that psychiatric classifications classify *disorders*) begs the question since the status of concepts like "disease" and "disorder" remains obscure. It is unlikely that Sydenham's view of diseases as independent natural entities causing illnesses would find many adherents today. As pointed out by Scadding [11], the concept of "a disease" has evolved with the advance of medical knowledge and, at present, is no more than "a convenient device by which we can refer succinctly to the conclusion of a diagnostic process which starts from recognition of a pattern of symptoms and signs, and proceeds, by investigation of varied extent and complexity, to an attempt to unravel the chain of causation". The diagnostic process in psychiatry has been summarized succinctly by Shepherd *et al.* [15]: "the psychiatrist interviews the patient, and chooses from a system of psychiatric terms a few words or phrases which he uses as a label for the patient, so as to convey to himself and others as much as possible about the aetiology, the immediate manifestations, and the prognosis of the patient's condition." Disease, therefore, is an *explanatory construct* integrating information about: (a) statistical deviance of structure and/or function from the population "norm"; (b) characteristic clinical (including behavioral) manifestations; (c) characteristic pathology; (d) underlying causes; and (e) extent of "harmful dysfunction" or reduced biological fitness. For a constellation of observations to be referred to as "a disease", these parameters must be shown to form a "real-world correlational structure" [16] which is stable and also distinct from other similar structures. This multivariate set of criteria (which can be extended and elaborated further) implies a polythetic definition of the disease concept, i.e. some, but not necessarily all, of the criteria must be met. Two issues are of relevance here. First, the typical progression of knowledge begins with the identification of the clinical manifestations (the *syndrome*) and the deviance from the "norm"; understanding of the pathology and aetiology usually comes much later. Secondly, there is no fixed point or agreed threshold of description beyond which a syndrome can be said to be "a disease". Today, Alzheimer's disease, with dementia as its clinical manifestation, specific brain morphology, tentative pathophysiology, and at least partially understood causes, is one of the few conditions appearing in psychiatric classifications that meet the above criteria. Schizophrenia, however, is still better described as a syndrome.

Thoughtful clinicians are aware that diagnostic categories are simply concepts, justified only by whether or not they provide a useful framework for organizing and explaining the complexity of clinical experience in order to derive predictions about outcome and to guide decisions about treatment. Unfortunately, once a diagnostic concept like schizophrenia has come into general use, it tends to become "reified"—people too easily assume that it is an entity of some kind which can be invoked to explain the patient's symptoms and whose validity need not be questioned. And even though the authors of nomenclatures like DSM-IV may be careful to point out that "there is no assumption that each category of mental disorder is a completely discrete entity with absolute boundaries dividing it from other mental disorders or from no mental disorder" [4], the mere fact that a diagnostic concept is listed in an official nomenclature and provided with a precise operational definition tends to encourage this insidious reification.

For most of the diagnostic rubrics of DSM-IV and ICD-10 (which clearly do not qualify as diseases), both classifications avoid discussing precisely what is being classified. DSM-IV explicitly rejects (presumably to avoid the implication of labeling) the "misconception that a classification of mental disorders classifies people" and states that "actually what are being classified are *disorders* that people have" [4]. The term "disorder", first introduced as a generic name for the unit of classification in DSM-I in 1952, has no clear correspondence with either the concept of disease or the concept of syndrome in medical classifications. It conveniently circumvents the problem that the material from which most of the diagnostic rubrics are constructed consists primarily of reported subjective experiences and patterns of behavior. Some of those rubrics correspond to syndromes in the medical sense, but many appear to be sub-syndromal and reflect isolated symptoms, habitual behaviors, or personality traits.

This ambiguous status of the classificatory unit of "disorder" has two corollaries that may create conceptual confusion and hinder the advancement of knowledge. Firstly, there is the "reification fallacy"—the tendency to view the DSM-IV and ICD-10 "disorders" as quasi-disease entities. Secondly, the fragmentation of psychopathology into a large number of "disorders"—of which many are merely symptoms—leads to a proliferation of comorbid diagnoses which clinicians are forced to use in order to describe their patients. This blurs the important distinction between true comorbidity (co-occurrence of aetiologically independent disorders) and spurious comorbidity masking complex but essentially unitary *syndromes*. It is not surprising, therefore, that recent epidemiological and clinical research leads to the conclusion that disorders, as defined in the current versions of DSM and ICD, have a strong tendency to co-occur, which suggests that "fundamental assumptions of the dominant diagnostic schemata may be incorrect" [17].

Psychopathological syndromes are dynamic patterns of intercorrelated symptoms and signs that have a characteristic evolution over time. Although the range and number of possible aetiological factors—genetic, toxic, metabolic, or experiential—that may give rise to psychiatric disorders is practically unlimited, the range of psychopathological syndromes is limited. The paranoid syndrome, the obsessive-compulsive syndrome, the depressive syndrome—to mention just a few major symptom clusters— occur with impressive regularity in different individuals and settings, although in each case their presentation is imprinted by personality and cultural differences. Since a variety of aetiological factors may produce the same syndrome (and conversely, an aetiological factor may give rise to a spectrum of different syndromes), the relationship between aetiology and clinical syndrome is an indirect one. In contrast, the relationship between the syndrome and the underlying pathophysiology, or specific brain dysfunction, is likely to be much closer. This was recognized long ago in the case of psychiatric illness associated with somatic and brain disorders where clinical variation is subsumed by a limited number of "organic" brain syndromes, or "exogenous reaction types" [18]. In the complex psychiatric disorders, where aetiology is multifactorial, future research into specific pathophysiological mechanisms could be considerably facilitated by a sharper delineation of the syndromal status of many current diagnostic categories.

In addition to their clinical utility, syndromes can also serve as a gateway to elucidating the pathogenesis of psychiatric disorders. This provides a strong rationale for reinstating the concept of the *syndrome* as the basic Axis I unit of future versions of psychiatric classifications. Indeed, this was proposed by Essen-Möller, the original advocate of multiaxial classification:

...at the present state of knowledge, there appears to be a much closer connection between aetiology and syndrome in somatic medicine than in psychiatry...while in somatic medicine it is an advantage that aetiologic diagnoses take the place of syndromes, in psychiatric classification, aetiology can never be allowed to replace syndrome...a system of double diagnosis, one of aetiology and one of syndrome, has to be used [19].

Can the Classification of Mental Disorders be a Biological Classification?

In this era of unprecedented advances in genetics, molecular biology and neuroscience, theoretical thinking in psychiatry tends increasingly towards biological explanatory models of mental disorders. Accordingly, biological classifications are increasingly seen as a model for the future evolution of psychiatric classification.

Classifying involves forming categories, or taxa, for ordering natural objects or entities, and assigning names to these. Ideally, the categories of a classification should be jointly exhaustive, in the sense of accounting for all possible entities, and mutually exclusive, in the sense that the allocation of an entity to a particular category precludes the allocation of that entity to another category of the same rank. In biology, despite continuing arguments between proponents of evolutionary systematics, numerical taxonomy and cladistics, there is agreement that classifications reflect fundamental properties of biological systems and constitute "natural" classifications. However, psychiatric classifications and biological classifications are dissimilar in important respects. First, as pointed out above, the objects that are being classified in psychiatry are explanatory constructs, i.e. abstract entities rather than physical organisms. Secondly, the taxonomic units of "disorders" in DSM-IV and ICD-10 do not form hierarchies and the current psychiatric classifications contain no supraordinate, higher-level organizing concepts.

DSM-IV and ICD-10 are certainly not systematic classifications in the usual sense in which that term is applied in biology. A closer analogue to current psychiatric classifications can be found in the so-called indigenous or "folk" classifications of living things (e.g. animals in traditional rural cultures) or other material objects. "Folk" classifications do not consist of mutually exclusive categories and have no single rule of hierarchy (but may have many rules that can be used *ad hoc*). Such naturalistic systems seem to retain their usefulness alongside more rigorous scientific classifications because they are pragmatic and well adapted to the needs of everyday life [16]. Essentially, they are augmented *nomenclatures*, i.e. lists of names for conditions and behaviors, supplied with explicit rules about how these names should be assigned and used. As such, they are useful tools of communication and should play an important role in psychiatric research, clinical management and teaching.

Can Psychiatric Classification be Atheoretical?

The claim that the classification of mental disorders ought to be atheoretical originated with DSM-III, which was constructed with the explicit aim of being free of the aetiological assumptions (mainly psychodynamic) that had characterized its predecessors. It was stated, correctly, that "clinicians can agree on the identification of mental disorders on the basis of their clinical manifestations without agreeing on how the disturbances came about" [1]. However, the extension of this argument to the exclusion of theoretical considerations from the design of classifications of psychiatric disorders is a *non-sequitur*, as noted by many critics. According to Millon [10], "the belief that one can take positions that are free of theoretical bias is naïve, if not nonsensical" since "it is theory that provides the glue that holds a classification together and gives it both its scientific and its clinical relevance". It is, therefore, important to highlight the theoretical underpinning of existing classifications, as well as to identify the theoretical inputs that might be helpful in the development of future classifications.

WHAT CONSTITUTES A "GOOD" CLASSIFICATION OF MENTAL DISORDERS?

The use of current classifications in clinical research and practice raises a number of issues concerning the "goodness of fit" between diagnostic concepts and clinical reality. Much of the foregoing discussion has concerned theoretical issues. The following overview of tentative desiderata for a "good" classification is based on critical questions about the nature of mental disorders and on assumptions about the purposes and functions of their classification.

The Vexing Issue of the Validity of Psychiatric Diagnoses

While the reliability of psychiatrists' diagnoses is now substantially improved, due to the general acceptance and use of explicit diagnostic criteria, the more important issue of their validity remains contentious. It is increasingly felt that if future versions of ICD and DSM are to be a significant improvement on their predecessors, it will be because the validity of the diagnostic concepts they incorporate has been enhanced. However, what is meant by the validity of a diagnostic concept, or of a system of classification in psychiatry, is rarely discussed and few studies have addressed this question explicitly and directly. The term "valid" (Lat. *validus*, "sound, defensible, well grounded, against which no objection can fairly be brought" —*The Shorter Oxford English Dictionary*) has no precise definition when applied to diagnostic categories in psychiatry. There is no simple measure of the validity of a diagnostic concept that is comparable to the reasonably well-established procedures for the assessment of reliability. Four types of validity are often mentioned in the discourse on psychiatric diagnosis—construct, content, concurrent and predictive—all of them being borrowed off the shelf of psychometric theory where they apply to the validation of psychological tests. A diagnostic category which (a) is based on a coherent, explicit set of defining features (construct validity); (b) has empirical referents, such as verifiable observations for establishing its presence (content validity); (c) can be corroborated by independent procedures such as biological or psychological tests (concurrent validity); and (d) predicts future course of illness or treatment response (predictive validity) is more likely to be useful than a category failing to meet these criteria. However, few diagnostic concepts in psychiatry meet these criteria at the level of stringency normally required of psychometric tests, and many of them are of uncertain applicability outside the setting or culture in which they were generated.

Despite these ambiguities, a number of *procedures* have been proposed with a view to enhancing the validity of psychiatric diagnoses in the absence of a simple *measure*. Thus, Robins and Guze [20] outlined a program with five components: (a) clinical description (including symptomatology, demography and typical precipitants); (b) laboratory studies (including psychological tests, radiology and post mortem findings); (c) delimitation from other disorders (by means of exclusion criteria); (d) follow-up studies (including evidence of stability of diagnosis); and (e) family studies. This schema was subsequently elaborated by Kendler [21] who distinguished between antecedent validators (familial aggregation, premorbid personality, precipitating factors); concurrent validators (including psychological tests); and predictive validators (diagnostic consistency over time, rates of relapse and recovery, response to treatment). More recently, Andreasen [22] has proposed "a second structural program for validating psychiatric diagnosis" which includes "additional" validators such as molecular genetics and molecular biology, neurochemistry, neuroanatomy, neurophysiology and cognitive neuroscience. While making the important and, in our view, correct, statement that "the goal is not to link a single abnormality to a single diagnosis, but rather to identify the brain systems that are disrupted in the disease", she nevertheless concludes that "the validation of psychiatric diagnoses establishes them as 'real entities'".

The weakness of these procedural criteria and schemata is that they implicitly assume that psychiatric disorders are distinct entities, and that the role of the criteria and procedures is to determine whether a putative disorder, like "good prognosis schizophrenia" or "borderline personality disorder", is a valid entity in its own right or a variant of some other entity. The possibility that disorders might merge into one another with no valid boundary in between—what Sneath [23] called a "point of rarity" but is better regarded as a "zone of rarity"—is simply not considered. Robins and Guze [20] commented, for example, that "the finding of an increased prevalence of the same disorder among the close relatives of the original patients strongly indicates that one is dealing with a valid entity". In reality, such a finding is equally compatible with continuous variation, and it seems that the possibility of an increased prevalence of more than one disorder in the patients' first degree relatives was overlooked. In fact, several DSM/ICD disorders have been found to cluster non-randomly among the relatives of individuals with schizophrenia, major depression and bipolar affective disorder, and this has given rise to the concepts of "schizophrenia spectrum" and "affective spectrum" disorders. There is also increasing evidence that at least one of the putative susceptibility loci associated with affective disorder (on chromosome 18) also contributes to the risk of schizophrenia [24] and that the genetic basis of generalized anxiety disorder is indistinguishable from that of major depression [25]. It will not be surprising if in time such findings of overlapping genetic predisposition to seemingly unrelated disorders become the rule rather than the exception. It is equally likely that the same environmental factors contribute to the genesis of several different syndromes [26].

Should future research replicate and extend the scope of such findings, a fundamental revision of the current nosology of psychiatric disorders will become inevitable. Widiger and Clark [27] have suggested that variation in psychiatric symptomatology may be better represented by "an ordered matrix of symptom-cluster dimensions" than by a set of discrete categories, and Cloninger [28] has stated firmly that "there is no empirical evidence" for "natural boundaries between major syndromes" and that "the categorical approach is fundamentally flawed". However, it would be premature at this time simply to discard the current categorical entities. Although there is a mounting assumption that most currently recognized psychiatric disorders are not disease entities, this has never been demonstrated, mainly because few studies of the appropriate kind have ever been designed and conducted. Statistical techniques like discriminant function analysis for testing whether related syndromes are indeed separated by a zone of rarity have existed for 50 years and it has been demonstrated that schizophrenia is distinguishable by this means from other syndromes [29]. Other more elaborate statistical techniques have been developed more recently. For example, a means of identifying clinical groupings by a combination of discriminant function analysis and admixture analysis was described by Sigvardsson *et al.* [30] and used to demonstrate two distinct patterns of somatization in Swedish men. Woodbury *et al.* [31] developed a "grade of membership" (GoM) model for identifying "pure types" of disorders and assigning individuals to these in a way which explicitly recognizes that natural classes have fuzzy boundaries and therefore allows individuals to have partial membership in more than one class [32]. Faraone and Tsuang [33] also proposed using "diagnostic accuracy statistics" (a variant of latent class analysis) to model associations among observed variables and unobservable, latent classes or continuous traits that mediate the association.

The central problem, therefore, is not that it has been demonstrated that there are no natural boundaries between our existing diagnostic categories, or even that there are no suitable statistical techniques, data sets or clinical research strategies for determining whether or not there are any natural boundaries within the main territories of mental disorder. The problem is that the requisite research has, for the most part, not yet been done. The resulting uncertainty makes it all the more important to clarify what is implied when a diagnostic category is described as being valid [34].

Clinical Relevance

The clinical relevance of a classification encompasses characteristics such as its representative scope (coverage), its capacity to describe attributes of individuals (such as clinical severity of the disorder, impairments and disabilities) and its ease of application in the various settings in which people with mental health problems present for assessment or treatment.

It is obvious that a classification should adequately cover the universe of mental and behavioral disorders that are of clinical concern. The list of diagnostic entities is open ended—new diagnoses may be added and obsolete ones deleted. There is no theoretical limit on the number of conditions and attributes to be included, but the requirement that new rubrics should only be added if they have adequate conceptual and empirical support, as well as practical considerations (e.g. ease of manipulation), calls for strict parsimony in any future revisions of the scope of the classification.

The system should be capable of discriminating not only between syndromes but also between degrees of their expression in individual patients and the severity of the associated impairments and disabilities. This implies that the multiaxial model of psychiatric diagnosis is likely to survive, subject to further refinement. By and large, a multiaxial arrangement allowing separate and independent assessment of psychopathological syndromes, personality characteristics, somatic morbidity, psychosocial precipitants or complicating factors, cognitive functioning and overall impairment or disability, should be capable of "individualizing" the diagnostic assessment sufficiently to satisfy most clinicians and researchers. However, the content and "packaging" of the information to be recorded on individual axes will require substantial refinement. For example, the axes that are particularly problematic in the present ICD and DSM multiaxial systems are those concerned with personality. Both ICD-10 and DSM-IV provide categories for personality disorders but lack provisions for assessing and recording clinically relevant personality traits or dimensions. The ICD-10 code Z73.1 "accentuation of personality traits" is clearly inadequate; DSM-IV offers no better alternative. While most contemporary clinicians are likely to explore aspects of premorbid or current personality in the clinical work-up of a case—because they appreciate the importance of personality traits as risk factors, modifiers of symptomatology, or predictors of outcome—they lack a conceptual framework and vocabulary to integrate this information into their diagnostic assessment.

Lastly, the system should be adaptable to different settings and should perform adequately in in- and out-patient services, primary care, emergencies, and the courtroom. In addition, it should be "user-friendly", i.e. sufficiently simple and clear in its overall organization to allow entry at different levels for different users, including non-professional health workers.

Reliability

Before the 1970s, psychiatric research and communication among clinicians were badly hampered by the low reliability of diagnostic assessment and by the fact that key terms like schizophrenia were used in different ways in different countries, or even in different centres within a single country [35]. The situation has changed radically since then, and particularly since the publication of DSM-III in 1980 and the research version of ICD-10 in 1993. Clearly, this has been largely the result of the introduction of explicit or "operational"* diagnostic criteria.

One of the earliest examples of explicit diagnostic criteria in medicine was the SNOP (Standardized Nomenclature of Pathology) adopted by the American Heart Association in 1923. In psychiatry, Bleuler's list of fundamental

---

* The term "operational" originates in modern physics [36] where the definition of the "essence" of an object has been replaced by a description of the operations (e.g. measurement) required to demonstrate the object's presence and identity in the context of an experiment. This term may be too demanding for psychiatry, where it may be more appropriate to speak of "explicit" rather than "operational" diagnostic criteria.

and accessory symptoms of schizophrenia [37] and Schneider's distinction between "first-rank" and "second-rank" symptoms in the differential diagnosis of schizophrenia and affective psychoses [38] can be regarded as early precursors of modern diagnostic criteria. The wide acceptance of the current DSM and ICD criteria is largely due to their derivation from an extensive knowledge base including recent clinical, biological and epidemiological research data. In addition, DSM-III and its successors DSM-III-R and DSM-IV, as well as ICD-10, have undergone extensive field trials and their final versions have been shown to be highly reliable. It can be assumed that the diagnostic criteria of future classifications will be similarly field-tested to remove or reword ambiguous elements in them, but it is unlikely that improving further the reliability of classification will remain a major goal—in contrast to issues of validity which are beginning to dominate the agenda. It is now recognized that the reliability of a diagnostic classification tells us little about the validity of its rubrics. In fact, a highly reliable diagnostic system can be of dubious validity, and in such a situation high reliability is of little value. On the other hand, a diagnostic concept of demonstrable validity—e.g. one with important external correlates like neurocognitive features, familial aggregation of cases, or prediction of treatment response, may command poor diagnostic agreement. This is particularly likely to occur if the diagnostic category is of low sensitivity but high specificity, as shown by Rice et al. [39] for the diagnosis of bipolar II affective disorder. By and large, however, reliability imposes a ceiling on the evaluation of validity in the sense that validity would be extremely difficult to determine if the diagnostic category was unreliable.

Structural Features: Categories Versus Dimensions

There are many different ways in which classifications can be constructed. The fundamental choice is between a categorical and a dimensional structure, and it is worth recalling the observation by the philosopher Carl Hempel 40 years ago that, although most sciences start with a categorical classification of their subject matter, they often replace this with dimensions as more accurate measurement becomes possible [40]. The requirement that the categories of a typology should be mutually exclusive and jointly exhaustive has never been fully met by any psychiatric classification, or, for that matter, by any medical classification. Medical, including psychiatric, classifications are eclectic in the sense that they are organized according to several different, coexisting classes of criteria (e.g. causes, presenting symptoms or traits, age at onset, course), without a clear hierarchical arrangement. One or the other among them may gain prominence as knowledge progresses or contextual (e.g. social, legal, service-related) conditions change. However, despite their apparent logical inconsistency, medical classifications survive and evolve because of their essentially pragmatic nature. Their utility is tested almost daily in therapeutic or preventive decision-making and in clinical prediction and this ensures a natural selection of useful concepts by weeding out impracticable or obsolete ideas.

Categorical models or typologies are the traditional, firmly entrenched form of representation for medical diagnoses. As such, they have many practical and conceptual advantages. They are thoroughly familiar, and most knowledge of the causes, presentation, treatment and prognosis of mental disorder was obtained, and is stored, in relation to these categories. They are easy to use under conditions of incomplete clinical information; and they have a capacity to "restore the unity of the patient's pathology by integrating seemingly diverse elements into a single, coordinated configuration" [10]. The cardinal disadvantage of the categorical model is its propensity to encourage a "discrete entity" view of the nature of psychiatric disorders. If it is firmly understood, though, that diagnostic categories do not necessarily represent discrete entities, but simply constitute a convenient way of organizing information, there should be no fundamental objection to their continued use—provided that their clinical utility can be demonstrated. Dimensional models, on the other hand, have the major conceptual advantage of introducing explicitly quantitative variation and graded transition between forms of disorder, as well as between "normality" and pathology. They therefore do away with the Procrustean need to distort the symptoms of individual patients to match a preconceived stereotype. This is important not only in areas of classification where the units of observation are traits (e.g. in the description of personality and personality disorders) but also for classifying patients who fulfil the criteria for two or more categories of disorder simultaneously, or who straddle the boundary between two adjacent syndromes. There are clear advantages, too, for the diagnosis of "sub-threshold" conditions such as minor degrees of mood disorder and the non-specific "complaints" which constitute the bulk of the mental ill-health seen in primary care settings. Whether psychotic disorders can be better described dimensionally or categorically remains an open, researchable question [41]. The difficulties with dimensional models of psychopathology stem from their novelty; lack of agreement on the number and nature of the dimensions required to account adequately for clinically relevant variation; the absence of an established, empirically grounded metric for evaluating severity or change; and, perhaps most importantly, the complexity and cumbersomeness of dimensional models in everyday clinical practice.

These considerations seem to preclude, at least for the time being, a radical restructuring of psychiatric classification from a predominantly categorical to a predominantly dimensional model. However, if psychiatric classification ought to be unashamedly eclectic and pragmatic, such restructuring may not be necessary or even desirable. Moreover, categorical and dimensional models need not be mutually exclusive, as demonstrated by so-called mixed or class-quantitative models [42] which combine qualitative categories with quantitative trait measurements. For example, there is increasing empirical evidence that should make it attractive to supplement a retained (and refined) categorical clinical description of the syndrome of schizophrenia with selected quantitative traits such as attention or memory dysfunction and volumetric deviance of cerebral structures.

Cognitive Ease of Use

As classifications are basically devices for reducing cognitive load, a diagnostic classification in psychiatry should also be examined from the point of view of its *parsimony*, i.e. its capacity to integrate diverse observations with a minimum number of assumptions, concepts and terms [10] and ease of evocation of its categories in clinical situations. The system should also be adaptable to the differing cognitive styles of its users. In particular, it should allow the clinician to use the type of knowledge usually described as clinical experience or judgement, and enable appropriate decisions to be made under conditions of uncertainty, incomplete data, and time pressure, which occur far more commonly than is assumed by the designers of diagnostic systems.

Applicability Across Settings and Cultures

Current classifications tend to obscure the complex relationships between culture and mental disorder. Although both ICD-10 and DSM-IV acknowledge the existence of cultural variation in psychopathology (and the inclusion of a gloss on "specific culture features" with many of the DSM-IV rubrics is a step forward), they essentially regard culture as a pathoplastic influence that distorts or otherwise modifies the presentation of the "disorders" defined in the classification. Both systems ignore the existence of "indigenous" languages in mental health [43] and this limits the relevance and value of the classification in many cultural settings. Characteristic symptoms and behaviors occurring in different cultural contexts should be directly identifiable, without the need for interpreting them in terms of "Western" psychopathology, and there should be provisions for diagnosing and coding the so-called culture-bound syndromes without forcing them into conventional rubrics.

Meeting the Needs of Various Users

The essentially pragmatic nature of psychiatric classification implies that both its content and presentation should meet the needs of a variety of potential users.

Needs of Clinicians

Assuming that clinicians are willing to use diagnostic criteria and classification schemes, they will expect such tools, first and foremost, to provide a "conceptual map", i.e. to articulate clinical observation into meaningful units that facilitate the treatment and management of patients, and discriminate reliably between real patients, rather than between idealized constructs. Secondly, a "good" classification should be easily adaptable to the cognitive style of clinical users. It should allow the clinician to use freely clinical experience or clinical judgement. Thirdly, the diagnostic decision rules should be set in such a way as to minimize the risk of serious treatment and management errors. Such errors can be of two types: (a) a misclassification leading to a treatment which is ineffective or even harmful; and (b) a misclassification excluding a treatment which is effective. These two types of error have different implications depending on the condition in question: failure to prescribe an antidepressant because a depressive illness was not recognized would be potentially more serious than, say, prescribing a benzodiazepine to a patient with depression.

Needs of the Users of Mental Health Services

A diagnostic system or a classification has far-reaching implications for the well-being and human rights of those who are being diagnosed or classified. Mental health services and psychiatry are increasingly under public scrutiny, and diagnostic classifications should be capable of serving as tools of communication between mental health professionals and the public. This means that the reasoning behind every psychiatric diagnosis, and the predictions and decisions based on it, should be amenable to presentation in lay terms, including terms that are meaningful within the particular culture. A final requirement which is rarely considered concerns the social needs and self-esteem of those who are diagnosed, i.e. the mental health care "consumers" and their families. Avoidance of the stigma associated with psychiatric diagnosis is an important concern that needs to be taken into account when developing, adapting, or translating diagnostic classifications.

Needs of Researchers

Both DSM-III and its successors and, to a lesser extent, ICD-10 were welcomed and quickly adopted by researchers as rigorous diagnostic standards. However, the performance of a classification as a research tool needs to be evaluated against a number of different requirements that are not always compatible—for example, the type of diagnostic criteria needed for clinical trials or for biological research may not be suitable for epidemiological surveys.

The use of restrictive DSM-IV or ICD-10 definitions, rather than broader clinical concepts, as sampling criteria in recruiting subjects for clinical or epidemiological research carries the risk of replacing random error (due to diagnostic inconsistencies) with systematic error (due to a consistent exclusion of segments of the syndrome). For example, the DSM-IV requirement of at least six months' duration of symptoms plus the presence of social or occupational dysfunction for a diagnosis of schizophrenia is likely to bias the selection of populations for biological, therapeutic, or epidemiological longitudinal studies. It would certainly make little sense to study the variation in course and outcome in a clinical population that had already been pre-selected for chronicity by applying the six-month duration criterion.

Major studies of the molecular genetics of psychoses, usually involving collaborative consortia of investigators and a considerable investment of resources, are predicated on the validity of DSM-III-R or DSM-IV criteria. However, so far no susceptibility genes have been identified and few of the reports of weak positive linkages have been replicated [44]. In addition to the likely genetic heterogeneity of psychiatric disorders across and within populations, it appears possible that "current nosology, now embodied in DSM-IV, although useful for other purposes, does not define phenotypes for genetic study" [45]. In the absence of genes of major effect, the chances of detecting multiple genes of small or moderate effect depend critically on the availability of phenotypes defining a characteristic brain dysfunction or morphology. The "disorders" of current classifications, defined by polythetic criteria, are probably surface phenomena, resulting from multiple pathogenetic and pathoplastic interactions. They may also be masking substantial phenotypic variation in symptomatology and outcome. Such variation would hinder genetic analysis and might nullify the power of the sample to generate high-resolution data. In addition to a better syndromal definition at the clinical symptom and course level, future developments of diagnostic systems for research are likely to involve supplementing the clinical diagnosis with measures of brain morphology and quantitative traits such as cognitive or neurophysiological dysfunction. Such enriched syndromes or "correlated phenotypes" may substantially increase the informativeness of patient samples for genetic and other biological research.

Classification, Stigma and the Public Image of Psychiatry

Reducing the stigma associated with psychiatric concepts and terms should be an important long-term objective. In the past this has rarely been a primary consideration in the development of diagnostic classifications but there are good reasons to include "stigma avoidance" among the criteria on which the merits of psychiatric classifications and nomenclatures should be assessed. Both ICD-10 and DSM-IV reflect the tendency of psychiatry to oscillate, pendulum-like, between two contrasting views of the nature of mental disorders aptly described by Eisenberg [46] as "mindless" and "brainless" psychiatry. Coupled with misinterpretations of advances in biology and genetics in the form of simplistic determinism, this lack of internal conceptual coherence may again make psychiatry vulnerable to political ideologies, market forces and various forms of abuse. The risk of misuse of diagnostic categories and classifications for political or economic purposes is not buried with the past. Concepts concerning the nature and classification of psychiatric illness will always attract ideological and political attention that can translate into laws or policies that may have unforeseen consequences. For example, calls for a rationing of psychiatric care will also seek an "evidence-based" imprimatur in psychiatric classification. The theory and practice of psychiatric diagnosis and classification cannot be divorced from their social context [47].

FUTURE SCENARIOS

One Classification or Many?

For the last 20 years, there have been two widely used classifications of mental disorders, the World Health Organization (WHO)'s ICD and the American Psychiatric Association (APA)'s DSM, the former widely used in Europe, Africa and Asia, the latter used mainly in the Americas and for research purposes worldwide. Fundamentally, the two are very similar, though there are some important conceptual differences between them and many differences in the explicit definitions of individual disorders. It is also important to appreciate that the ICD is a comprehensive classification of all "diseases and related health problems" for worldwide use, and that every country is obliged to report basic morbidity data to WHO using its categories, whereas the DSM is a stand-alone classification of mental disorders designed, at least in the first instance, for use by American health professionals.

For a variety of political and financial reasons, both classifications will continue to produce new editions or revisions and in some respects to compete with one another. Radical changes are much more likely to be introduced by the APA than by the WHO, mainly because the former only has to persuade its own Board of Trustees, whereas the latter has to persuade the representatives of over 200 different countries at a formal Revision Conference. It is, of course, confusing to have two rival classifications, particularly because many of the differences between them are trivial, and in some cases accidental. On the other hand, the existence of two parallel nomenclatures and sets of explicit definitions does help to emphasize that most of psychiatry's illness concepts are still provisional and their definitions arbitrary. It is likely that both parent organizations will try to reduce the number of minor differences between their respective classifications in future revisions, and where irreconcilable conceptual differences are involved this will at least stimulate research to elucidate the advantages and disadvantages of the rival concepts or definitions. It is unlikely that any other national or international body will produce another comprehensive classification of mental disorders, but individual research groups may well produce novel concepts and definitions for specific purposes and should not be discouraged from doing so. Innovation is essential to progress and sooner or later radical changes are going to be needed.

The Immediate Future

When the time comes to produce the next versions of the DSM and ICD—and the APA is already contemplating a DSM-V—both the APA and the WHO will be confronted with a dilemma. The revision process is bound to generate requests to alter the explicit criteria defining many individual disorders and a variety of reasons will be cited—to improve reliability, to reduce ambiguity, to improve discrimination between related syndromes, to reduce variation in treatment response or outcome, to eliminate redundant criteria or phrases, and so on. In many cases these reasons, viewed in isolation, will seem cogent. On the other hand, all definitional changes have disadvantages: they are confusing to clinicians; they create a situation in which the relevance of all previous clinical and epidemiological research to the disorder as it is now defined is uncertain; and they involve tedious and sometimes costly changes in the content and detailed wording of diagnostic interviews and in the algorithms used to generate diagnoses from clinical ratings. Moreover, a series of such changes—from DSM-III to DSM-III-R to DSM-IV to DSM-V, for example—risks discrediting the whole process of psychiatric classification. Many difficult decisions about the balance of advantage and disadvantage will therefore be required. Because the disadvantages of minor changes will generally be as substantial as those of major changes, there ought, in our view, to be a prejudice against minor changes, even if this results among other things in perpetuating irritating differences between the ICD and DSM definitions of some individual disorders [48].

Perhaps the greatest weakness of DSM-IV and ICD-10 is their classification of personality disorders. Both provide a heterogeneous set of categories of disorder and in both cases individual patients commonly meet the criteria for two or three of these categories simultaneously. As there is much evidence that human personality is continuously variable, and all contemporary classifications of the variation in normal personality are dimensional, there is a strong case for a dimensional classification of personality disorders and it is possible that this will be provided by DSM-V.

Evolution of Concepts and the Language of Psychiatry

It is important to maintain awareness of the fact that most of psychiatry's disease concepts are merely working hypotheses and their diagnostic criteria are provisional. The present evolutionary classification in biology would never have been developed if the concept of species had been defined in rigid operational terms, with strict inclusion and exclusion criteria. The same may be true of complex psychobiological entities like psychiatric disorders. Perhaps both extremes—a totally unstructured approach to diagnosis and a rigid operationalization—should be avoided. Defining a middle range of operational specificity, which would be optimal for stimulating critical thinking in clinical research, but also rigorous enough to enable comparisons between the results of different studies in different countries, is probably a better solution.

Impact of Neuroscience and Genetic Research on Psychiatric Classification

It has been suggested that clinical neuroscience will eventually replace psychopathology in the diagnosis of mental disorders, and that phenomenological study of the subjective experience of people with psychiatric illnesses will lose its importance. Such a transformation of clinical psychiatry would replicate developments in other medical disciplines where molecular, imaging and computational tools have largely replaced traditional clinical skills in making a diagnosis. In time, such developments might result in a completely redesigned classification of mental disorders, based on genetic aetiology [49]. The categories of such a classification and their hierarchical ordering may disaggregate and recombine our present clinical categories in quite unexpected ways, and eventually approximate to a "natural" classification of psychiatric disorders.

This, indeed, is already happening in general medicine where molecular biology and genetics are transforming medical classifications. New organizing principles are producing new classes of disorders, and major chapters of neurology are being rewritten to reflect novel taxonomic groupings such as diseases due to nucleotide triplet repeat expansion or mitochondrial diseases [50]. The potential of molecular genetic diagnosis in various medical disorders is increasing steadily and is unlikely to bypass psychiatric disorders. Although the majority of psychiatric disorders appear to be far more complex from a genetic point of view than was assumed until recently, molecular genetics and neuroscience will play an increasing role in the understanding of their aetiology and pathogenesis. However, the extent of their impact on the diagnostic process and the classification of psychiatric disorders is difficult to predict. The eventual outcome is less likely to depend on the knowledge base of psychiatry *per se*, than on the social, cultural and economic forces that shape the public perception of mental illness and determine the clinical practice of psychiatry. A possible but unlikely scenario is the advent of an eliminativist "mindless" psychiatry which will be driven by biological models and jettison psychopathology. It is much more likely in our view that clinical psychiatry will retain psychopathology (i.e. the systematic analysis and description of subjective experience and behavior) at its core. It is also likely that classification will evolve towards a system with at least two major axes: one aetiological, using neurobiological and genetic organizing concepts, and another syndromal or behavioral–dimensional. The mapping of two such axes onto one another would provide a stimulating research agenda for psychiatry for the foreseeable future.

REFERENCES

1. American Psychiatric Association (1980) *Diagnostic and Statistical Manual of Mental Disorders*, 3rd edn (DSM-III). American Psychiatric Association, Washington.
2. American Psychiatric Association (1987) *Diagnostic and Statistical Manual of Mental Disorders*, 3rd edn, revised (DSM-IIIR). American Psychiatric Association, Washington.
3. World Health Organization (1992) *The ICD-10 Classification of Mental and Behavioural Disorders. Clinical Descriptions and Diagnostic Guidelines*. World Health Organization, Geneva.

4. American Psychiatric Association (1994) *Diagnostic and Statistical Manual of Mental Disorders*, 4th edn (DSM-IV). American Psychiatric Association, Washington.
5. World Bank (1993) *World Development Report 1993: Investing in Health*. Oxford University Press, New York.
6. Sokal R.R. (1974) Classification: purposes, principles, progress, prospects. *Science*, **185**: 115–123.
7. Kant I. (1970) *The Essential Kant* (Ed. A. Zweig). Mentor Books, New York.
8. Nelson K. (1973) Some evidence for the cognitive primacy of categorization and its functional basis. *Merril-Palmer Quarterly of Behavior and Development*, **19**: 21–39.
9. Rosch G., Mervis C.B., Gray W., Johnson D., Boyes-Braem P. (1976) Basic objects in natural categories. *Cogn. Psychol.*, **8**: 382–439.
10. Millon T. (1991) Classification in psychopathology: rationale, alternatives, and standards. *J. Abnorm. Psychol.*, **100**: 245–261.
11. Scadding G. (1993) Nosology, taxonomy and the classification conundrum of the functional psychoses. *Br. J. Psychiatry*, **162**: 237–238.
12. Horowitz L.M., Post D.L., French R. de S., Wallis K.D., Siegelman E.Y. (1981) The prototype as a construct in abnormal psychology: 2. Clarifying disagreement in psychiatric judgments. *J. Abnorm. Psychol.*, **90**: 575–585.
13. Cantor N., Smith E.E., French R., Mezzich J. (1980) Psychiatric diagnosis as prototype categorization. *J. Abnorm. Psychol.*, **89**: 181–193.
14. Feinstein A.R. (1972) Clinical biostatistics. XIII: On homogeneity, taxonomy and nosography. *Clin. Pharmacol. Ther.*, **13**: 114–129.
15. Shepherd M., Brooke E.M., Cooper J.E., Lin T.Y. (1968) An experimental approach to psychiatric diagnosis. *Acta Psychiatr. Scand.* Suppl. 201.
16. Rosch E. (1975) Cognitive reference points. *Cogn. Psychol.*, **7**: 532–547.
17. Sullivan P.F., Kendler K.S. (1998) Typology of common psychiatric syndromes. *Br. J. Psychiatry*, **173**: 312–319.
18. Bonhoeffer K. (1909) Zur Frage der exogenen Psychosen. *Zentralblatt für Nervenheilkunde*, **32**: 499–505.
19. Essen-Möller E. (1961) On the classification of mental disorders. *Acta Psychiatr. Scand.*, **37**: 119–126.
20. Robins E., Guze S.B. (1970) Establishment of diagnostic validity in psychiatric illness: its application to schizophrenia. *Am. J. Psychiatry*, **126**: 983–987.
21. Kendler K.S. (1980) The nosologic validity of paranoia (simple delusional disorder). A review. *Arch. Gen. Psychiatry*, **37**: 699–706.
22. Andreasen N.C. (1995) The validation of psychiatric diagnosis: new models and approaches. *Am. J. Psychiatry*, **152**: 161–162.
23. Sneath P.H.A. (1975) A vector model of disease for teaching and diagnosis. *Med. Hypotheses*, **1**: 12–22.
24. Crow T.J., DeLisi L.E. (1998) The chromosome workshops at the 5th International Congress of Psychiatric Genetics—the weight of the evidence from genome scans. *Psychiatr. Genet.*, **8**: 59–61.
25. Kendler K.S. (1996) Major depression and generalised anxiety disorder: same genes, (partly) different environments—revisited. *Br. J. Psychiatry*, **168** (Suppl. 30): 68–75.
26. Brown G.W., Harris T.O., Eales M.J. (1996) Social factors and comorbidity of depressive and anxiety disorders. *Br. J. Psychiatry*, **168** (Suppl. 30): 50–57.
27. Widiger T.A., Clark L.A. (2000) Toward DSM-V and the classification of psychopathology. *Psychol. Bull.*, **126**: 946–963.

28. Cloninger C.R. (1999) A new conceptual paradigm from genetics and psychobiology for the science of mental health. *Aust. N. Zeal. J. Psychiatry*, **33**: 174–186.
29. Cloninger C.R., Martin R.L., Guze S.B., Clayton P.J. (1985) Diagnosis and prognosis in schizophrenia. *Arch. Gen. Psychiatry*, **42**: 15–25.
30. Sigvardsson S., Bohman M., von Knorring A.L., Cloninger C.R. (1986) Symptom patterns and causes of somatization in men: I. Differentiation of two discrete disorders. *Genet. Epidemiol.*, **3**: 153–169.
31. Woodbury M.A., Clive J., Garson A. (1978) Mathematical typology: a grade of membership technique for obtaining disease definition. *Computers and Biomedical Research*, **11**: 277–298.
32. Manton K.G., Korten A., Woodbury M.A., Anker M., Jablensky A. (1994) Symptom profiles of psychiatric disorders based on graded disease classes: an illustration using data from the WHO International Pilot Study of Schizophrenia. *Psychol. Med.*, **24**: 133–144.
33. Faraone S.V., Tsuang M.T. (1994) Measuring diagnostic accuracy in the absence of a "gold standard". *Am. J. Psychiatry*, **151**: 650–657.
34. Kendell R.E. (1989) Clinical validity. *Psychol. Med.*, **19**: 45–55.
35. Stengel E. (1959) Classification of mental disorders. *WHO Bull.*, **21**: 601–663.
36. Bridgman P.W. (1927) *The Logic of Modern Physics*. Macmillan, New York.
37. Bleuler E. (1950) *Dementia Praecox, or the Group of Schizophrenias*. International Universities Press, New York.
38. Schneider K. (1959) *Clinical Psychopathology*. Grune & Stratton, New York.
39. Rice J.P., Rochberg N., Endicott J., Lavori P.W., Miller C. (1992) Stability of psychiatric diagnoses: an application to the affective disorders. *Arch. Gen. Psychiatry* **49**: 824–830.
40. Hempel C.G. (1961) Introduction to problems of taxonomy. In *Field Studies in the Mental Disorders* (Ed. J. Zubin), pp. 3–22. Grune & Stratton, New York.
41. Grayson D.A. (1987) Can categorical and dimensional views of psychiatric illness be distinguished? *Br. J. Psychiatry*, **26**: 57–63.
42. Skinner H.A. (1986) Construct validation approach to psychiatric classification. In *Contemporary Directions in Psychopathology* (Eds T. Millon, G.L. Klerman), pp. 307–330. Guilford Press, New York.
43. Fabrega H. (1992) Diagnosis interminable: toward a culturally sensitive DSM-IV. *J. Nerv. Ment. Dis.*, **180**: 5–7.
44. Hyman S.E. (1999) Introduction to the complex genetics of mental disorders. *Biol. Psychiatry*, **45**: 518–521.
45. Ginsburg B.E., Werick T.M., Escobar J.I., Kugelmass S., Treanor J.J., Wendtland L. (1996) Molecular genetics of psychopathologies: a search for simple answers to complex problems. *Behav. Genet.*, **26**: 325–333.
46. Eisenberg L. (2000) Is psychiatry more mindful or brainier than it was a decade ago? *Br. J. Psychiatry*, **176**: 1–5.
47. Jablensky A. (1999) The nature of psychiatric classification: issues beyond ICD-10 and DSM-IV. *Aust. N. Zeal. J. Psychiatry*, **33**: 137–144.
48. Andrews G., Slade T., Peters L. (1999) Classification in psychiatry: ICD-10 versus DSM-IV. *Br. J. Psychiatry*, **174**: 3–5.
49. Kendell R.E. (2000) The next 25 years. *Br. J. Psychiatry*, **176**: 6–9.
50. Grodin M.A., Laurie G.T. (2000) Susceptibility genes and neurological disorders. *Arch. Neurol.*, **57**: 1569–1574.

2

International Classifications and the Diagnosis of Mental Disorders: Strengths, Limitations and Future Perspectives

T. Bedirhan Üstün[1], Somnath Chatterji[1] and Gavin Andrews[2]

[1]Department of Evidence for Health Policy, World Health Organization, Geneva, Switzerland
[2]School of Psychiatry, University of New South Wales at St. Vincent's Hospital, Darlinghurst, Australia

INTRODUCTION

The classification of mental disorders improved greatly in the last decade of the twentieth century and now provides a reliable and operational tool. A common way of defining, describing, identifying, naming, and classifying mental disorders was made possible by the *International Classification of Diseases (ICD)*, Mental Disorders chapter [1, 2] and the *Diagnostic and Statistical Manual of Mental Disorders (DSM)* [3]. General acceptance of the ICD and DSM rests on the merits of their descriptive and "operational" approach towards diagnosis [4]. These classifications have greatly facilitated practice, teaching and research by providing better delineation of the syndromes. The absence of aetiological information linked to brain physiology, however, has limited understanding of mental illness and has been a stumbling block to the development of better classifications. This chapter reviews the strengths and limitations of the ICD system as a common classification for different cultures and explores the issues around future revisions given the expectations of scientific advances in the fields of genetics, neurobiology, and cultural studies.

Psychiatric Diagnosis and Classification. Edited by Mario Maj, Wolfgang Gaebel, Juan José López-Ibor and Norman Sartorius. © 2002 John Wiley & Sons, Ltd.

Limits of Our Knowledge about Mental Disorders

Classification of mental disorders creates great interest because it offers a synthesis of our current knowledge of those disorders. A classification reflects both the nature of mental disorders (i.e. ontology) and our approach to know them (i.e. epistemology). Like the periodic table of elements which displays properties of atoms in meaningful categories, the classification of mental disorders may yield some knowledge about the "essence" of underlying mechanisms of mental disorders. At the same time, organization of the classification may reflect the conceptual path of how we know and group various mental disorders. Having all this knowledge organized in a classification presents a challenge for consistency and coherence. It also helps us to identify shortcomings of our knowledge and leads to further research on unresolved issues.

Classification of mental disorders has traditionally started from a practical effort to collect statistical information and make comparisons among patient groups. Today its greatest use is for administrative and reimbursement purposes. However, it has also gained importance as a "guide" in teaching and clinical practice, because of its special nature of bringing mental disorders into mainstream medicine. Since earlier practice of psychiatry and behavioral medicine was mainly based on clinical judgement and speculative theories about aetiology, the introduction of operational diagnostics allowed for demystification of non-scientific aspects of various practices.

Current classification systems mainly remain "descriptive". They aim to define the pathology in terms of clinical signs or symptoms and formulate them as operational diagnostic criteria. These criteria are a logically coherent set of quantifiable descriptors that aim to identify the presence of a psychopathology. Our knowledge today, with a few exceptions, does not allow us to elucidate the underlying mechanism as to what actually constitutes the disorder or produces the symptom. The path from appearances to essence depends on the progress of scientific knowledge.

As scientific knowledge advances, we become aware that the current "descriptive" system of classifications, however, does not fully map on the neurobiology in terms of its pathophysiological groupings. For example, obsessive-compulsive disorder, which has been shown to have a totally different neural circuit, has been grouped together with anxiety disorders [5–7]. Similarly, despite the hair-splitting categorizations of anxiety and depressive disorders with complex exclusion rules, clinical and epidemiological studies indicate high rates of comorbidity and similar psychopharmacological agents prove efficacious in their treatment [8–11]. Despite the belief of distinct genetic mechanisms between schizophrenia and bipolar disorders, family studies have shown the concurrent heritability [12]. Such examples will inevitably accumulate to identify paradoxes between the appearance and the essence (i.e. the underlying mechanisms).

The classification of mental disorders is built on observation of pathological human behaviors. It identifies patterns of signs or symptoms that are stable over time and across different cultural settings, and can be informed by new knowledge of the way the mind and brain work. Such a classification is a reflection of (a) natural observable "phenomena", (b) cultural ways of understanding these, and (c) the social context in which these experiences occur. Since one of the major purposes of a diagnostic classification is to help clinicians communicate with each other by identifying patterns linked to disability, interventions and outcomes, these classifications have often evolved based on the "sorting techniques" that clinicians use. All psychiatric classifications are therefore human tools intended for use within a social system. Therefore, in thinking about the classification of mental disorders, multiple factors need to be taken into account, simply because our understanding of genetics, physiology, individual development, behavioral patterns, interpersonal relations, family structures, social changes, and cultural factors all affect how we think about a classification. The twentieth century has been marked by several distinct phases in the way mental phenomena and disorders have been understood. The determinism of psychoanalysis and early behaviorism has been superseded by the logical empiricism of biological psychiatry that is searching for the underpinnings of human behavior in the brain in particular, and in human biology in general. Our current knowledge of mental disorders remains limited because of the lack of disease-specific markers, and is largely based on observation of concurrent behavioral and psychological phenomena, on response to pharmacological and other treatments and on some data on familial aggregation of these elements. The task of creating an international classification of mental disorders is, therefore, a very challenging multiprofessional and multicultural one that seeks to integrate a variety of findings within a unifying conceptual framework.

STRENGTHS OF ICD-10: A RELIABLE INTERNATIONAL OPERATIONAL SYSTEM

The ICD is the result of an effort to create a universal diagnostic system that began at an international statistical congress in 1891 with an agreement to prepare a list of the causes of death for common international use. Subsequently, periodic revisions took place and in 1948, when the World Health Organization was formed, the sixth revision of the ICD was produced. Member states since then have decided to use the ICD in their national health statistics. The sixth revision of the ICD for the first time contained a separate section on mental disorders. Since then extensive efforts have been undertaken to better define the mental disorders. There has been a synchrony between ICD-6 and DSM-I, ICD-8 and DSM-II, ICD-9 and DSM-III and ICD-10 and DSM-IV with increasing harmony and consistency thanks to the international collaboration.

In the most recent tenth revision of the ICD (ICD-10), the mental disorders chapter has been considerably expanded and several different descriptions are available for the diagnostic categories: the "clinical description and diagnostic guidelines" (CDDG) [1], a set of "diagnostic criteria for research" (DCR) [2], "diagnostic and management guidelines for mental disorders in primary care" (PC) [13], "a pocket guide" [14], a multiaxial version [15] and a lexicon [16]. These interrelated components all share a common foundation of ICD grouping and definitions, yet differentiate to serve the needs of different users.

In the ICD-10, explicit diagnostic criteria and rule-based classification have replaced the art of diagnosis with a reliable and replicable system that has considerable predictive validity in terms of effective interventions. Its development has relied on international consultation and has been linked to the development of assessment instruments. The mental disorders chapter of the ICD-10 has undergone extensive testing in two phases to evaluate the CDDG as well as the DCR. The field trials of the CDDG [17] were carried out in 35 countries where joint assessments were made of 2460 different patients. For each patient, clinicians who were familiarized with the CDDG were asked to record one main diagnosis and up to two subsidiary diagnoses. Inter-rater agreements, as measured by the kappa statistic, for most categories in the "two-character groups" (e.g. F2, schizophrenic disorders) were over 0.74, indicating excellent agreement. It was lowest at 0.51 for the F6 category, which includes personality disorders, disorders of sexual preference, disorders of gender identity and habit and impulse disorders. At a more detailed level of diagnosis, agreement on individual personality disorders (except dyssocial personality disorder), mixed anxiety and depression states, somatization disorder and organic depressive disorder were below acceptable limits. As a result, the descriptions for these categories were improved and clarified. Some categories were omitted altogether from the ICD-10 due to poor reliability (e.g. the category of hazardous use of alcohol).

Based on the experience gathered from the field trials of the CDDG, the ICD-10 DCR were developed with the assistance of experts from across the world. Operational criteria with inclusion and exclusion rules were specified for each diagnostic category. For the DCR field trials [18], 3493 patients were assessed in a clinical interview by two or more clinicians across 32 countries. Once again, for the F6 category the kappa value of 0.65 (though improved from the CDDG field trials) was lower than for the other 9 two character categories, which all had kappas over 0.75. For the more detailed diagnoses, poor kappa values of <0.4 were obtained mainly for those categories that were either polymorphic syndromes (e.g. acute psychotic disorders) or were at the milder end of the spectrum (e.g. hypomania, mild depressive episode).

LIMITATIONS OF CLASSIFICATION OF MENTAL DISORDERS IN THE ICD

The new classification systems have generally greatly facilitated teaching, clinical practice, scientific research, and communication. What then are the problems?

Classification by Syndromal Similarity

The ICD categories are grouped by their syndromal similarity, i.e. the common clustering of a set of symptoms and signs in clinical practice with no other organizing principle deemed to be necessary. This approach may, however, not always be valid, since a higher order rule may override apparent similarities or differences. For example, given external character-istics, one may intuitively classify sharks and dolphins as fish, based on the similarities in appearance and the nature of the habitat. Yet, this would obviously be false as a higher order rule dictates that dolphins are mammals and sharks are not. Categories in the ICD (and DSM) having passed the test of expert consensus (and therefore providing the face validity that they are indeed commonly identifiable patterns in clinical patients) do not always make scientific sense and may have created boundaries where none exists. For example, it appears arbitrary (and therefore unacceptable) to classify the severe end of the psychosis spectrum as a "disorder" while classifying the milder version within the personality disorder group. In fact the current criteria for schizophrenia in both DSM and ICD have been viewed as having serious limitations as they rely heavily on psychotic symptoms that may be the final common pathway for a variety of disorders. Features occurring before the advent of psychosis that are clinical, biological, and/or neuro-psychological in nature may provide more information about the genetic, pathophysiological, and developmental origins of schizophrenia [19].

The separation of the diagnostic criteria from aetiological theories was an explicit approach undertaken to avoid being speculative, since these theor-ies about causation had not been empirically tested. However, this "atheore-tical" approach has also been severely criticized because, if one takes a totally atheoretical and solely operational approach, it may be possible to classify normal but statistically uncommon phenomena as psychiatric dis-orders [20]. Diagnostic categories have been proposed and accepted merely because of recognizable patterns of co-occurring symptoms rather than because of a true understanding of their distinctive nature that would make them discrete categories within a classification.

What Defines a Mental Disorder?

While ICD is a classification of diseases (or "disorders" in the context of mental illness), there is no explicit agreement on the definition of a mental disorder. Despite the call for a definition [21], no agreement has been forthcoming and this ambiguity creates a fuzzy boundary between disorder and wellness. At the lowest level, a mental disorder is an identifiable and distinct set of signs and symptoms that commonly produce disability, and that the healers in the society claim to be able to ameliorate through various interventions. While practical, such a definition can lead to error, e.g. homosexuality was once defined as a disorder.

The answer to the question "What is a disorder?" needs to be evaluated against rigorous scientific standards rather than just from societal or personal points of view. A disorder may be defined by a set of general principles that characterize a specific entity, such as common aetiology, signs and symptoms, course, prognosis and outcome. It may then have other correlates, such as familial aggregation (due to genetic or contextual factors), a pattern of distress or disability, and a predictable range of outcomes following a variety of specific interventions. Robins and Guze [22], in their classic paper, proposed five phases for establishing the validity of psychiatric diagnosis: clinical description, laboratory studies, delimitation from other disorders, follow-up study to show diagnostic homogeneity over time, and family study to demonstrate the familial aggregation of the syndrome. Experience gathered since then shows that some of these criteria lead to contradictory conclusions. For example, if one wants to define schizophrenia by its diagnostic stability over time, the best approach is to define the illness at the very outset by a duration criterion of six months of continuous illness, which tends to select for subjects with a poor outcome. In contrast, the familial aggregation of schizophrenia is best demonstrated when the notion of the disorder is broadened to include the notion of "schizotaxia"— a broad spectrum notion that views the predisposition to schizophrenia to be characterized by negative symptoms, neuropsychological impairment and neurobiological abnormalities and schizophrenia to be a psychotic neurotoxic end-point in the process. The latter approach suggests that narrowing the definition of schizophrenia using the former strategy may in fact hinder progress in identifying the genetic causes of the disorder [19].

The lack of a definition of what is a disorder also creates an ambiguity about so-called "sub-threshold" disorders. Many have shown the presence of cases that have significant distress and disability and with clinically significant signs or symptoms who fail to fulfil the criteria for a disorder in the present diagnostic classifications [23]. How one should define such conditions has been left to arbitrary decisions, mainly based on relaxing the diagnostic criteria. A good illustration is "sub-threshold" depression. Perhaps the most common of psychiatric presentations in primary care, subjects with this diagnosis do not meet the diagnostic criteria for any depressive disorder in the classification systems and yet are associated with sufficient distress to lead to a consultation and have an impact on the person's functioning [24]. In other words, the boundaries between "sub-threshold" and "subclinical" are not drawn at the same place. It is unclear if these disorders are quantitatively or qualitatively different from the supra-threshold categories within the diagnostic systems, such as adjustment disorders, dysthymia and depressive episodes. Perhaps there is a need to focus on these conditions in primary care settings in order to understand what distinguishes them from normal mood fluctuations given the life experience of people, and to appreciate what they mean for the reorganization of the current categories within the diagnostic system such as, for example, the broadening of the notion of dysthymia to include both acute, sub-acute and chronic states.

How "clinical significance" ought to be defined has been the subject of recent debate [25, 26], mainly based on tightening the diagnostic criteria. It has been suggested that the notion of "harmful dysfunction" be used to define psychiatric disorders. A dysfunction is construed as a failure of an internal mechanism to perform one of the functions for which it is naturally designed, i.e. a function the mechanism and form of which is understood in evolutionary theory terms. Harm, on the other hand, is understood as a value that is ascribed to that dysfunction depending on individual circumstances transforming the dysfunction into a disorder. For example, though a dysfunction of the brain may exist that interferes with reading ability, it would not be a disorder in preliterate societies. The approach acknowledges the combining of a factual scientific notion with a value component in the creation of a "disorder". It must be noted though that this is not a problem unique to mental disorders. A male with azoospermia may not receive a diagnosis (of primary infertility) and may be considered to be healthy until he is required to procreate. Hence, while the concept of "dysfunction" is a useful construct, the descriptor of "harmful" is not.

Separation of Diagnosis from Functioning and Distress

Diagnosis of a disease or disorder should be uncoupled from disability. Disease process and disability or distress are distinct phenomena and their presence for a diagnosis is neither necessary nor sufficient. Each one of the ICD and DSM diagnostic entities is defined by three rubrics: (a) specific phenomenology, (b) signs and symptoms and (c) rules that exclude the diagnosis being made in certain circumstances. The DSM definition, in addition, calls for "clinically significant impairment or distress", meaning that disruption in social, occupational, or other areas of functioning must accompany the set of observable phenomena. While the intent of this criterion was to distinguish mental disorders from daily experiences of distress and broaden the clinical focus beyond symptoms, this criterion blurs the construct of functioning with the definition of mental disorder. For so-called "physical disorders" (e.g. diabetes or tuberculosis), clinical significance is not required for diagnosis. Putting "distress" or "impairment in functioning" as a necessary prerequisite for diagnosis of a mental disorder is of little use if these are not operationalized or independently assessed [27]. Besides, this approach has major implications for receiving treatment or services. The lack of "distress or impairment" would preclude a diagnosis, and would disallow early provision of care that could prevent the disorder worsening. It would impair research and subjects without impairment would be excluded from studies to identify the cause or treatment of the disorder.

Many patients in primary care settings fall into sub-threshold diagnostic categories, particularly those with depression as noted above. In deciding when to initiate treatment, functional change may be even more important than discrete symptom profiles. Recognizing and treating depression as a comorbid condition in patients with other medical illnesses represents an additional challenge for the primary care physician. In anxiety disorders, it remains questionable whether the current ICD-10 diagnosis of generalized anxiety disorder, defined by a six month minimum duration and four associated symptoms, is the most appropriate option. Using this definition a substantial proportion of disabled subjects with lesser levels of anxiety, tension and worrying remain outside the diagnostic criteria, and hence may go untreated.

The uncoupling of disability from diagnosis would allow the examination of the unique prognostic significance of disability and the interactive relationship and direction of change in symptomatology and functioning following interventions. It would allow the development of more rational forms of intervention, including rehabilitation strategies, which are specifically targeted to improving functioning by altering individual capacity or modifying the environment in which the person lives in order to improve real life performance. It would also underscore efforts to make changes at the level of health policy and the need to deal with larger social issues such as stigma in order to improve access to care and social participation of psychiatric patients.

The development of the International Classification of Functioning, Disability and Health (ICF) [28] is an important landmark in this regard. Disability related research suggested the need for a revision of the ICF framework that would focus on an "aetiology neutral" and "universal" model that would also then allow the development of a common metric to compare "physical" with "mental" and alcohol or other drug use disorders and allow for arguments for parity of these conditions. In recognition of the need to define disability in a manner consistent with a clear conceptual framework, the current revision of the ICF has focused on providing operational definitions of all dimensions and for all terms. The ICF classifies functioning at the level of body or body part, the whole person, and the whole person in a social context. Disability thus involves dysfunctioning at one or more of these same levels: impairments, activity limitations and participation restrictions. Activity and participation can be described further in terms of capacity (what a person can do given a uniform environment, i.e. the environment adjusted ability of the person) and performance (what happens in the person's real life environment, i.e. what the person does in actual life). Having access to both performance and capacity data enables the ICF user to determine the "gap" between capacity and performance. If capacity is less than performance, then the person's current environment has enabled him or her to perform better than the data about capacity would predict: the environment has facilitated performance. On the other hand, if capacity is greater than performance, then some aspect of the environment is a barrier to performance.

The distinction between environmental "barriers" and "facilitators", as well as the extent to which an environmental factor acts in one way or another, is also captured by the qualifier for coding environmental factors in the ICF.

In summary, the assessment and classification of disability in a different system is a strong theoretical and practical requirement to refine the definition of mental disorders. The separate classification of disease and disability phenomenon in ICD and ICF is likely to lead to better understanding of the underlying body function impairments for mental disorders and associated disability. In this way we would be able to describe and delineate more clearly the features of mental illness.

Mind, Brain or Context?

Recent progress in the cognitive sciences, developmental neurobiology and real time *in vivo* imaging of the intact human brain has provided us with new insights into the basic correlates of emotions and cognitions that should inform a new psychopathology. A better understanding of the neural circuitry involved in complex emotional and cognitive functions will accelerate the development of testable hypotheses about the exact pathophysiological bases of mental disorders.

Genetic sciences emphasize the interaction between the genome and the environment and hopefully will lead to a better understanding of the plasticity of the human brain and how it malfunctions in mental disorders. This approach is different from seeking a molecular pathology for every mental sign, and the progress of gene expression through central nervous system function to emotional and cognitive constructs will always describe multilinear processes.

Progress in the neural sciences is already blurring the boundaries of the brain and mind, yet such a mind–body dualism as expressed in the organic vs. non-organic distinction in the ICD (but not in DSM) does have a utility. It directs the clinician to pay special attention to an underlying "physical" state as the cause of the "mental" disturbance. However, the term "organic" implies an outmoded functional vs. structural and mind vs. body dualism. Similarly, at the other end of the spectrum, cultural relativism can undermine efforts towards the meaningful diagnosis of mental disorders. The view that stigma and labelling can wrongly define a person as ill implies that mental illnesses are "myths" created by society. This has resulted in a devaluation of insights that are inherent in a cultural perspective. A similar danger of further dismissing the role of cultural factors in the causation, maintenance and outcome of mental disorders exists when culture is seen as antithetical to neurobiology.

International Use: Need for Universalism and Diversity

As an international classification of diseases, the ICD must contain a culturally neutral list of all possible disease entities. The frequencies with which these conditions occur in different settings cannot be a principle used to include or exclude conditions. The need to find a "common language" of mental disorders must be balanced with the need to keep local sensitivities in mind, and to allow users of the classification to find the appropriate conceptual equivalents and to identify variations in their culture.

Culture

Although some cultural elements have been included in the ICD and DSM, much remains to be done. There is a need to move beyond "culture-bound syndromes", the inclusion of which perhaps does little more than pay lip service to the recognition of the role that culture plays in the manifestation of mental disorders. These conditions reflect an extreme, and provide little if any understanding of the complex interaction between culture and mental phenomena. There is a need for a better cultural formulation of diagnosis and for informed research to address the impact of culture on the explanatory, pathoplastic and therapeutic processes. Unless typologies are formulated on the basis of careful research, sound theory, and clinical relevance, they are likely to be relegated to the status of historical artefacts.

"Etic" versus "Emic" Approaches

There is a fundamental dilemma with all international cross-cultural comparisons: the need to provide an international common language while not losing sight of the unique experiences that occur as a feature of living in different social and cultural contexts. There is need to look for global, universal features of mental conditions—an approach that is driven by analysis and emphasizes similarities rather than differences. The "etic" approach relies on multi-group comparisons and is often carried out from a viewpoint that is located outside of the system. Equally, it is important to understand the diverse nature of human experience that needs to be discovered within a culture-specific system, and to emphasize the differences from one culture to another (the "emic" approach). A balance between the two approaches is in the interest of an international classification.

For example, a Dutch psychiatrist, with three of his Dutch colleagues, classified 40 Ethiopian visitors to a psychiatric outpatient clinic in Addis Ababa. In spite of the culture-specific way in which Ethiopians present their complaints, the diagnostic criteria of DSM appeared to be useful and the inter-rater reliability was comparable with that from America. The results were congruent for the categories that are well defined, like psychotic and affective disorders. This agreement did not apply to the somatoform and factitious disorders [29].

Conversely, the Explanatory Model Interview Catalogue (EMIC) was used to elicit indigenous explanations of illness and patterns of prior help seeking, and generated the popular humoral theories of mental disorder. Even though most laypersons are unfamiliar with the content of the classical treatises of Ayurveda, the humoral traditions which they represent still influence current perceptions. While case vignettes written in this tradition can clarify the nature of the relationship between cultural, familial and personal factors that influence the experience of illness, and can provide unique insights for care [30], the underlying aetiological explanation is not informative.

Unique national classificatory systems, such as the Chinese Classification of Mental Disorders, third edition (CCMD-3), often attempt to strike a balance between retaining the categories of international systems while making particular additions (e.g. traveling psychosis, qigong induced mental disorders) and deletions (e.g. somatoform disorders, pathological gambling, and a number of personality and sexual disorders). Such systems reveal the changing notions of illness in contemporary China [31]. The main discrepancies between Chinese and American diagnostic systems are in neurasthenia and hysterical neuroses. Such discrepancies may have resulted from differential labeling, e.g. depression being labeled as neurasthenia, or from creating a new disorder entity, such as "Eastern gymnastic exercises-induced mental disorder". *Shenjing shuairuo* (neurasthenia), a ubiquitous psychiatric disease in China prior to 1980, is now reconstituted as the popular Western disease of depression among academic psychiatrists in urban China. It is argued that this new-found disease of depression is based not only on empirical evidence but also on a confluence of historical, social, political, and economic forces.

Taijin kyofusho (TKS), a common Japanese psychiatric disorder character-ized by a fear of offending or hurting others through one's awkward social behavior or an imagined physical defect, is similar to dysmorphophobia or social phobia in ICD-10. Nevertheless, TKS can be understood as an ampli-fication of culture-specific concerns about the social presentation of self within the Japanese context. Cultural studies focusing on these disorders are urgently needed to understand the nature of the phenomenon, the cultural influences on diagnosis, the relationship of culture-bound syn-dromes to psychiatric disorders, and the social and psychiatric history of the syndrome in the life course of the sufferer. Such research will enhance the international classifications of mental disorders.

The cultural applicability of international classification warrants careful consideration in future comparative research. For example, WHO's research on drinking norms definitely shows differences in terms of thresholds of problem drinking and dependence in "wet" and "dry" cultures [32]. Cul-tural differences in the meaning of mental distress may vary in different ways: (a) in terms of threshold, the point at which respondents from differ-ent societies recognize a disorder as something serious; (b) in whether the entities described in international classifications count as problems in all cultures; (c) in causal assumptions about how mental problems arise; and (d) in the extent to which there exist culture-specific manifestations of symptoms not adequately captured by official disease nomenclature.

Categorical and Dimensional Models

There are two quite different ways of conceptualizing mental disorders: as dimensions of symptoms or as categories, often by identifying a threshold on the dimension. Clinicians are obliged to use categorical concepts, as they must decide who is sufficiently ill to justify treatment. But, in our efforts to understand the relationships between social and biological variables, dimensional models are far more appropriate [33]. Dimensional models are more consistent with the polygenic (or oligogenic) models of inheritance favored for most mental disorders. These models assume that a number of genes combine with one another and interact with the environmental factors to cause the disorder. Persons can thus have various doses of the risk factors that predispose to the illness and, depending on the dose, the severity of the manifest condition may vary along a continuum. Such approaches have been shown to provide important clinical advantages with psychotic illnesses [34] and personality disorders.

Though psychiatric disorders are construed to be disorders of brain chemistry, a fundamental notion underpinning the classification systems is that different disorders represent different classes of disturbance of mental life. These categories thus must be understood as being distinct not only among themselves but also from "normality". In psychiatric classification, therefore, categories can be seen as mathematical sets which, based on their properties, can be reliably and meaningfully placed in valid classes of similar objects. These categories are often nominated by means of descriptive parameters which then lead to categories that are big or small depending on our purpose, as noted earlier. Psychiatric classifications attempt to define classes not just by positive defining parameters but also by excluding other possibilities. In other words, categories are defined according to the principle that members of each category are more similar to each other than to members of other categories. The attempt is thus to make the categories more internally consistent. In addition, to separate or distance the category from others we employ exclusion criteria in order to prevent overlap between categories. However, it is not sufficient just to have categories that are internally consistent. They must also be meaningful, and membership of a category must also be able to predict more about the member than what is said in the inclusion rules alone. Further, once an exhaustive list of categories has been achieved, they must be sorted according to some larger principle in order to make such a list more manageable and identify a purpose. This also ensures the comparison of like with like, i.e. the comparison of categories that are understood to be at the same level of complexity. This, however, means that at the same level of hierarchy we cannot have categories that are determined according to totally unrelated parameters. In any categorical system it is imperative to ensure that the elements sort into discrete groups; otherwise, the implication is that either the sorting rules were incorrect or the categories did not exist.

Especially with regard to the categories of personality disorders, this problem becomes exemplified when researchers assess every criterion in every subject in a rigorous manner. In a study of 110 outpatient subjects where all the 112 criteria for DSM-III-R personality disorder were scored, 68 patients met the criteria for a total of 155 diagnoses. The presumption was that none of the subjects could be considered to have a normal personality since all met a substantial number of criteria for personality disorders [35].

The concept of comorbidity becomes important when the classification logic posits discrete categories. Comorbidity, the concurrence of more than one diagnosis, does occur but it can be an artefact of hierarchical rules used in classification systems. Excessive splitting of classical syndromes into subtypes of disorders with overlapping boundaries and indefinite thresholds adds to the confusion. Though the co-occurrence of pathology in different subsystems of the body (or mind) is indeed contingent, it can be attributed either to the same underlying etiological cause affecting different body systems (as is the case, for example, with diabetes causing hyperglycemia, peripheral neuropathy and nephropathy) or to distinct causes that just happen to co-occur (as is the case with diabetes and a lacerated wound following an injury). Further, the notion of comorbidity can only be accepted when the categories are not mutually exclusive, in order to avoid category errors. For example, one can be classified as a friend and an enemy provided it is not to the same person at the same time as these would be contradictory categories.

We need to address the issue of comorbidity with novel research strategies in experimental psychiatry. The challenge lies in determining when co-occurring conditions are derived from the same underlying etiology, where they are contradictory category errors and therefore must be disallowed, and where they have an interactive effect on course and outcomes. Systematic studies are required to understand the frequencies with which comorbid mental disorders occur, the impact that this has on outcomes and responses to interventions and on functioning and disability. Commonly occurring comorbid conditions need to be further evaluated to understand if they share a common etiology or if they are downstream effects of one another or modulating or predisposing factors for each other. For example, if depression and alcohol use disorders occur commonly, are these the result of a common "hyposerotonergic" state in the brain brought about by a confluence of genetic factors or is being depressed a psychological state that then leads on to the behavior of drinking as a coping mechanism that soon becomes uncontrollable due to the independent physiological effects of alcohol and in turn depletes serotonin in the brain setting up a cycle? The answers to such questions from the study of comorbid conditions will then help categorize such multiple conditions using an organizing principle that may be quite different from that in the current classificatory systems.

FUTURE PERSPECTIVES

WHO's network on the family of international classifications has not planned for an overall revision of the classification of diseases before 2010. This period will allow for a more extensive knowledge base to develop and build up mechanisms so that such a knowledge base informs the ICD revision. In particular, new information on genetics, neurobiology and epidemiology can be used in an iterative process to update the categories, criteria and grouping of disorders. To achieve this aim, a mechanism should be identified to build up this process and criteria should be identified to shape the content.

A sound epistemological approach should be identified towards evidence so as to identify the disorder, disease and disability. Bounds of normality in universal human functioning should be operationally and empirically defined so as to set up the thresholds for identification of disease process. Future classifications should go beyond a common language and reliability. Expert-opinion-based alterations to the classification should be stopped and future changes should be based only on research specifically designed to resolve issues pertinent to the classification.

We should go beyond the comparison of diagnostic traditions or schools of psychiatry. The utility of comparisons of non-affective functional psychoses, such as the French bouffée dèlirante that is not diagnosed in Great Britain, is useful but limited without further neurobiological evidence. The British divide these psychoses into schizophrenic and non-schizophrenic disorders, particularly using Schneiderian criteria for the diagnosis of schizophrenia. Curiously, it is precisely these criteria, referred to as "automatisme mental" which are used in France to diagnose the "chronic hallucinatory psychoses". This diagnosis is unknown in Great Britain, yet in France is classed firmly among the non-schizophrenic psychoses [36]. It is unlikely that both are correct.

An evidence-based review mechanism and focused empirical testing for specific categorizations should be started. Underlying physiological mechanisms should be preferred for disease grouping instead of traditional conventions. Applicability and reliability of the new proposals for classification should be tested in field trials. Operationalization and reliability are merely useful guides for diagnosis, but they are not sufficient for validity. Clinical utility is frequently used as an argument for the relevance of a classification. This construct mainly deals with the precision with which a disorder could be identified to benefit from known interventions. If criteria and categorization are useful, clinical utility will naturally follow given the function of correct identification of cases.

In this context, the future steps will depend basically on the planned revisions and process around the ICD and other national classifications, particularly DSM. In the evolution of DSM and ICD, since the sixth version of ICD and first version of DSM, there has been a constant effort to get closer. ICD-8 and DSM-II, ICD-9 and DSM-III and ICD-10 and DSM-IV have displayed greater similarity and consistency thanks to the international collaboration.

The ICD and DSM in their current forms are both descriptive, non-aetiological classifications with operationally defined criteria and rule-based approaches to generating diagnoses. The efforts to harmonize the two classifications have left minor differences between the two systems. Currently these systems are not entirely homologous, but in a large majority of criteria they are identical or differ in non-significant ways. Differences are most marked in the case of near-threshold, mild or moderate conditions. Discordance is particularly high with categories such as post-traumatic stress disorder and harmful use or abuse of substances [37–40].

The Australian national mental health survey [37] that compared the two diagnostic systems revealed that the disagreements between the systems lead to widely varying estimates of burden from different mental health conditions. In other words, these differences do matter. It showed that though the intention of the two sets of criteria for several of the disorders appeared to be very similar, trivial differences in the words used or in the number of symptoms often accounted for the dissonance. These differences are needless and best avoided. A more substantial reason for difference appeared to be the way the exclusion rules are used by the two classifications. There is a need to agree on a common set of principles that will dictate these exclusion rules.

On the other hand, substantive differences between ICD and DSM also exist. ICD uncouples disability from diagnosis. ICD does not put personality disorders or physical disorders in a different axis.

Both the ICD and DSM have been subjected to extensive field testing and are in wide use. Prior to the next revisions of these classifications, after removing the non-essential differences in the two classifications, the remaining conceptual distinctions should be identified and subjected to further empirical testing in order to reduce the dissonance. Ideally, this testing would be carried out in an international manner, since this is the mandate of the WHO. It would be desirable to then further harmonize the two classifications, so that diagnoses in which there are conceptual agreement have identical criteria and, where differences exist after examination of the empirical data, users should be informed about the differences in the concepts and about the best practical resolution of the differences perhaps depending on the purpose as gathered from the foregoing studies.

Future Research Agenda to Inform Classification Revision

The major strides that have been undertaken in neuroscience and molecular genetics provide exciting new opportunities for refining our classification and, if the promise of these technologies bears fruit, we may soon be able to validate and refine our current descriptive categories [41]. The current available evidence supports multiple candidate regions for schizophrenia as possible susceptibility sites, particularly chromosomes 1q, 4q, 5p, 5q, 6p, 6q, 8p, 9q, 10p, 13q, 15q, 22q, and Xp [42]. Similarly, for bipolar disorders, several genetic loci on chromosomes 4p, 12q, 13q, 18, 21q, 22q and Xq have been reported [43]. The chromosomal regions implicated are large. However, the use of data sets that have detailed phenotypic information, of marker-intensive genome-wide searches for linkage and association, of novel technologies such as DNA pooling, DNA chip methods and high speed SNP (single nucleotide polymorphism) testing, and of advanced statistical tools, may lead to the discovery of the schizophrenia and bipolar disorder gene(s). For the present, however, the data are insufficient, and we must continue in the painstaking way that we had for the past 100 years.

Failure to obtain convincing results in psychiatric genetics can be attributed partly to the fact that progress in molecular biology and genetic epidemiology has not been followed by an equivalent development in the phenotypic description of these disorders themselves. Defining better endophenotypes using imaging (such as magnetic resonance imaging) and electrophysiological techniques (such as evoked responses, eye movements, etc.) may lead to the identification of more heritable and homogeneous forms of the disorders. Instead of relying entirely on classical nosological approaches, identifying more homogeneous forms of diseases through a "candidate symptom approach" among affected subjects, as well as an endophenotype approach looking for subclinical traits among non-affected relatives, might yield better results. Focusing on vulnerability traits might stimulate the redefinition of traditional psychiatric syndromes and help to bridge the gap between clinical and experimental approaches [44, 45].

ICD and DSM currently rely heavily on models of adult psychopathology and use identical diagnostic criteria for some disorders for both adults and children. Besides the questionable appropriateness of this approach, it is imperative to identify changing psychopathology over the lifespan. This will allow the early detection in childhood of potentially damaging conditions yet to arise in adulthood and might lead to preventive interventions. It would be very valuable to identify if the manifestation of deviant behavior in childhood is a "forme fruste" of an adult onset disorder, or if it heralds the development of a different category of illness in adulthood. For example, research has shown an association between childhood attention deficit hyperactivity disorder (ADHD) and adult onset substance use and bipolar disorders [46, 47]. Family members of children with ADHD and bipolar disorder are more likely to have bipolar disorder and to be socially impaired. The co-occurrence of these disorders seems to happen significantly more often than by chance alone. Similarly, ADHD was associated with a twofold increased risk for substance use disorders. ADHD subjects are significantly more likely to make the transition from an alcohol use disorder to a drug use disorder. Cross-sectional and longitudinal studies will clarify whether the criteria for some disorders need to be modified for their application in children.

A numerical taxonomic approach has been in the literature since the early 1960s. Development of naturally occurring, empirically defined classes rather than expert defined categories is an option. Statistical clustering techniques are limited by the quality of the data. Newer statistical techniques, such as Rasch analysis, which place subjects and items on a single unidimensional scale, have been applied to categories such as substance dependence. They can be used to redefine disorders (or latent constructs) in a uniform manner across settings and validate them against a theory derived from data that are accrued from neurobiological and genetic studies [48]. Novel computational techniques such as fuzzy logic neural networks may also improve our understanding of patterns that exist in the universe of psychopathology. Research should avoid the quicksands of quantitative psychopathology and circular validation and should instead focus on comprehensive assessment strategies like the Schedules for Clinical Assessment in Neuropsychiatry (SCAN) combined with biological markers to contribute to new classificatory models. In addition, hierarchical or weighed approaches that accord different levels of salience to different features of a diagnostic category may also provide solutions to the dimensional vs. categorical problem, as well as creating categories with varying degrees of homogeneity.

These, combined with statistical analytical techniques, such as grade of membership (GoM) analysis, will allow the measurement of the degree to which a given subject belongs to a specified category. The GoM model, based on fuzzy-set theoretic concepts, is a classification procedure that uses a pattern recognition approach and allows a person to be a member of more than one diagnostic class. It simultaneously quantifies the degrees of membership in classes while generating the discrete symptom profiles or "pure types" describing these classes. The GoM method has been explicitly applied to diagnostic systems by quantitatively identifying and characterizing subpatterns of illness within a broad class. It has been used to examine the classification of schizophrenia, dementia, personality disorders and several other diagnostic conditions [35, 49, 50]. The evolution of Alzheimer's disease is a highly ordered sequential process with a pathology characterized by neurofibrillary tangles, diffuse plaques and neuritic plaques. The GoM method has been shown recently to be useful in better defining the process of progression from normal ageing to severe dementia. With regard to personality disorders, the GoM method provides a more parsimonious handling of the criteria than provided by classifying according to DSM categories. In an application of this method in 110 psychiatric outpatients examining the 112 diagnostic criteria from DSM-III-R, the method revealed the presence of four pure types and failed to confirm the natural occurrence of any single specific Axis II personality disorder or cluster. A GoM based psychiatric classification might more clearly identify core disease processes than conventional classification models, by filtering the confounding effects of individual heterogeneity from pure type definitions.

A related issue is the relative importance attached to the individual criteria within diagnostic categories. Future work ought to focus on the evaluation of whether prevalent symptoms are present in random or predictable combinations, whether there exists a specific hierarchy of severity of symptoms, and whether symptoms are accumulated in a predictable pattern. The search for a universal criteria set for disorders must continue. We must perhaps strive to find those variables that are universally applicable with culture-specific thresholds and cross-cultural transformations that translate local language and experience into comparable diagnostic approaches. A complex algorithm that may then weight these sets of criteria differently and locally derived combinatorial rules might pave the way for a true cross-cultural epidemiology.

CONCLUSIONS

The expectations from a classification of mental disorders are many. A classification is expected to be useful in clinical settings as well as being valid for legal and financial purposes. It has to respond to the cultural reality of the users while providing comparability across diverse populations. The current classification needs to be revised to incorporate these multiple utilities. Consideration of developmental issues across the life-span and cultural issues in diverse countries or populations should be included and combined with scientific rigor. We need better tools to respond to the legitimate expectations of users.

Future classifications should go beyond a common language and reliability. A system based on consensus opinion can never be acceptable to everyone. Expert-opinion-based alterations to the classification should be stopped and future changes should be based only on research specifically designed to resolve issues pertinent to the classification. We need to build a scientific research agenda that brings a multicultural and multidisciplinary approach to a series of focused field trials. In organizing, conducting and funding such a collaborative, goal-directed effort, the WHO should and could play a seminal role. With international research we could build better classifications that can lead to better understanding of mental disorders.

REFERENCES

1. World Health Organization (1992) *The ICD-10 Classification of Mental and Behavioural Disorders: Clinical Descriptions and Diagnostic Guidelines*. World Health Organization, Geneva.
2. World Health Organization (1993) *The ICD-10 Classification of Mental and Behavioural Disorders: Diagnostic Criteria for Research*. World Health Organization, Geneva.
3. American Psychiatric Association (1994) *Diagnostic and Statistical Manual of Mental Disorders*, 4th edn. American Psychiatric Association, Washington.
4. Stengel E. (1959) Classification of mental disorders. *WHO Bull.*, **21**: 601–603.
5. Montgomery S.A. (1993) Obsessive compulsive disorder is not an anxiety disorder. *Int. Clin. Psychopharmacol.*, **8** (Suppl. 1): 57–62.
6. Liebowitz M.R. (1998) Anxiety disorders and obsessive compulsive disorder. *Neuropsychobiology*, **37**: 69–71.
7. Lucey J.V., Costa D.C., Busatto G., Pilowsky L.S., Marks I.M., Ell P.J., Kerwin R.W. (1997) Caudate regional cerebral blood flow in obsessive-compulsive disorder, panic disorder and healthy controls on single photon emission computerised tomography. *Psychiatry Res.*, **74**: 25–33.
8. Mineka S., Watson D., Clark L.A. (1998) Comorbidity of anxiety and unipolar mood disorders. *Annu. Rev. Psychol.*, **49**: 377–412.
9. Boerner R.J., Moller H.J. (1999) The importance of new antidepressants in the treatment of anxiety/depressive disorders. *Pharmacopsychiatry*, **32**: 119–126.
10. Kaufman J., Charney D. (2000) Comorbidity of mood and anxiety disorders. *Depress. Anxiety*, **12** (Suppl. 1): 69–76.
11. Kessler R.C., Keller M.B., Wittchen H.U. (2001) The epidemiology of generalized anxiety disorder. *Psychiatr. Clin. North Am.*, **24**: 19–39.
12. Kendler K.S., Karkowski L.M., Walsh D. (1998) The structure of psychosis: latent class analysis of probands from the Roscommon Family Study. *Arch. Gen. Psychiatry*, **55**: 492–499.
13. World Health Organization (1996) *Diagnostic and Management Guidelines for Mental Disorders in Primary Care: ICD-10 Primary Care Version*. Hogrefe and Huber, Bern.
14. Cooper J.E. (1994) *Pocket Guide to the ICD-10 Classification of Mental and Behavioural Disorders, with Glossary and Diagnostic Criteria for Research*. Churchill Livingstone, Edinburgh.
15. World Health Organization (1997) *Multiaxial Presentation of the ICD-10 for Use in Adult Psychiatry*. Cambridge University Press, Cambridge.
16. World Health Organization (1989) *Lexicon of Psychiatric and Mental Health Terms*. World Health Organization, Geneva.
17. Sartorius N., Kaelber C.T., Cooper J.E., Roper M.T., Rae D.S., Gulbinat W., Üstün T.B., Regier D.A. (1993) Progress toward achieving a common language in psychiatry. Results from the field trial of the clinical guidelines accompanying the WHO classification of mental and behavioral disorders in ICD-10. *Arch. Gen. Psychiatry*, **50**: 115–124.
18. Sartorius N., Üstün T.B., Korten A., Cooper J.E., van Drimmelen J. (1995) Progress toward achieving a common language in psychiatry. II: Results from the International Field Trials of the ICD-10 Diagnostic Criteria for Research for Mental and Behavioral Disorders. *Am. J. Psychiatry*, **152**: 1427–1437.
19. Tsuang M.T., Stone W.S., Faraone S.V. (2000) Toward reformulating the diagnosis of schizophrenia. *Am. J. Psychiatry*, **157**: 1041–1050.

20. Bentall R.P. (1992) A proposal to classify happiness as a psychiatric disorder. *J. Med. Ethics*, **18**: 94–98.

21. Kendler K.S., Neale M.C., Kessler R.C., Heath A.C., Eaves L.J. (1992) A population based study of major depression in women—The impact of varying definitions of illness. *Arch. Gen. Psychiatry*, **49**: 257–265.

22. Robins E., Guze S.B. (1970) Establishment of diagnostic validity in psychiatric illness: its application to schizophrenia. *Am. J. Psychiatry*, **126**: 983–987.

23. Hasin D., Paykin A. (1999) Dependence symptoms but no diagnosis: diagnostic "orphans" in a 1992 national sample. *Drug Alcohol Depend.*, **53**: 215–222.

24. Pincus H.A., Davis W.W., McQueen L.E. (1999) "Subthreshold" mental disorders. A review and synthesis of studies on minor depression and other "brand names". *Br. J. Psychiatry*, **174**: 288–296.

25. Regier D.A., Kaelber C.T., Rae D.S., Farmer M.E., Knaupfer B., Kessler R.C., Norquist G.S. (1998) Limitations of diagnostic criteria and assessment instruments for mental disorders: implications for research and policy. *Arch. Gen. Psychiatry*, **55**: 109–115.

26. Spitzer R.L., Wakefield J.C. (1999) DSM-IV criteria for clinical significance. Does it help solve the false positive problem? *Am. J. Psychiatry*, **156**: 1856–1864.

27. Üstün T.B., Chatterji S., Rehm J. (1998) Limitations of diagnostic paradigm: it doesn't explain "need". *Arch. Gen. Psychiatry*, **55**: 1145–1146.

28. World Health Organization (2001) *International Classification of Functioning, Disability and Health (ICF)*. World Health Organization, Geneva.

29. Kortmann F. (1988) DSM-III in Ethiopia: a feasibility study. *Eur. Arch. Psychiatry Neurol. Sci.*, **237**: 101–105.

30. Weiss M.G., Raguram R., Channabasavanna S.M. (1995) Cultural dimensions of psychiatric diagnosis. A comparison of DSM-III-R and illness explanatory models in south India. *Br. J. Psychiatry*, **166**: 353–359.

31. Lee S. (1995) The Chinese classification of mental disorders. *Br. J. Psychiatry*, **167**: 117–118.

32. Room R., Janca A., Bennett L.A., Schmidt L., Sartorius N. (1996) WHO cross-cultural applicability research on diagnosis and assessment of substance use disorders: an overview of methods and selected results. *Addiction*, **91**: 199–220.

33. Goldberg D. (2000) Plato versus Aristotle. Categorical and dimensional models for common mental disorders. *Compr. Psychiatry*, **41**(Suppl. 1): 8–13.

34. van Os J., Gilvarry C., Bale R., van Horn E., Tattan T., White I., Murray R. (2000) Diagnostic value of the DSM and ICD categories of psychosis: an evidence-based approach. *Soc. Psychiatry Psychiatr. Epidemiol.*, **35**: 305–311.

35. Nurnberg H.G., Woodbury M.A., Bogenschutz M.P. (1999) A mathematical typology analysis of DSM-III-R personality disorder classification: grade of membership technique. *Compr. Psychiatry*, **40**: 61–71.

36. Pull C.B., Pull M.C., Pichot P. (1984) French empiric criteria for psychoses. I. Situation of the problem and methodology. *Encephale*, **10**: 119–123.

37. Andrews G., Slade T., Peters L. (1999) Classification in psychiatry: ICD-10 versus DSM-IV. *Br. J. Psychiatry*, **174**: 3–5.

38. First M.B., Pincus H.A. (1999) Classification in psychiatry: ICD-10 v. DSM-IV. A response. *Br. J. Psychiatry*, **175**: 205–209.

39. Farmer A., McGuffin A. (1999) Comparing ICD-10 and DSM-IV. *Br. J. Psychiatry*, **175**: 587–588.

40. Üstün B., Compton W., Mager D., Babor T., Baiyewu O., Chatterji S., Cottler L., Gogus A., Mavreas V., Peters L. *et al.* (1997) WHO study on the reliability and

validity of the alcohol and drug use disorder instruments: overview of methods and results. *Drug Alcohol Depend.*, **47**: 161–169.

41. Henderson A.S., Blackwood D.H. (1999) Molecular genetics in psychiatric epidemiology: the promise and challenge. *Psychol. Med.*, **29**: 1265–1271.

42. Baron M. (2001) Genetics of schizophrenia and the new millennium: progress and pitfalls. *Am. J. Hum. Genet.*, **68**: 299–312.

43. Kelsoe J.R., Spence M.A., Loetscher E., Foguet M., Sadovnick A.D., Remick R.A., Flodman P., Khristich J., Mroczkowski-Parker Z., Brown J.L. *et al.* (2001) A genome survey indicates a possible susceptibility locus for bipolar disorder on chromosome 22. *Proc. Natl. Acad. Sci. USA*, **98**: 585–590.

44. Leboyer M., Bellivier F., Nosten-Bertrand M., Jouvent R., Pauls D., Mallet J. (1998) Psychiatric genetics: search for phenotypes. *Trends Neurosci.*, **21**: 102–105.

45. Iacono W.G., Carlson S.R., Malone S.M. (2000) Identifying a multivariate endophenotype for substance use disorders using psychophysiological measures. *Int. J. Psychophysiol.*, **38**: 81–96.

46. Faraone S.V., Biederman J., Mennin D., Wozniak J., Spencer T. (1998) Attention-deficit hyperactivity disorder with bipolar disorder: a familial subtype? *J. Am. Acad. Child. Adolesc. Psychiatry*, **37**: 459–460.

47. Biederman J., Wilens T.E., Mick E., Faraone S.V., Spencer T. (1998) Does attention-deficit hyperactivity disorder impact the developmental course of drug and alcohol abuse and dependence? *Biol. Psychiatry*, **44**: 269–273.

48. Kan C.C., Breteler M.H., van der Ven A.H., Zitman F.G. (1998) An evaluation of DSM-III-R and ICD-10 benzodiazepine dependence criteria using Rasch modelling. *Addiction*, **93**: 349–359.

49. Manton K.G., Korten A., Woodbury M.A., Anker M., Jablensky A. (1994) Symptom profiles of psychiatric disorders based on graded disease classes: an illustration using data from the WHO International Pilot Study of Schizophrenia. *Psychol. Med.*, **24**: 133–144.

50. Corder E.H., Woodbury M.A., Volkmann I., Madsen D.K., Bogdanovic N., Winblad B. (2000) Density profiles of Alzheimer disease regional brain pathology for the Huddinge brain bank: pattern recognition emulates and expands upon Braak staging. *Exp. Gerontol.*, **35**: 851–864.

The American Psychiatric Association (APA) Classification of Mental Disorders: Strengths, Limitations and Future Perspectives

Darrel A. Regier[1,2], Michael First[3], Tina Marshall[1] and William E. Narrow[1,2]

[1]*Division of Research, American Psychiatric Association, Washington, DC, USA*
[2]*American Psychiatric Institute for Research and Education, Washington, DC, USA*
[3]*Department of Psychiatry, Columbia University, and Biometrics Research Department, New York State Psychiatric Institute, New York, NY, USA*

INTRODUCTION

This volume is being prepared during a period of relative quiescence for developers of the two major classification systems for mental, behavioral, and addictive disorders—the fourth edition of the *Diagnostic and Statistical Manual (DSM-IV)* [1] and the tenth edition of the *International Classification of Diseases (ICD-10)* [2]. We are at a point where the clinical and research communities have had 8–10 years of experience with these systems and can expect another similar period of time before major revisions appear. Hence, at this time it is useful to review where we have come in the history of creating reliable and valid diagnostic criteria for mental disorders, and to consider the potential for improving their specificity and clinical utility.

The following discussion has been developed to facilitate an historical perspective for future work in defining the boundaries and characteristics of psychopathology. The chapter begins with an historical overview of the American Psychiatric Association (APA)'s classification systems, that started with efforts to collect statistics about the population at large (i.e. US census), which would be consistent with statistics on the diagnostic composition of patients in mental hospitals. Next, there is a review of the history of international collaboration that has allowed for the ongoing coordination of

Psychiatric Diagnosis and Classification. Edited by Mario Maj, Wolfgang Gaebel, Juan José López-Ibor and Norman Sartorius. © 2002 John Wiley & Sons, Ltd.

efforts to develop classification systems by both the APA and the international scientific community. After a review of the strengths and limitations of the DSM-IV, the chapter concludes with a look ahead to future efforts to improve the validity and clinical utility of diagnostic criteria for psychopathology, and the arrangement of such diagnoses into a system of classification. The roots of the fifth edition of the *Diagnostic and Statistical Manual (DSM-V)* developmental process are described as are options for future efforts to ensure continued collaboration between US and international developers of the DSM and ICD systems.

HISTORICAL DEVELOPMENT

The natural predilection to categorize (and consequently to understand) mental illness dates back to at least 3000 BC, with a description of senile dementia in Prince Ptahhotep, followed by various terminology and classification approaches that have been proposed by philosophers and physicians throughout history [3]. The many proposed nomenclatures have differed based on their relative focus on phenomenology, aetiology, anatomical pathology, and course as central defining features of the disorders. One of the main purposes for developing a classification in the United States was for the collection of statistical information about the population at large (i.e. US census), which would be consistent with statistics on the diagnostic composition of patients in mental hospitals. The first official attempt to gather statistics about mental disorders in the United States started with the 1840 census, where a single category (idiocy/insanity) was included to count the number of individuals with a mental disorder or mental retardation. By the time of the 1880 census, seven distinct categories were recognized: mania, melancholia, monomania, paresis, dementia, dipsomania, and epilepsy [4].

In addition to this official federal effort as part of the census, individual insane asylums developed their own local classifications. By the turn of the twentieth century, there were almost as many statistical classifications in use as there were mental hospitals, thus preventing accurate comparisons among patient groups in different institutions. In 1918, spurred on by concern that the lack of a uniform classification would discredit the science of psychiatry, the Committee on Statistics of the American Medico-Psychological Association (which later became the American Psychiatric Association) introduced a 22-item list of disorders. This list could be used in every hospital in the country and also for detecting the prevalence of mental disorders in the 1920 census. This list was adopted by most mental hospitals until 1935, when a revised and expanded version was incorporated into the second edition of the American Medical Association (AMA)'s *Standard Classified Nomenclature of Diseases*.

This 1935 AMA classification proved to be inadequate when used in settings other than the chronic inpatient one. In particular, the significant number of acute psychiatric problems which developed among servicemen during World War II (10% of premature discharges during the war were for psychiatric reasons) prompted the Armed Forces to develop their own classification systems. By the end of the war, there were four major competing systems: the 1935 AMA Nomenclature, the US Army classification, the US Navy classification, and a system developed for use in the Veterans Administration hospitals. The emergence of multiple systems demonstrated the lack of a uniform classification that hampered comparisons among different settings. Furthermore, other sources of heterogeneity in the classification of mental disorders came from the attempts being made, around the same time, at developing an official international classification of mental disorders.

In 1948, the World Health Organization (WHO) took responsibility for the sixth revision of the *International List of Causes of Death*, and renamed it the *International Classification of Diseases, Injuries, and Causes of Death (ICD-6)* [5]. It added for the first time a section for the classification of mental disorders, which contained 10 categories of psychosis, nine categories of psychoneurosis, and seven categories of disorders of character, behavior, and intelligence. However, problems with the classification rendered it unsatisfactory for use in the United States and other countries (only five countries, including the United Kingdom, officially adopted it). First, several important categories, such as the dementias, many personality and adjustment disorders, were not included. In addition, many diagnostic terms had aetiologic implications that were at odds with the various schools of psychiatry in the United States.

For these reasons, an alternative to the mental disorders section of ICD-6 was developed in 1952 as the *Diagnostic and Statistical Manual, Mental Disorders (DSM-I)* [6], which, for the first time in an official classification, provided a glossary of definitions. It included many concepts that were influential in American psychiatry at the time, like the term "reaction", reflecting Adolph Meyer's perspective that mental disorders represented reactions of the person to psychological, social, and biologic factors.

In recognition of the lack of widespread international acceptance of the mental disorder sections of ICD-6 and ICD-7, the WHO asked Erwin Stengel, a British psychiatrist, to offer recommendations as to how the next revision of the ICD should proceed. He recommended the adoption of operational definitions of disorders that were independent of any aetiologic theories [7]. Although these suggestions were not adopted in time for ICD-8, they did foreshadow the introduction of explicit diagnostic criteria into the DSM-III.

In 1959, the WHO (with the assistance of psychiatrists in the United States) began work on the next revision of the ICD with the goal of creating a system that would represent a consensus of concepts and terms acceptable to all of its member nations. In 1965, the APA started preparing a second edition of the DSM based on early drafts of ICD-8 [8], but with definitions of each disorder for use in the United States [9]. Such definitions were necessary because ICD-8 (which came into effect in 1968) was initially published without an accompanying glossary. A glossary was eventually published in 1974, six years after the introduction of DSM-II [10]. DSM-II dropped the term "reaction", and, unlike DSM-I, encouraged clinicians to make multiple diagnoses, even if one diagnosis was causally related to another (e.g. alcoholism secondary to depression).

The precedent for developing "local" adaptations of the ICD system goes back to ICD-6. Adaptations of ICD were originally developed starting in 1950 for use in indexing hospital medical records [11], a purpose for which ICD-6 was not particularly well suited. After independent efforts were made by a number of different institutions, the US National Committee on Vital and Health Statistics proposed that uniform changes in the ICD be made. The major users of the ICD for hospital indexing purposes consolidated their experiences, and an adaptation of ICD-6 (called the ICDA) was first published in December 1959. Although the 1965 International Conference for the Revision of the ICD noted that ICD-8 (unlike ICD-6) had been constructed with hospital indexing in mind and suggested that it would, therefore, be suitable for hospital use in some countries, it also recognized that it might provide inadequate detail for diagnostic indexing in other countries.

After study of ICD-8 by a group of consultants in the United States, it was decided that further detail was needed for coding hospital morbidity data and that an ICDA continued to be needed [12]. In order to preserve international compatibility, complete correspondence between the ICDA and the parent ICD classification was maintained at the three digit level. This principle of adaptation to suit the needs of healthcare providers and institutions has continued in the United States, as evidenced by the development and ongoing maintenance of "Clinical Modifications" of the ICD by a consortium of US Government and professional organizations. Updates to this version of the ICD (currently ICD-9-CM in the United States) are made on a yearly basis, in response to proposals made by healthcare professionals, organizations and institutions.

The early 1970s saw the introduction of diagnostic criteria for research in the United States. Although the DSM-II glossary definitions were an improvement over just having a list of diagnostic terms, these brief paragraphs were too vague to assist in identifying homogeneous groups for research studies. Researchers responded to this problem by developing their own explicit diagnostic criteria for the particular disorders they were studying. In 1972, a group of researchers at the Washington University School of

Medicine, led by Eli Robins and Samuel Guze, developed the first set of St. Louis diagnostic criteria for research, named the "Feighner Criteria", after the senior author of the paper presenting the criteria [13]. Going back to the Kraepelinian principles of classifying patients based on a description of symptoms that co-occur across groups of patients, diagnostic criteria were provided for 16 diagnostic categories. A few years later, as part of the National Institute of Mental Health (NIMH) collaborative project on the psychobiology of depression, Robert L. Spitzer and colleagues modified the Feighner criteria and added criteria for several additional disorders. The resulting classification was called the Research Diagnostic Criteria (RDC) [14].

In order to facilitate the reliable application of these newly defined diagnostic criteria, structured interviews were developed to help researchers elicit the symptoms necessary for determining whether criteria were met. For the Feighner criteria, an interview called the Renard Diagnostic Interview was developed [15]; for the RDC, the interview was known as the Schedule for Affective Disorders and Schizophrenia (SADS) [16]. Both the RDC and the associated interview schedules became popular among researchers and were frequently used in research on psychotic and mood disorders.

To develop the mental disorders section for ICD-9, WHO initiated an intensive program aiming to identify problems encountered by psychiatrists in different countries in the use of the mental disorders section of ICD-8 and to formulate recommendations for their solutions. A series of eight international seminars were held annually from 1965 to 1972, each of which focused on a recognized problem in psychiatric diagnosis. The outcome of the seminars formed the basis for the recommendations made for ICD-9, which was ultimately published in 1978.

In 1974, after reviewing early drafts of ICD-9, the APA opted to develop a third edition of the *Diagnostic and Statistical Manual (DSM-III)* because of concerns that the specificity and subtyping were inadequate, and that the glossary of ICD-9 did not take advantage of the then-recent innovations, such as explicit diagnostic criteria and a multiaxial system [17]. Under the leadership of Robert L. Spitzer, successive drafts of DSM-III were prepared by 14 advisory committees composed of professionals with special expertise. The drafts were distributed among American and international psychiatrists for comments and review. Many of the DSM-III criteria sets were based on the RDC criteria, with additional criteria sets developed based on expert clinical consensus.

The improvement in reliability over DSM-II (which provided only glossary definitions) was demonstrated by a large NIMH supported field trial in which clinicians were asked to independently evaluate patients using drafts of the DSM-III criteria (Appendix F: pp. 467–481). The two main innovations introduced by DSM-III were the provision of explicit diagnostic criteria for each of the disorders in the classification and a multiaxial system for recording the diagnostic evaluation. The multiaxial system facilitated the use of a biopsychosocial model of evaluation by separating (and thereby calling attention to) developmental and personality disorders (Axis II), physical conditions (Axis III), stressors (Axis IV), and degree of adaptive functioning (Axis V) from the usually more florid presenting diagnoses (Axis I).

Despite initial opposition among some psychiatrists (most especially those with a psychoanalytic orientation), DSM-III proved to be a great success. Soon after its publication, it became widely accepted in the United States as the common language of mental health clinicians and researchers for communicating about mental disorders. Although it was intended primarily for use in the United States, it was translated into 13 languages and widely used by the international research community.

Experience with the DSM-III in the few years after its publication in 1980 revealed a number of inconsistencies and lack of clarity in the diagnostic criteria sets. Furthermore, research conducted in the early 1980s demonstrated errors in some of the assumptions that went into the construction of the DSM-III criteria sets [18–20]. For example, the DSM-III prohibition against giving an additional diagnosis of panic disorder to individuals with major depressive disorder and panic attacks was shown to be incorrect, based on data demonstrating that relatives of individuals with both major depressive disorder and panic attacks can have either major depressive or panic disorder. For this reason, work began on a revision of the DSM-III, which was published as DSM-III-R in 1987 [21].

The APA started work on the development of DSM-IV [1] shortly afterward, spurred on by the need to coordinate its development with the already ongoing development of ICD-10. There were three main innovations in the DSM-IV developmental process [22]:

1. Its reliance on a comprehensive review of the literature and other empirical data as a justification for making changes.
2. Efforts made to solicit and incorporate input and guidance from the widest variety of sources (i.e. from national and international panels of advisors, from various organizational bodies, and from clinicians and others via widespread dissemination of drafts).
3. Documentation of the empirical basis for changes in a four-volume *DSM-IV Sourcebook* [23–26].

In conjunction with the publication of DSM-IV in 1994, an "international version" of DSM-IV was published in 1995 [27]. This version of DSM-IV was identical in content except for its use of ICD-10 diagnostic codes in place of the ICD-9-CM codes appearing in the North American version. For a number of reasons, implementation of ICD-10 has been delayed in the United States, necessitating the continued use of ICD-9-CM codes. In the United States, reimbursement to healthcare providers and institutions by the Health Care Financing Administration (HCFA) is tied to medical diagnosis through a complex system known as diagnosis-related groupings (DRGs). Thus, the cost of implementing ICD-10-CM is potentially much more than simply substituting alphanumeric codes for the current numeric codes in ICD-9. Reticence about allocating the considerable funds for reprogramming the DRG system, combined with the decision to allocate most programming resources to fix "Y2K bugs" during the latter half of the 1990s, has resulted in significant delays in ICD-10-CM implementation. Although progress has been slow, it appears that ICD-10-CM implementation in the United States should be a reality over the next several years.

INTERNATIONAL COLLABORATION ON DIAGNOSTIC CRITERIA AND INSTRUMENTS

Impact of DSM-III on Diagnostic Instrument Development

The availability of explicit criteria for defining specific types of mental disorder in the DSM-III led immediately to their incorporation into several diagnostic assessment instruments for research studies. The previous DSM-II and ICD-9 classifications contained general descriptions or "thumbnail sketches" of disorder concepts that were aided by glossaries that defined clinical terms in greater detail. However, because of the lack of precision in defining diagnostic syndromes, actual clinical experience was considered necessary to fully understand the nature of the diagnostic entities. Since clinical experience and traditions for evaluating potential causes for disorders vary widely, the reliability of diagnoses across different national boundaries was found to be low.

A cross-national United States/United Kingdom (US/UK) study, conducted in the late 1960s [28], demonstrated that the application of a semi-structured diagnostic assessment instrument, the Present State Examination (PSE), which forced clinicians in both countries to use identical criteria and methods, could eliminate the wide national variations in hospital inpatient rates of schizophrenia and manic-depressive disorder that had been found when diagnoses were based only on clinician judgement [29]. However, until the emergence of the DSM-III, widely accepted official diagnostic criteria were not sufficiently explicit for incorporation into a highly structured interview that could be administered by non-clinicians in large-scale epidemiological studies of general populations.

With the emergence of the DSM-III criteria in the late 1970s, the NIMH initiated a collaborative process between the chief editor of the DSM-III, Robert Spitzer, and Lee Robins, the lead author of the Renard Diagnostic Interview, which was designed to incorporate the St. Louis criteria for use in epidemiological studies. The resultant NIMH Diagnostic Interview Schedule (DIS) [30] incorporated the new DSM-III criteria for use as the diagnostic assessment instrument of the Epidemiologic Catchment Area (ECA) study—a five-site study of 20 000 community and institutionalized residents to determine prevalence, incidence, and mental health service rates in the United States [31, 32].

In addition to the DIS, which has been widely used in many national and international epidemiological studies, Robert Spitzer and colleagues [33] also developed a semi-structured clinical interview, the Structured Clinical Interview for DSM (SCID), which became a standardized assessment instrument for most clinical research studies in the United States and in many international studies.

Impact of DSM-III on International Classification

After significant differences between the ICD-9 and emerging DSM-III were recognized in the late 1970s, scientific leaders of the US Alcohol, Drug Abuse, and Mental Health Administration (ADAMHA) and the WHO initiated a process to bring these major diagnostic systems closer together. Gerald Klerman, Administrator of ADAMHA, and Norman Sartorius, Director of the Mental Health Division of WHO, began a multi-phase project that was initiated in 1980–1981 with a series of international task forces to prepare position papers and reviews of the different approaches taken by national "schools" of psychiatry in describing specific mental and addictive disorders [34]. The second phase (1981–1982) was the planning and execution of a major International Conference on Diagnosis and Classification of Mental Disorders and Alcohol- and Drug-Related Problems, which took place in April 1982 in Copenhagen, Denmark, involving 150 invited participants from 47 different countries [35]. It was at this conference that an international consensus was reached to adopt an operational approach to describing clinical disorders with explicit diagnostic criteria—without aetiological implications—for the ICD-10 [36].

Although Erwin Stengel had recommended such an approach as far back as 1959, the DSM-III exemplified the feasibility of breaking with nationalistic theoretical traditions in favor of an approach that transformed diagnostic criteria into testable hypotheses. Rather than having diagnostic constructs containing untestable aetiological assumptions (e.g. anxiety, depressive or psychotic states were reactive to environmental stress/unconscious conflicts or biologically determined), it became possible to focus on the degree to which a constellation of observable signs and symptoms, of specified duration and intensity, could predict clinical course, response to treatment, genetic aggregation, and other external laboratory-based indicators of diagnostic validity and clinical utility [37].

A third phase (1982–1994) of international collaboration was supported by a continuous cooperative agreement between the WHO and three US ADAMHA/National Institutes of Health (NIH)—the NIMH, the National Institute of Drug Abuse (NIDA), and the National Institute on Alcoholism and Alcohol Abuse (NIAAA). The strategy employed in this collaboration, co-chaired through most of this period by Norman Sartorius at the WHO and Darrel Regier at the NIMH, was to develop diagnostic assessment instruments for epidemiological and clinical studies that would permit cross-national data collection to expand the empirical base of diagnosis and classification for DSM-IV and ICD-10. Since useful criteria needed to be sufficiently clear and explicit to be incorporated into these instruments for empirical testing, less testable and vague concepts, contained in previous versions of the ICD or other national classifications, were systematically eliminated by the multinational collaborative group. Three instruments were developed under this project: the Composite International Diagnostic Interview (CIDI) [38, 39], which was based on the DIS, for epidemiological study; the Schedules for Clinical Assessment in Neuropsychiatry (SCAN) [40], which was based on the PSE, for clinical research; and the International Personality Disorders Examination (IPDE) [41].

As a result of clinical and epidemiological research with the resulting diagnostic assessment instruments, it became apparent that the increased specificity of diagnostic criteria had not eliminated wide ranges of disability and impairment within diagnostic groups. Attention was then turned toward the collaborative development of a revised version of the *International Classification of Impairments, Disabilities and Handicaps (ICIDH)* [42], to increase the reliability with which these dimensions of illness could be classified. Although the lead for this activity has been with the WHO staff led by Bedirhan Üstün [43], substantial support and collaborative research expertise was provided by the NIH. A disability assessment schedule (WHO-DAS) linked to the ICIDH was also developed and tested as part of the WHO/NIH cooperative agreement.

Collaborative Development of DSM-IV and ICD-10

At the same time that the various international workgroups were developing the three instruments and subjecting them to multi-site reliability testing, a series of diagnostic-specific consensus conferences between

DSM-IV (led by Allen Frances) and ICD-10 workgroups (led by Norman Sartorius) were convened and coordinated by Darrel Regier under the sponsorship of ADAMHA. These workgroups, guided by emerging epidemiological and clinical research findings from studies using most of the above instruments, were able to obtain consensus on the overall framework of the diagnostic system and on the great majority of explicit criteria for specific disorders. The few remaining discrepancies in criteria are being subjected to empirical tests to determine the impact of such differences on prevalence and service use rates [44, 45].

Finally, testing for the clarity, clinical utility, and reliability of the diagnostic criteria for both DSM-IV and ICD-10 took place in international field trials, which greatly increased the acceptability and use of both diagnostic systems. The ICD-10 field trials followed a similar approach to that used in the early DSM-III trials to assess acceptability, clinical utility, and reliability of raters—involving over 200 centers in 50 countries [46, 47]. The exceptional congruence between DSM-IV and ICD-10 has permitted the development of a cumulative body of knowledge that has greatly advanced research on both psychosocial and pharmacological treatments for these disorders.

STRENGTHS OF THE DSM SYSTEM

The numerous strengths of the DSM system, particularly since the publication of DSM-III, have been covered in the historical narrative presented in the previous sections, and will be summarized here. Undoubtedly the most important strength of the DSM system is its widespread acceptance by clinicians, researchers, administrators, and others as a common language for describing psychopathology. This acceptance comes as a result of several factors. The "atheoretical" stance of the DSM-III helped to ensure that diagnostic criteria would not be tied to any particular school of thought regarding aetiology, allowing use by persons with different clinical experience and traditions. Diagnostic criteria, based solely on descriptive phenomenology, were specified with a greater degree of precision than with previous diagnostic systems, increasing the reliability of diagnosis between diagnosticians in various settings. Efforts to improve congruence with the ICD system, and the translation of DSM into multiple languages have facilitated international use of the system.

Beyond providing a readily usable common language for mental disorders, the DSM has several other strengths. The precise, descriptive diagnostic criteria in DSM-III and its successors have contributed to a new era in psychiatric research through the development of reliable structured and semi-structured research instruments. Another strength of the DSM, particularly the DSM-IV and its text revision (DSM-IV-TR), was the commitment of its developers to having an empirical basis for all further revisions [48]. The development of the DSM-IV, described above, entailed a three-stage empirical review process, and to avoid bias consulted review panels comprised of diverse national and international experts. This rigorous process, documented in the *DSM-IV Sourcebook* [23–26], further enhanced scientific credibility and acceptance of the diagnostic criteria. The DSM-IV-TR reflected recent advances in epidemiology, clinical research, and other contextual areas, underscoring the importance of empirical evidence to the ongoing development of the diagnostic system, and providing up-to-date information for students, clinicians, family members, and others.

LIMITATIONS OF THE DSM SYSTEM

DSM-III's use of explicit diagnostic criteria based on symptoms, relatively free of aetiologic assumptions and subject to direct observation and measurement, fostered a renewed optimism for psychiatric research in the United States. Such objective criteria, it was hoped, would facilitate the validation of psychiatric diagnoses, much in the way described by Robins and Guze [37], i.e. through an increasingly precise clinical description, laboratory studies, delimitation of disorders, follow-up studies of outcome, and family studies. Once validated, the classification would form the basis for the identification of standard, homogeneous groups for aetiologic and treatment studies.

Over the succeeding 20 years, however, fulfilling the Robins and Guze validity criteria has remained an elusive goal. Laboratory indices pathognomonic for the major DSM disorders have not been found. Epidemiologic and clinical studies have shown high rates of non-specific comorbidities among the disorders, making a clear delimitation of disorders difficult [18, 49]. Long-term follow-up studies have been relatively rare, due to their complexity and cost, but epidemiologic studies have shown a high degree of short-term diagnostic instability for many disorders [50, 51].

There is not strong evidence that treatment response is indicative of the specificity of individual diagnoses. Many of the new psychotropic medications that have been developed, such as the selective serotonin reuptake inhibitors, are efficacious across different diagnoses, such as major depression, obsessive-compulsive disorder, panic disorder, binge-eating disorder, and post-traumatic stress disorder. Furthermore, family studies have shown that many DSM disorders are familial in origin, with strong genetic components, but also that a wide variety of disorders may be expressed in a single family, for example, schizophrenia with schizophrenia-spectrum disorders and certain affective disorders [52].

To date, the aetiologies of the major DSM disorders have not been elucidated, although variably strong evidence exists for genetic, neuroanatomical, infectious, traumatic, and developmental factors. The problems in establishing the aetiology of DSM disorders may in part be related to the difficulties in establishing the validity of the diagnostic categories mentioned above. It has been suggested that aetiologic research should venture beyond the current descriptive diagnostic boundaries of the DSM, and that resulting advances in genetics, neurobiology, and epidemiology be used in an iterative process to update diagnostic criteria. This will help prevent premature reification of current DSM categories and ensure a dynamic interaction between research and the refinement of diagnoses [53–56].

Despite its many advances, the DSM-IV has limitations, many of which have been acknowledged by its developers [57, 58]. A growing literature from a range of disciplines—such as psychology, nursing, marital and family therapy, anthropology, and philosophy—has also documented limitations in the DSM-IV [59–62]. Some of the criticisms of DSM-IV stem from general criticisms of a categorical approach to mental disorders; some are targeted to specific criteria or specific disorders. The limitations can be broadly grouped into four categories:

1. Problems with the DSM definition of a mental disorder.
2. Problems with the research base for many disorders.
3. Gaps in classification.
4. Problems with the use of DSM in diverse populations and settings.

A major underlying concept with all of the limitations is a concern for the validity of the classification.

DSM-IV Definition of Mental Disorder

DSM-IV states:

> Each of the mental disorders is conceptualized as a clinically significant behavioral or psychological syndrome or pattern that occurs in an individual and that is associated with present distress (e.g. a painful symptom) or disability (i.e. impairment in one or more important areas of functioning) or with a significantly increased risk of suffering death, pain, disability, or an important loss of freedom. In addition, this syndrome or pattern must not be merely an expectable and culturally sanctioned response to a particular event, for example, the death of a loved one. Whatever its original cause, it must currently be considered a manifestation of a behavioral, psychological or biological dysfunction in the individual. Neither deviant behavior (e.g. political, religious or sexual) nor conflicts that are primarily between the individual and society are mental disorders unless the deviance or conflict is a symptom of a dysfunction in the individual as described above.

The authors of the DSM-IV were straightforward about the limitations of this definition, and of any definition of mental disorder. A major concern is that the boundary between normal experiences of life and a pathological condition cannot be clearly stated, giving rise to criticisms that DSM "pathologizes the normal". In practical terms, this problem is most pronounced in "threshold" cases, which barely meet diagnostic criteria, are of mild severity, or associated with only mild distress or impairment in functioning. The clinical significance or need for treatment in such cases is a hotly debated issue [63].

Alternative definitions of mental disorder have been proposed. For example, Wakefield [64] argues for a definition of mental disorder based on the concept of "harmful mental dysfunction", which requires both evidence that the symptoms are a manifestation of a mental dysfunction—the failure of a mental mechanism to perform its natural (i.e. evolutionarily selected) function—and that the symptoms cause harm to the individual (e.g. lead to impairment in social or occupational functioning). While this definition is appealing, because it combines both scientific/factual elements (i.e. the requirement for dysfunction) as well as social values (i.e. requirement for harm) into the definition, in practical terms it is usually limited by insufficient understanding of the aetiology of disorders, which prevents a determination of the mental mechanism that is disordered. The adoption in DSM-V of a revised definition of mental disorder that satisfactorily reduces potential false positives, would be most useful in setting the diagnostic thresholds for the various criteria sets of individual DSM disorders.

The concepts of present distress and disability took on new importance in DSM-IV, as they were embedded in the diagnostic criteria of many disorders. It can be argued that the inclusion of such a criterion increases the likelihood that cases meeting symptom criteria have a clinically significant disorder, or are "true cases", at least for health policy and planning purposes [63]. On the other hand, it has been argued that the syndrome, composed of symptoms, should remain uncoupled from disability and distress in making a diagnosis, which is the model used by the WHO [65, 66]. The developmental trajectories and interrelationships of psychiatric symptoms and associated disabilities are not yet clear. It is well-known, for example, that significant disability and mental health service use can occur in persons with symptoms that do not meet criteria for major depressive disorder [67–69]. Also, symptom patterns, regardless of disability, are important for aetiologic research such as genetic epidemiology [70].

Research Base for DSM-IV Disorders

Two types of problems have been pointed out regarding the research base for DSM-IV, one concerned with the revision process itself and the other concerned with the amount and type of research underlying the diagnoses [71]. The revision process of DSM-IV was explicitly guided by the empirical database available for each disorder, and was accomplished through comprehensive literature reviews, secondary data analyses and field trials. Still, it has been argued that the DSM-IV workgroups, comprised overwhelmingly of psychiatrists, neglected the potential value of basic behavioral and social sciences in reaching their decisions. This argument has been particularly pointed in the child and adolescent field, in which the discipline of developmental psychopathology has sought an increased role [72]. Higher visibility and increased participation of researchers in neuroscience, genetics, epidemiology, anthropology, and sociology in future revisions of the DSM have also been advocated.

Ideally, a research base for mental disorder nosology and classification should include studies representing epidemiology, genetics, clinical research, basic brain research, social and behavioral science, and psychometrics. The current research base varies widely from this ideal, both in quality and quantity. For example, in the child and adolescent field, research on disability and its relationship to symptoms has outpaced the same research for adult populations [73, 74]. There is a fast-growing body of work in basic child development and its relationship to psychopathology. Yet treatment research has lagged for children, and there is still no widely generalizable epidemiological study of mental disorders for this population in the United States [75, 76]. A relative lack of data has prevented a needed overhaul of the personality disorder diagnoses which are universally agreed to be unsatisfactory, and there are virtually no data on the "not otherwise specified" diagnoses. A weak database undermines confidence in the reliability and validity of a diagnosis among clinicians and scientists. Among other users of the DSM—such as the legal system, insurers, government officials, and the public at large—diagnoses can be assigned an uncritical equivalence in validity, leading to inappropriate usage.

Gaps in Classification

The DSM-IV diagnostic categories, as mentioned above, were set up with varying degrees of research to support them. As the research base grows, and as the classification is used and scrutinized by clinicians, limitations inevitably emerge, as well as opportunities for modification. Personality disorders have received considerable attention [77]. Although in DSM-IV they are categorical entities and their criteria are generally met by symptom counts, the DSM-IV "general diagnostic criteria for a personality disorder" seem to lend themselves to a scalar or dimensional approach. For example, a person with a personality disorder must have inner experiences and behaviors that deviate markedly from his or her cultural expectations. Further, the personality pattern must occur in areas that are not generally thought of as categorical: cognition (i.e. perception and interpretation of self, others and events), affectivity, interpersonal functioning, or impulse control. DSM-IV further characterizes personality disorders as occurring when "personality traits are inflexible and maladaptive and cause significant functional impairment or subjective distress", the notion of traits further supporting a scalar or dimensional approach [1]. The placement of several disorders on Axis II rather than Axis I has also been questioned. Several personality disorders have been implicated as "spectrum disorders" of Axis I conditions in genetic studies—for example, schizotypal personality disorder with schizophrenia [78]. The rationale for schizotypal personality disorder's placement on Axis II is not clear, particularly when other spectrum disorders such as cyclothymic disorder appear on Axis I.

Suggestions have been made to integrate two areas, relational problems and high-risk conditions, into the DSM system [61]. Relational problems are now included in DSM-IV as "other conditions that may be a focus of clinical attention", and are coded on Axis I or Axis IV. Specific criteria were not provided, due to a lack of relevant data, although research has been accumulating. A better conceptualization of relational problems may help elucidate some Axis I disorders, for example oppositional defiant disorder. Inclusion of relational problems into the DSM system has implications for clinical assessment by expanding the focus of diagnostic assessments from the individual to a relationship.

DSM-IV shows a lack of attention to high-risk conditions, reflecting a general focus on treatment rather than prevention. This has been due in part to a lag in research to accurately and efficiently identify persons at high risk for mental disorders and a paucity of rigorously tested, effective interventions. Issues of stigmatization are also a concern. Current research with depressed mothers and their children [79], and with persons having the syndrome of schizotaxia [80], have shown promise as targets for preventive interventions. Whether the field of prevention will develop in time for consideration in DSM-V remains to be seen, but ultimately, high-risk conditions should be identified and operationalized, and interventions, including regular "mental health check-ups", could be instituted.

Use of DSM in Diverse Populations and Settings

DSM-IV has become the *de facto* classification system for mental disorders in the United States and much of the world, a testimony to its ease of use, generalizability, and utility in a variety of clinical and non-clinical settings. The classification does fall short for patients at either end of the lifespan, for minorities and for non-Western cultures. Also, practitioners in non-specialty settings may not be able to make full use of the DSM.

DSM-IV presents a number of problems in the classification of child and adolescent disorders. Several of these have been alluded to above, including gaps in the research base and insufficient attention to the vicissitudes of normative and pathological development, the contributions of relational problems and other contextual factors, and high-risk conditions. DSM-IV gives minimal guidance on the diagnosis of "child onset" disorders in adults, e.g. attention deficit/hyperactivity disorder (ADHD) [81], and on the diagnosis of "adult onset" disorders in children, e.g. bipolar disorder [82]. High rates of mental disorder comorbidity in this population call into question the adequacy of the individual DSM-IV diagnoses to accurately represent psychopathology [83]. Disorders of infants and very young children are not covered well in DSM-IV, which has led to the development of a separate diagnostic system called *Diagnostic Classification of Mental Health and Developmental Disorders of Infancy and Early Childhood*, better known as DC: 0–3 [84]. The field's understanding of the significance of developmental changes beyond young adulthood has come relatively late, and this is also reflected in DSM-IV. Little attention has been paid to changes in the diagnostic picture as an individual ages, and with a rapidly aging population in the United States, the phenomenology of mental disorders in the elderly is of crucial importance [85].

The United States continues to increase in its ethnic, racial and cultural diversity. Western or Euro-American social norms, meanings of illness and treatment, and idioms of distress cannot be assumed for other cultural groups. DSM-IV tends to reflect a Western model of mental disorders, but does give attention to culture in several places: in the introduction ("Issues in the use of DSM-IV"); in its definitions of disorder; in the "specific culture features" sections of the text; and in Appendix I, "Outline for cultural formulation and glossary of culture-bound syndromes". It does not, however, provide guidance on applying specific cultural features to specific disorders. This is a tall order indeed, considering the wide diversity of cultural groups in the United States, encompassing those identified by language, color, religion, sexual orientation, disability, and a host of other factors [86–90].

Finally, another important limitation of the DSM-IV is its difficulty of use in non-specialty treatment settings, in particular primary care settings. This limitation is particularly important in rural areas with low concentrations of specialty providers, and in areas where primary care providers do the majority of mental health care. Many aspects of the DSM criteria require clinical judgement that is best obtained by specialty training, for example diagnosing personality disorders. Time limitations on general practitioners may impede the full psychiatric evaluation that DSM-IV requires. The psychiatric interview also relies on the verbal self-report of symptoms by the patient; DSM-IV gives no guidance on laboratory tests, rating scales or other mechanisms that may aid in the evaluation of many of these problems [27]. More research and training are needed to fully integrate mental health evaluations into primary care settings.

DEVELOPMENTAL PROCESS FOR DSM-V

Update of Text Revision—DSM-IV-TR

Since the publication of DSM-III in 1980, the average interval between major revisions of the DSM has been seven years. DSM-III-R, which was published in 1987, came shortly after DSM-III because its goal was to correct those errors and problems identified in the DSM-III. Work began on DSM-IV almost immediately afterward because of the need to convene work groups that could work collaboratively with the previously mentioned WHO working groups who were aiming toward a 1992 target date for publication of ICD-10. After the publication of DSM-IV in 1994, with no externally driven timeline for DSM-V, the APA decided to considerably lengthen the gap between DSM-IV and DSM-V, in order to allow for a more extensive knowledge base to develop that would inform the DSM-V revision process.

One potential effect of the lengthened interval is its effect on the currency of the DSM-IV text. Each disorder in DSM-IV is accompanied by 1–10 pages of explanatory text that is designed to educate clinicians, researchers, students, interns, residents, patients, and family members about the clinical presentation, course, prevalence, familial risk, and other aspects of the disorder. Like the DSM-IV diagnostic criteria, the DSM-IV text was prepared based on a comprehensive review of the literature dating up to mid-1992. Thus, as each year passes, the information presented in the text runs the risk of becoming increasingly out of date with the large volume of research published each year. Therefore, the APA decided to undertake a revision of the DSM-IV text to ensure that it continues to be informative and clinically useful during the years prior to the release of DSM-V.

Two overriding principles governed the preparation of a text revision of DSM-IV. First, no major changes were allowed in the DSM-IV criteria sets or structure of the DSM-IV. Criteria set changes are disruptive to both researchers and clinicians in terms of the costs of revamping the myriad of assessment tools, the cost of the educational efforts, and its effect on complicating the comparison of studies that used different versions of the criteria sets. A few small changes in criteria sets to correct known DSM-IV errors were permitted, however [91]. The second principle was that the text revision be empirically based. Thus, changes to the DSM-IV were based on a literature review that covered the research database from 1992 until 1999. The DSM-IV text revision, referred to as DSM-IV-TR to distinguish it from DSM-IV, was published in July 2000 [4].

DSM-V Research Planning Process

In preparation for the DSM-V revision, the APA has initiated a process to stimulate research that might enrich the empirical database in psychiatry. The DSM-V research planning process began in September 1999 with a conference sponsored by the APA and the NIMH. The conference resulted in a series of forums to identify gaps within the current classification systems and to develop a research agenda to be pursued over the coming years. Many of the strengths and limitations outlined above were discussed in the forums, which led to the identification of six topic areas: nomenclature, disability and impairment, DSM-IV "gaps" (i.e. personality and relational disorders and the role of racism in DSM), developmental disorders, neuroscience, and cross-cultural issues. Workgroups corresponding to the six topic areas were comprised of leading experts in the field and were charged with the task of writing research recommendations in the form of white papers. In addition to writing a separate white paper on core cross-cultural issues and gender-specific issues that span all diagnostic criteria, cross-cultural workgroup members were also involved in the remaining workgroups to contribute recommendations on cross-cultural issues and gender-specific issues as they specifically related to the other five topic areas.

Nomenclature

The Nomenclature workgroup discussed many of the limitations outlined above regarding the DSM-IV definition of mental disorder. The group recommended exploring viable definitions of mental disorders and evaluating their effectiveness using a range of currently available theoretical approaches such as the previously described Wakefield's proposal [64].

The Nomenclature workgroup also contributed research recommendations intended to increase the compatibility between the DSM-V and the ICD-11 and, accordingly, increase the applicability of criteria across different cultures. The workgroup recommended a stepwise approach for future research, starting with a replication of the present DSM and ICD dissonance estimates to identify minor differences that may be easily resolved. For example, minor differences in the exclusionary criteria for the DSM and ICD may explain some of the variance found in comparison studies. Defining clear principles to govern exclusion criteria would be a useful step for improving comparability. Subsequently, a research strategy would also be required to address substantive differences between the DSM and ICD.

To enhance the usefulness of the DSM-IV in non-psychiatric treatment settings, the Nomenclature workgroup contributed a set of recommendations to facilitate the diagnostic process in such settings. These were to promote research examining the degree to which diagnostic criteria can be reliably and validly rated using self-report, and the degree to which biological tests or psychometrically sound rating scales may be used in the diagnostic process to screen subjects that can benefit from different types of intervention.

Disability and Impairment

As mentioned above, the inclusion of the concepts of disability and impairment in the DSM definition of mental disorders and the multiaxial approach strengthen the diagnostic process by broadening the clinical focus beyond symptoms to the assessment of psychosocial issues and functioning. However, inconsistencies in the association between symptoms and functioning raise the question of whether the current axial system is the best approach. To examine the complex interaction between symptoms and disability, the Disability and Impairment workgroup recommended research on the conceptual and operational definitions of functioning, disability and impairment. These studies should assess the potential for incorporating contextual, environmental, lifespan and cultural considerations into the assessment of disability and impairment. These factors may help form distinctions between individuals who are unable to function due to the disability as opposed to those experiencing deficits in functioning due to a lack of opportunity or discrimination. In addition to alternative frameworks for measuring disability, new tools to assess disability and impairment were also recommended.

Gaps in Classification

The Gaps workgroup contributed research recommendations to address gaps in diagnostic criteria for personality disorders and relational problems. The group is also recommending that research be considered to address whether racism should be more prominently featured in the DSM. Recommendations to inform the diagnosis and treatment of personality disorders were focused on clarifying the relationship between personality disorders and Axis I disorders. The workgroup recommended further investigations of whether some of the current DSM-IV personality disorders may be better viewed as on a spectrum with current Axis I disorders rather than by the current categorical approach.

The Gaps workgroup recommended exploring alternative conceptualizations for describing maladaptive personality patterns, such as dimensional models of personality. Studies comparing the validity (particularly documenting that the pattern is stable and of long duration), reliability and clinical usefulness of various dimensional models are recommended. Additionally, the workgroup recommended longitudinal research to explore the interaction between temperaments and environment in the development of personality disorders.

While important advances have been made in understanding biological mechanisms for antisocial, borderline, and schizotypal personality disorders, more biogenetic and heritability research is needed for these and other personality disorders. Furthermore, the workgroup highlighted the need to identify neurophysiological mechanisms that would explain the heritability of maladaptive personality patterns.

Future research may explore ways to define specific relational disorders and how relational problems interact with Axis I disorders. These issues may also be informed by research examining the development of diagnostic criteria for relational disorders and by research that determines the effects of differences in criteria on the expression and prevalence of relational disorders. Categorical and dimensional criteria may be tested for reliability, validity and clinical utility.

The workgroup also recommended research that allows for the examination of cultural variations in the application of diagnostic criteria for personality disorders and relational problems. Further research evaluating the effectiveness of current personality assessment instruments and the development of new culturally sensitive assessment tools is needed. Finally, the workgroup also recommended research that examines how and if some forms of racism should be integrated into the diagnostic classification. Options include incorporating racism as a symptom in certain diagnostic criteria sets, adding racism as a disorder (or as a subtype of narcissistic personality disorder), and examining the relational aspects of racism.

Developmental Aspects

Advances in clinical science indicate that changes in brain structure and function are exhibited throughout childhood and into early adulthood. Such work emphasizes the need for a developmental approach to examining psychopathology. For example, longitudinal studies indicate associations between tic disorders and obsessive-compulsive disorder. Increased understanding of developmental changes in normal and abnormal brain functioning may provide insight on changing symptom manifestations across the lifespan. The Developmental workgroup recommended research that may inform expressions of psychopathology across the lifespan, including genetic research, neurocircuitries research and prospective follow-up studies with representative samples of children with well-described behaviors.

Recommendations to promote research on early intervention and primary and secondary prevention were also made by the workgroup. Research identifying environmental risk factors and associated impairments in functioning is needed to inform early intervention strategies.

With respect to Axis II, the workgroup recommended research on mental retardation and antisocial personality disorders. Developmental psychopathology studies, which include samples of subjects with both mental retardation and psychiatric disorders, are needed to inform the development of future diagnostic criteria that are valid, reliable and clinically useful. While antisocial personality disorder appears in Axis II for adults, the diagnosis is included on Axis I for children. The workgroup recommended research to examine effectiveness and the clinical utility of this conceptualization.

Limited data exist regarding the similarities and differences in assessing psychosocial and environmental problems in children as compared with adults. The workgroup recommended further research to support future DSM guidelines in this area and the development and evaluation of instruments for assessment purposes.

Neuroscience

Major breakthroughs in neuroscience are expected to inform the development of the DSM-V, much more than previous DSM editions. New genomic technologies, such as high-throughput genotyping via mass spectrometry, may further our understanding of how genes interact with each other and the environment in producing vulnerability to mental disorders. Further identification of reliable neurobiological markers will continue to inform diagnosis and prognosis, and lead to new techniques for treating mental disorders.

The Neuroscience workgroup recommended research examining the links between genetics, imaging and neuroepidemiology. Over the next five years, imaging data are expected to help delineate between clusters and large diagnostic categories. Links between neuroscience and basic research in cognition, emotion and behavior could clarify the processes underlying mental disorder symptoms and disabilities, leading to new conceptualizations of diagnoses.

Pharmacogenetic and pharmacodynamic research examining differences in metabolism, drug absorption and tissue response is expected to inform the development of a biologically based nosology with great implications for treatment. Such findings may lead to the development of diagnostic subtypes and pharmacogenomic tools designed to assist psychiatrists in developing individualized treatment regimens.

While research has documented the universality of human genetic codes, ethnic variations are substantial for the genes potentially associated with mental disorders. The Neuroscience workgroup recommended further research to examine cross-ethnic variations for neurobiological markers and other neurobiological parameters.

The challenge for DSM-V will be to incorporate the advances in neuroscience into the diagnostic criteria. The Neuroscience workgroup emphasized the need to develop an integrative approach that may be used over the next five to ten years.

Cross-cultural Aspects

The Cross-cultural workgroup recommended research to inform the future development of diagnostic criteria applicable to all cultures and cross-cultural variants in definitions of symptoms, distress, dysfunction, impairment, and disability. Ethnographic research may lead to the development of alternative definitions, which may be integrated into diagnostic criteria to improve their cultural sensitivity.

The workgroup also recommended further epidemiological research that encompasses specialty groups such as legal and illegal immigrants, and refugee groups to further study the effect of contextual factors in the manifestation of the disorder or as a potential cause for a different type of psychopathology. Epidemiological research in the United States and internationally is expected to clarify cultural factors associated with risk, course and treatment outcomes for mental disorders. Additionally, the workgroup identified stigma, racism and acculturation as potential culturally based risk factors for psychopathology. Further research examining the effects of these risk factors for different racial/ethnic groups was recommended.

The DSM-IV included Cultural Formulation Guidelines to assist clinicians in collecting information regarding patients' cultural background to inform the diagnostic process. The workgroup recommended research to evaluate the clinical utility of these guidelines, and other studies to examine how clinicians incorporate information regarding culture, race and ethnicity into the diagnostic process. They also recommended the development of alternative procedures to guide clinicians in their efforts to combine cultural information collected for the purpose of diagnosis and treatment.

The workgroup highlighted the need to develop culturally sensitive standardized instruments for assessing mental disorders. Further research assessing the validity, reliability, and clinical usefulness of currently available assessment instruments for individuals of different racial and ethnic backgrounds is also needed. Collaboration with professionals from various fields may facilitate and strengthen this process. Professionals may include anthropologists, sociologists, or linguists who may pinpoint communication or translation barriers.

The Cross-cultural workgroup emphasized the importance of including subjects of different racial/ethnic backgrounds into neurobiological research protocols. Systematic examinations of racial and ethnic variations are expected to inform the understanding of how culture influences the development, the natural course, and treatment outcomes for persons with mental disorders.

ALTERNATIVES FOR FUTURE DIRECTIONS

The DSM-V revision process will remain firmly committed to being empirically based. Given our expectation that the DSM-V will be published no sooner than 2010, we have the opportunity over the next 10 years to develop a strong empirical database to guide decisions of the future DSM-V workgroups. There are many possible options for enriching the empirical database in advance of the DSM-V process. One such effort, described in the previous section and currently underway, was to set up groups of multidisciplinary researchers to review the current state-of-the-art in psychiatry to identify new research directions that might inform the most significant questions underlying nosology and classification, e.g. the impact of neurobiology and genetics on the nosology.

We anticipate that research proposals emanating from the efforts of the DSM-V research development groups will be reviewed and refined by many international investigators. It is our hope that they will stimulate a broad base of support from research funding agencies in many countries with the interest and capacity to advance our understanding of mental disorders. The World Psychiatric Association, in particular, can be of assistance in facilitating the review of gaps in our knowledge that could usefully be addressed by colleagues in many parts of the world. It appears probable that the time frame for the resulting research agenda will be long-term, with much of the research likely to bear fruit over the next 10 to 20 years. As a result, much of the research generated by these developmental efforts may have its greatest impact on DSM-VI or DSM-VII rather than on DSM-V or ICD-11.

Another possible direction would focus more on the near term and would attempt to fortify the empirical database that will be available to the future

DSM-V workgroups. Major constraints impacting on the DSM-IV revision process were caused by gaps and inadequacies in the empirical database at the time. The DSM-IV revision process consisted of a three-stage empirically based review, which was comprised of a comprehensive review of the literature, data set reanalyses, and focused field trials. Although many gaps were identified in the existing literature, there were only limited options available to the workgroups for filling in these gaps. One such mechanism was the MacArthur Foundation-funded data reanalysis process in which existing data sets were combined and reanalyzed in order to try to answer certain diagnostic questions. Although useful in some cases, many of the data reanalyses were seriously hampered by incompatibilities in the data sets and by the fact that the data necessary to answer a particular diagnostic question often had not been collected. The only studies conducted specifically for the DSM-IV revision process were the 15 NIMH-funded focused field trials. Because of limited resources and time to conduct the trials, the goals of these field trials were fairly modest. Most typically, the goals were to compare different criteria sets in terms of reliability, user acceptability and/or comparison to a clinical standard as opposed to the more rigorous Robins–Guze validity criteria.

The proposed research effort entails the convening of a number of diagnostic planning conferences organized by diagnostic grouping, i.e. each conference would be devoted to one of the major diagnostic areas (e.g. mood disorders, anxiety disorders, psychotic disorders, etc.). The goal of each of these conferences would be to establish a research agenda focusing on the near term (i.e. the next five years) rather than the long term. Participants at these conferences would consist of the leading experts from North America as well as internationally in each of the diagnostic areas.

In advance of the actual conference, participants would be assigned specific topic areas to review the literature for the purpose of identifying gaps. At the actual conference, participants would present their reviews and the group would discuss and formulate potential short-term research agendas addressing these gaps. Collaborative studies pooling the efforts of different North American or international research centers might be suggested and/or, in some cases, field trials of competing criteria sets or definitions might be appropriate. For example, one controversial issue in the area of mood disorders concerns the nosology of antidepressant-induced mania. Do such episodes indicate that the patient has a bipolar diathesis and thus should be considered to be in the bipolar spectrum or should such episodes continue to be diagnosed as analogous to substance-induced mania? Participants at the conference could be assigned in advance the task of reviewing the existing literature relevant to this bipolar III disorder and present suggestions for collaborative studies or reanalyses of existing data sets that might elucidate the issue. The white papers resulting from each conference might serve as starting points for collaborative projects undertaken by participants at the conference as well as encourage other researchers to incorporate some of the research agenda into their own existing or proposed research projects. We envision that laying this groundwork will greatly enhance the eventual DSM-V workgroups' efforts in making empirically informed decisions about changes in DSM-V.

Given past experience with DSM revisions, the following timetable might be advisable (assuming a 2010 publication date). Participants to the conferences would be invited in 2001–2002, with several conference calls convened in advance of the meeting in order to assign tasks to review the current empirical database relevant to the diagnostic areas. The actual conferences would then be convened during 2002–2003, with the goal being a series of white papers that would appear in the scientific literature. This would allow a period of at least five years for studies to be undertaken to address some of the issues identified in these white papers. The actual DSM-V workgroups could then be formed in the second half of the decade so that there would be sufficient time to conduct the careful empirical review and set up prospective field trials to test out alternative suggestions for DSM-V changes.

CONCLUSIONS

In addition to tracing mental disorder classification efforts back to early-recorded history, we also note that the APA and its predecessors have been engaged in this activity for more than a century. The interaction between diagnostic classifications and diagnostic assessment tools for epidemiologic research is traced back to the early 1800s but became particularly intertwined for a wide range of clinical research in the 1970s. Although some of the strengths and weaknesses of the current DSM-IV-TR edition are reviewed, it is important to recognize that major advances in diagnosis and treatment effectiveness over the past century are reflected in the existing criteria, which will in turn facilitate further research advances.

The interaction between the United States and international colleagues in the development of diagnostic classifications has a long history, which includes particularly productive collaborative activities over the past 20 years. As a result of the international collaborative efforts between the developers of both the DSM-IV and the ICD-10, we now have a common international language for communicating about the nature of mental disorders found in multiple cultures. This achievement has resulted in an increasingly cumulative outpouring of basic, epidemiologic and clinical research investigations over the past decade, which have used similar diagnostic criteria. In addition to increasing our understanding of the characteristics of mental disorders, including their prevalence, risk factors, course of illness and treatment response, we have also learned a great deal about the shortcomings of existing diagnostic criteria.

The next 8–10 year period prior to DSM-V or ICD-11 revisions offers an opportunity to address some of the known limitations of our existing diagnostic criteria with empirically based research investigations. It is anticipated that investments in this research enterprise will involve many international funding agencies that have a demonstrated interest in improving the quality of research and clinical practice for persons with mental, behavioral and addictive disorders. Those of us at the APA who are involved with the coordination of future DSM-V revisions look forward to a collaborative effort with members of the World Psychiatric Association and the WHO in providing a focus on areas where research may be most promising in improving the validity of new diagnostic criteria. We hope that this chapter will facilitate that collaborative process.

ACKNOWLEDGEMENT

The authors wish to express their appreciation to Dr Maritza Rubio-Stipec for her critical review and contribution to improvements in the manuscript.

REFERENCES

1. American Psychiatric Association (1994) *Diagnostic and Statistical Manual of Mental Disorders*, 4th edn. American Psychiatric Association, Washington.
2. World Health Organization (1992) *The ICD-10 Classification of Mental and Behavioural Disorders. Clinical Descriptions and Diagnostic Guidelines*. World Health Organization, Geneva.
3. Mack A.H., Forman L., Brown R., Frances A. (1994) A brief history of psychiatric classification. From the ancients to DSM-IV. *Psychiatr. Clin. North Am.*, **17**: 515–523.
4. American Psychiatric Association (2000) *Diagnostic and Statistical Manual of Mental Disorders*, 4th edn, text revision. American Psychiatric Association, Washington.
5. World Health Organization (1948) *Manual of the International Statistical Classification of Diseases, Injuries and Causes of Death*, 6th revision, vol. 1. World Health Organization, Geneva.
6. American Psychiatric Association (1952) *Diagnostic and Statistical Manual of Mental Disorders*, 1st edn. American Psychiatric Association, Washington.
7. Stengel (1959) Classification of mental disorders. *WHO Bull.*, **21**: 601–603.
8. World Health Organization (1969) *Manual of the International Statistical Classification of Diseases, Injuries and Causes of Death*, 8th revision, vol. 1. World Health Organization, Geneva.
9. American Psychiatric Association (1968) *Diagnostic and Statistical Manual of Mental Disorders*, 2nd edn. American Psychiatric Association, Washington.

10. World Health Organization (1974) *Glossary of Mental Disorders and Guide to Their Classification for Use in Conjunction With The International Classification of Diseases*, 8th revision. World Health Organization, Geneva.
11. US Public Health Service (1968) *International Classification of Diseases, adapted for use in the United States (ICDA)*, 8th revision, PHS Publication No. 1693. US Government Printing Office, Washington.
12. Commission on Professional and Hospital Activities (1973) *Hospital Adaptation of ICDA (H-ICDA)* 2nd edn, vol. 1, tabular list. Commission on Professional and Hospital Activities, Ann Arbor.
13. Feighner J.P., Robins E., Guze S.B., Woodruff R.A., Jr., Winokur G., Munoz R. (1972) Diagnostic criteria for use in psychiatric research. *Arch. Gen. Psychiatry*, **26**: 57–63.
14. Spitzer R.L., Endicott J., Robins E. (1978) Research diagnostic criteria: rationale and reliability. *Arch. Gen. Psychiatry*, **35**: 773–782.
15. Helzer J.E., Robins L.N., Croughan J.L., Welner A. (1981) Renard diagnostic interview. Its reliability and procedural validity with physicians and lay interviewers. *Arch. Gen. Psychiatry*, **38**: 393–398.
16. Spitzer R.L., Endicott J. (1978) *Schedule for Affective Disorders and Schizophrenia, SADS*. New York State Psychiatric Institute, Biometrics Research Division, New York.
17. American Psychiatric Association (1980) *Diagnostic and Statistical Manual of Mental Disorders*, 3rd edn. American Psychiatric Association, Washington.
18. Boyd J.H., Burke J.D., Jr., Gruenberg E., Holzer C.E., III, Rae D.S., George L.K., Karno M., Stoltzman R., McEvoy L., Nestadt G. (1984) Exclusion criteria of DSM-III. A study of co-occurrence of hierarchy-free syndromes. *Arch. Gen. Psychiatry*, **41**: 983–989.
19. Boyd J.H., Burke J.D., Gruenberg E., Holzer C.E., Rae D.S., George L.K., Karno M., Stolzman R., McEvoy L.M., Nestadt G. (1987) The exclusion criteria of DSM-III, a study of the co-occurrence of hierarchy-free syndromes. In *Diagnosis and Classification in Psychiatry: A Critical Appraisal of DSM-III* (Ed. G.L. Tischler), pp. 403–424. Cambridge University Press, Cambridge.
20. Breier A., Charney D.S., Heninger G.R. (1984) Major depression in patients with agoraphobia and panic disorder. *Arch. Gen. Psychiatry*, **41**: 1129–1135.
21. American Psychiatric Association (1987) *Diagnostic and Statistical Manual of Mental Disorders*, 3rd edn, revised. American Psychiatric Association, Washington.
22. Widiger T.A., Frances A.J., Pincus H.A., Davis W.W., First M.B. (1991) Toward an empirical classification for the DSM-IV. *J. Abnorm. Psychol.*, **100**: 280–288.
23. Widiger T.A., Frances A.J., Pincus H.A., Ross R., First M.B., Davis W.W. (1994) *DSM-IV Sourcebook*, vol 1. American Psychiatric Association, Washington.
24. Widiger T.A., Frances A.J., Pincus H.A., Ross R., First M.B., Davis W.W. (1996) *DSM-IV Sourcebook*, vol. 2. American Psychiatric Association, Washington.
25. Widiger T.A., Frances A.J., Pincus H.A., Ross R., First M.B., Davis W.W. (1997) *DSM-IV Sourcebook*, vol. 3. American Psychiatric Association, Washington.
26. Widiger T.A., Frances A.J., Pincus H.A., Ross R., First M.B., Davis W.W., Kline M. (1998) *DSM-IV Sourcebook*, vol. 4. American Psychiatric Association, Washington.
27. American Psychiatric Association (1995) *Diagnostic and Statistical Manual of Mental Disorders*, 4th edn, international version. American Psychiatric Association, Washington.

28. Cooper J.E., Kendell R.E., Gurland B.J., Sharpe L., Copeland J.R.M., Simon R. (1972) *Psychiatric Diagnosis in New York and London*. Oxford University Press, London.
29. Wing J.K., Nixon J.M., Mann S.A., Leff J.P. (1977) Reliability of the PSE (ninth edition) used in a population study. *Psychol. Med.*, 7: 505–516.
30. Robins L.N., Helzer J.E., Croughan J., Ratcliff K.S. (1981) National Institute of Mental Health Diagnostic Interview Schedule. Its history, characteristics, and validity. *Arch. Gen. Psychiatry*, **38**: 381–389.
31. Regier D.A., Myers J.K., Kramer M., Robins L.N., Blazer D.G., Hough R.L., Eaton W.W., Locke B.Z. (1984) The NIMH Epidemiologic Catchment Area program. Historical context, major objectives, and study population characteristics. *Arch. Gen. Psychiatry*, **41**: 934–941.
32. Robins L.N., Regier D.A. (1991) *Psychiatric Disorders in America: The Epidemiologic Catchment Area Study*. Free Press, New York.
33. Spitzer R.L., Williams J.B., Gibbon M., First M.B. (1992) The Structured Clinical Interview for DSM-III-R (SCID). I: History, rationale, and description. *Arch. Gen. Psychiatry*, **49**: 624–629.
34. Sartorius N., Jablensky A., Regier D.A., Burke J.D., Hirschfeld R.M.A. (Eds) (1990) *Sources and Traditions of Classification in Psychiatry*. Huber, Lewiston.
35. WHO/ADAMHA (1985) *Mental Disorders; Alcohol- and Drug-Related Problems. International Perspectives on Their Diagnosis and Classification*. Elsevier, Amsterdam.
36. World Health Organization (1994) *The International Statistical Classification of Diseases and Related Health Problems*, 10th revision. World Health Organization, Geneva.
37. Robins E., Guze S.B. (1970) Establishment of diagnostic validity in psychiatric illness: its application to schizophrenia. *Am. J. Psychiatry*, **126**: 983–987.
38. Robins L.N., Wing J., Wittchen H.U., Helzer J.E., Babor T.F., Burke J., Farmer A., Jablensky A., Pickens R., Regier D.A. et al. (1988) The Composite International Diagnostic Interview. An epidemiologic instrument suitable for use in conjunction with different diagnostic systems and in different cultures. *Arch. Gen. Psychiatry*, **45**: 1069–1077.
39. Wittchen H.U., Robins L.N., Cottler L.B., Sartorius N., Burke J.D., Regier D. (1991) Cross-cultural feasibility, reliability and sources of variance of the Composite International Diagnostic Interview (CIDI). The Multicentre WHO/ADAMHA Field Trials. *Br. J. Psychiatry*, **159**: 645–653.
40. Wing J.K., Babor T., Brugha T., Burke J., Cooper J.E., Giel R., Jablensky A., Regier D., Sartorius N. (1990) SCAN. Schedules for Clinical Assessment in Neuropsychiatry. *Arch. Gen. Psychiatry*, **47**: 589–593.
41. Loranger A.W., Sartorius N., Andreoli A., Berger P., Buchheim P., Channabasavanna S.M., Coid B., Dahl A., Diekstra R.F., Ferguson B. (1994) The International Personality Disorder Examination. The World Health Organization/Alcohol, Drug Abuse, and Mental Health Administration international pilot study of personality disorders. *Arch. Gen. Psychiatry*, **51**: 215–224.
42. World Health Organization (1980) *International Classification of Impairments, Disabilities, and Handicaps: A Manual of Classification Relating to the Consequences of Disease*. World Health Organization, Geneva.
43. Üstün T.B., Cooper J.E., Duuren-Kristen S., Kennedy C., Hendershot G., Sartorius N. (1995) Revision of the ICIDH: mental health aspects. WHO/MNH Disability Working Group. *Disabil. Rehabil.*, **17**: 202–209.

44. Andrews G., Slade T., Peters L. (1999) Classification in psychiatry: ICD-10 versus DSM-IV. *Br. J. Psychiatry*, **174**: 3–5.
45. Slade T., Andrews G. (2001) DSM-IV and ICD-10 generalized anxiety disorder: discrepant diagnoses and associated disability. *Soc. Psychiatry Psychiatr. Epidemiol.*, **36**: 45–51.
46. Sartorius N., Kaelber C.T., Cooper J.E., Roper M.T., Rae D.S., Gulbinat W., Üstün T.B., Regier D.A. (1993) Progress toward achieving a common language in psychiatry. Results from the field trial of the clinical guidelines accompanying the WHO classification of mental and behavioral disorders in ICD-10. *Arch. Gen. Psychiatry*, **50**: 115–124.
47. Regier D.A., Kaelber C.T., Roper M.T., Rae D.S., Sartorius N. (1994) The ICD-10 clinical field trial for mental and behavioral disorders: results in Canada and the United States. *Am. J. Psychiatry*, **151**: 1340–1350.
48. Spitzer R.L., Williams J.B. (1988) Having a dream. A research strategy for DSM-IV. *Arch. Gen. Psychiatry*, **45**: 871–874.
49. Vella G., Aragona M., Alliani D. (2000) The complexity of psychiatric comorbidity: a conceptual and methodological discussion. *Psychopathology*, **33**: 25–30.
50. Regier D.A., Narrow W.E., Rupp A., Rae D.S., Kaelber C.T. (2000) The epidemiology of mental disorder treatment need: community estimates of "medical necessity". In *Unmet Need in Psychiatry* (Eds G. Andrews, S. Henderson), pp. 41–58. Cambridge University Press, Cambridge.
51. Nelson E., Rice J. (1997) Stability of diagnosis of obsessive-compulsive disorder in the Epidemiologic Catchment Area study. *Am. J. Psychiatry*, **154**: 826–831.
52. Kendler K.S., Karkowski L.M., Walsh D. (1998) The structure of psychosis: latent class analysis of probands from the Roscommon Family Study. *Arch. Gen. Psychiatry*, **55**: 492–499.
53. Frances A.J., Egger H.L. (1999) Whither psychiatric diagnosis. *Aust. N.Z. J. Psychiatry*, **33**: 161–165.
54. Jablensky A. (1999) The nature of psychiatric classification: issues beyond ICD-10 and DSM-IV. *Aust. N.Z. J. Psychiatry*, **33**: 137–144.
55. van Praag H.M. (1997) Over the mainstream: diagnostic requirements for biological psychiatric research. *Psychiatry Res.*, **72**: 201–212.
56. Follette W.C., Houts A.C. (1996) Models of scientific progress and the role of theory in taxonomy development: a case study of the DSM. *J. Consult. Clin. Psychol.*, **64**: 1120–1132.
57. Frances A.J., First M.B., Widiger T.A., Miele G.M., Tilly S.M., Davis W.W., Pincus H.A. (1991) An A to Z guide to DSM-IV conundrums. *J. Abnorm. Psychol.*, **100**: 407–412.
58. Widiger T.A., Clark L.A. (2000) Toward DSM-V and the classification of psychopathology. *Psychol. Bull.*, **126**: 946–963.
59. Crowe M. (2000) Constructing normality: a discourse analysis of the DSM-IV. *J. Psychiatr. Ment. Health Nurs.*, **7**: 69–77.
60. Sadler J.Z., Hulgus Y.F., Agich G.J. (1994) On values in recent American psychiatric classification. *J. Med. Philos.*, **19**: 261–277.
61. Kaslow F.W. (1993) Relational diagnosis: an idea whose time has come? *Fam. Process*, **32**: 255–259.
62. Carson R.C. (1991) Dilemmas in the pathway of the DSM-IV. *J. Abnorm. Psychol.*, **100**: 302–307.
63. Regier D.A., Kaelber C.T., Rae D.S., Farmer M.E., Knauper B., Kessler R.C., Norquist G.S. (1998) Limitations of diagnostic criteria and assessment instruments

for mental disorders. Implications for research and policy. *Arch. Gen. Psychiatry*, **55**: 109–115.

64. Wakefield J.C. (1992) Disorder as harmful dysfunction: a conceptual critique of DSM-III-R's definition of mental disorder. *Psychol. Rev.*, **99**: 232–247.

65. World Health Organization (2000) ICIDH-2: *International Classification of Functioning, Disability and Health*. Prefinal draft, full version. World Health Organization, Geneva.

66. Üstun T.B., Chatterji S., Rehm J. (1998) Limitations of diagnostic paradigm: it doesn't explain "need". *Arch. Gen. Psychiatry*, **55**: 1145–1146.

67. Narrow W.E., Regier D.A., Rae D.S., Manderscheid R.W., Locke B.Z. (1993) Use of services by persons with mental and addictive disorders. Findings from the National Institute of Mental Health Epidemiologic Catchment Area Program. *Arch. Gen. Psychiatry*, **50**: 95–107.

68. Magruder K.M., Calderone G.E. (2000) Public health consequences of different thresholds for the diagnosis of mental disorders. *Compr. Psychiatry*, **41**: 14–18.

69. Olfson M., Broadhead W.E., Weissman M.M., Leon A.C., Farber L., Hoven C., Kathol R. (1996) Subthreshold psychiatric symptoms in a primary care group practice. *Arch. Gen. Psychiatry*, **53**: 880–886.

70. Kendler K.S. (1999) Setting boundaries for psychiatric disorders. *Am. J. Psychiatry*, **156**: 1845–1848.

71. Meehl P.E. (1995) Bootstraps taxometrics. Solving the classification problem in psychopathology. *Am. Psychol.*, **50**: 266–275.

72. Zeanah C.H. (1996) Beyond insecurity: a reconceptualization of attachment disorders of infancy. *J. Consult. Clin. Psychol.*, **64**: 42–52.

73. Bird H.R., Davies M., Fisher P., Narrow W.E., Jensen P.S., Hoven C., Cohen P., Dulcan M.K. (2000) How specific is specific impairment? *J. Am. Acad. Child Adolesc. Psychiatry*, **39**: 1182–1189.

74. Narrow W.E., Regier D.A., Goodman S.H., Rae D.S., Roper M.T., Bourdon K.H., Hoven C., Moore R. (1998) A comparison of federal definitions of severe mental illness among children and adolescents in four communities. *Psychiatr. Serv.*, **49**: 1601–1608.

75. US Department of Health and Human Services (2001) *Report of the Surgeon General's Conference on Children's Mental Health: A National Action Agenda*. US Department of Health and Human Services, Washington.

76. US Department of Health and Human Services (1999) *Mental Health: A Report of the Surgeon General*. US Department of Health and Human Services, Washington.

77. Westen D., Shedler J. (2000) A prototype matching approach to diagnosing personality disorders: toward DSM-V. *J. Personal. Disord.*, **14**: 109–126.

78. Kendler K.S., Gardner C.O. (1997) The risk for psychiatric disorders in relatives of schizophrenic and control probands: a comparison of three independent studies. *Psychol. Med.*, **27**: 411–419.

79. Field T. (1998) Early interventions for infants of depressed mothers. *Pediatrics*, **102**: 1305–1310.

80. Tsuang M.T., Stone W.S., Faraone S.V. (2000) Towards the prevention of schizophrenia. *Biol. Psychiatry*, **48**: 349–356.

81. Faraone S.V., Biederman J., Feighner J.A., Monuteaux M.C. (2000) Assessing symptoms of attention deficit hyperactivity disorder in children and adults: which is more valid? *J. Consult. Clin. Psychol.*, **68**: 830–842.

82. Wozniak J., Biederman J., Kiely K., Ablon J.S., Faraone S.V., Mundy E., Mennin D. (1995) Mania-like symptoms suggestive of childhood-onset bipolar dis-

order in clinically referred children. *J. Am. Acad. Child Adolesc. Psychiatry*, **34**: 867–876.

83. Pliszka S.R. (2000) Patterns of psychiatric comorbidity with attention-deficit/ hyperactivity disorder. *Child Adolesc. Psychiatr. Clin. North Am.*, **9**: 525–540.

84. Zero to Three (1994) *Diagnostic Classification 0–3: Diagnostic Classification of Mental Health and Developmental Disorders of Infancy and Early Childhood.* National Center for Clinical Infant Programs, Arlington.

85. Martin R.L. (1997) Late-life psychiatric diagnosis in DSM-IV. *Psychiatr. Clin. North Am.*, **20**: 1–14.

86. Mezzich J.E., Kirmayer L.J., Kleinman A., Fabrega H., Jr., Parron D.L., Good B.J., Lin K.M., Manson S.M. (1999) The place of culture in DSM-IV. *J. Nerv. Ment. Dis.*, **187**: 457–464.

87. Hartung C.M., Widiger T.A. (1998) Gender differences in the diagnosis of mental disorders: conclusions and controversies of the DSM-IV. *Psychol. Bull.*, **123**: 260–278.

88. Lala F.J., Jr. (1998) Is there room in the DSM for consideration of deaf people? *Am. Ann. Deaf*, **143**: 314–317.

89. Alarcon R.D. (1995) Culture and psychiatric diagnosis. Impact on DSM-IV and ICD-10. *Psychiatr. Clin. North Am.*, **18**: 449–465.

90. Lukoff D., Lu F., Turner R. (1992) Toward a more culturally sensitive DSM-IV. Psychoreligious and psychospiritual problems. *J. Nerv. Ment. Dis.*, **180**: 673–682.

91. First M.B., Pincus H.A. (2001) Bridging the gap between DSM-IV and DSM-V: the DSM-IV text revision. *Psychiatr. Serv.*, in press.

4

Implications of Comorbidity for the Classification of Mental Disorders: The Need for a Psychobiology of Coherence

C. Robert Cloninger

Department of Psychiatry, Washington University School of Medicine, St. Louis, Missouri, USA

INTRODUCTION

The classification of mental disorders is currently based on a descriptive approach that attempts to be atheoretical. This descriptive approach is basically a refinement and extension of categorical diagnosis as advocated by Emil Kraepelin and others for schizophrenic and mood disorders [1–3]. The current diagnostic approach in the International Classification of Diseases and in the American Psychiatric Association's *Diagnostic and Statistical Manual* was stimulated by the work of Robins and Guze [4] on the establishment of diagnostic validity for mental disorders. Consequently, it is revealing to examine the initial assumptions that influenced the development of the current diagnostic systems, particularly in order to appreciate the implications of comorbidity for the classification of mental disorders.

The neo-Kraepelinean approach of Robins and Guze [4] was based on the hopeful assumption that categorical diagnoses reflected underlying discrete disease entities that could be distinguished from one another based on clinical symptoms, age of onset, course of illness and family history [2]. Eli Robins frequently emphasized to his students that he expected that a person really had only one mental disorder, and that if there was evidence for more than one the patient should be considered as "undiagnosed", that is, as having an uncertain diagnosis [5]. Robins, Guze and their colleagues validated diagnostic criteria that allowed about 80% of all psychiatric patients to be assigned to one of 15 specific diagnostic groups. The diagnoses included

Psychiatric Diagnosis and Classification. Edited by Mario Maj, Wolfgang Gaebel, Juan José López-Ibor and Norman Sartorius. © 2002 John Wiley & Sons, Ltd.

neuroses (anxiety, phobic, obsessional, hysterical disorders), affective disorders (depressive or bipolar disorders), schizophrenia, organic brain syndromes, substance abuse disorders (alcoholism, other drugs), sexual disorders (homosexuality, transsexuality), eating disorders (anorexia, bulimia), and one personality disorder (antisocial personality) [6]. However, about one in every five psychiatric patients coming to clinical care could not be diagnosed with certainty because of "atypical" clinical features or co-occurrence of two or more syndromes at one time [5]. It was hopefully assumed that this remaining 20% would someday be diagnosable as a result of validation of other diagnostic categories or the development of laboratory tests.

The assumptions of Robins and Guze about discreteness and the absence of comorbidity certainly appear questionable today. Moreover, the addition of hundreds of further diagnostic categories has not reduced the frequency with which patients appear to be "atypical" or "not otherwise specified". The addition of other diagnoses may have helped to describe the heterogeneity that exists within broad categories like anxiety or mood disorders, but these subdivisions have seldom been well validated in the rigorous way recommended by Robins and Guze. Moreover, most patients who meet current criteria for any one mental disorder also fulfil the criteria for two or more disorders [7–11]. For mental disorders, comorbidity, defined as the increased risk of multiple mental disorders occurring together, is the rule rather than the exception.

Likewise, efforts to demonstrate the discreteness of different disorders have led to inconsistent results for psychoses and milder anxiety and depressive disorders [12, 13]. Even when it is replicably found that intermediate or combined syndromes are relatively rare, the separation of groups (e.g. schizophrenics vs. manics) has been only moderately complete [1, 14]. For personality disorders, there is no evidence whatsoever of discrete boundaries between categories or even clusters, and most patients with any personality disorder satisfy criteria for two or more putative categories [15–17].

Furthermore, no laboratory test for any mental disorder has practical clinical utility because such tests are all low in their sensitivity or specificity. At the molecular genetic level, genome-wide scans for major mental disorders that are clearly heritable, such as schizophrenia or bipolar disorder, have not yielded conclusive results that any single gene or set of a few genes accounts for a substantial proportion of cases or a large proportion of the variance in risk for the disorder [18]. This suggests that the disorders are polygenic, multifactorial and developmentally complex. Even at the level of underlying personality traits associated with vulnerability to psychopathology, there is only partial specificity of contributions from candidate genes associated with individual differences in temperament or character [19].

Finally, there is an underlying multidimensional architecture for psychiatric comorbidity, suggesting that comorbid disorders share some, but not all, of their vulnerability components in common. This architecture corresponds closely to the multidimensional structure of personality [13, 20–22]. For example, individuals who are high in harm avoidance are at increased risk for what used to be called neuroses, including anxiety disorders, phobic disorders, personality disorders. Individuals who are high in novelty seeking are at risk for substance dependence, bulimia, and cluster B personality disorders. Individuals who are low in reward dependence are at increased risk for schizophrenia and cluster A personality disorders. Various multidimensional configurations of temperament and character are related to subtypes of psychoses and mood disorders [23]. Yet there are no linear (one-to-one) relationships between personality and psychopathology [24]. Rather, the relationships are non-linear, with multidimensional configurations of personality traits having multiple alternative outcomes in terms of Axis I syndromes and each Axis I syndrome having multiple possible antecedent personality configurations [13, 20, 21, 25].

In summary, mental disorders generally can be characterized as manifestations of complex adaptive systems that are multidimensional descriptively, multifactorial in their origins, and non-linearly interactive in their development. In other words, they are clinically and etiologically heterogeneous with a complex epigenesis involving non-linear interactions among multiple genetic and environmental influences. Although there may be rare cases of discrete disorders with sharp causal or clinical boundaries, these are exceptional. Consequently, efforts to describe psychopathology in terms of categorical diagnoses result in extensive comorbidity [2, 26]. This is an indication of the inadequacy of current systems of classification for efficient case description or treatment planning. Current classifications simply do not characterize psychopathology well for understanding aetiology, treatment or clinical variability. A "top-down" strategy for classification, based on clinical variation and hoping to help understand aetiology and treatment, appears to be grossly inadequate because development is not linear and involves a complex adaptive system with many components that interact in a non-linear manner. Just as neuroscientists have abandoned the notion that the brain has discrete centers that regulate specific functions, so clinicians need to recognize that mental disorders are not composed of discrete disease entities. In fact, this has been rigorously demonstrated by detailed taxonomic analysis for many years, but was little understood or appreciated by most clinicians [13]. However, more recently, clinicians have recognized the absurdity of the assumptions underlying current classifications as a result of comorbidity. It is an inescapable fact of life for clinicians that most patients who satisfy the criteria for one putative category of mental disorder usually satisfy the criteria for others as well. In addition, evidence for discrete boundaries between disorders is lacking despite strenuous efforts to devise improved criteria and to develop laboratory markers for diagnostic confirmation.

MOLECULAR OR BOTTOM-UP STRATEGIES TO CLASSIFICATION

Some biological psychiatrists and neuroscientists have suggested the alternative of redefining mental disorders to correspond to variables defined at a molecular level. Hope for the feasibility of this bottom-up approach is based on the assumption of a linear chain of development from individual differences at a molecular level to a cellular level, and then from the cellular level to physiological and behavioral levels [27]. This reduction of behavioral variability to diagnosis based on molecular variants would be possible if and only if there is linear development from molecular genetic determinants up to clinical variation. However, it is already clear that that development is extremely non-linear and involves complex gene–gene and gene–environment interactions that are not predictable at the molecular level, even with information about initial conditions [19, 28]. In brief, the development of mental disorders is the consequence of a complex non-linear epigenesis from genotype to phenotype. In fact, there is not sufficient information in the entire genome to explain the information content of neural connections in the adult human brain [29]. This is simply another way of saying that cognitive and neural development are experience-dependent and cannot be reduced to genetic, molecular or cellular factors alone [30, 31].

Perhaps there are intermediate levels of molecular development that are more informative, but it is doubtful that laboratory tests at a molecular level can be sufficient to define clinical phenomena. This statement is justified for the exact same reason that "top-down" strategies are inadequate: any molecular variant simply lacks the necessary information content to define specific phenotypic features in the absence of a linear developmental sequence in which there are one-to-one correspondences between a particular molecular variant and a phenotypic feature of clinical importance. Furthermore, for most psychopathology, variation unique to the individual accounts for about half of phenotypic variability, so that genetic and cultural factors are incomplete accounts of the causes of mental disorders [32]. Also, lifespan developmental studies indicate that biological and cultural factors provide an incomplete account of human development in the sense that as we age biology and culture are unable to maintain a positive balance of developmental gains over developmental losses [33]. Again, factors unique to each individual result in morbidity and mortality.

It appears that neither mind-less nor brain-less approaches will be adequate for classification of mental disorders [30, 31]. Brain-less top-down strategies that consider only clinically observable behavior are inadequate for characterizing a non-linear adaptive system. Likewise, mind-less bottom-up strategies that consider only underlying molecular processes are inadequate for such complex systems. Both strategies fail for the same reason—the absence of linearity in development from genotype to phenotype, such that there are no one-to-one correspondences between genotype and phenotype. Comorbidity is the marker of the failure of the brain-less categorical approach of current classifications. Molecular non-specificity is the marker of the failure of mind-less molecular approaches. In fact, the complexity of mental health as a non-linear adaptive system is a coin with two sides—clinical comorbidity and molecular non-specificity. Fortunately, there is an alternative approach that integrates information about both brain and mind as a holistic functional psychobiology.

PRACTICAL IMPLICATIONS OF COMORBIDITY

Comorbidity has a significance for classification that is widely known by practicing clinicians but rarely acknowledged by academics. Prior to the introduction of explicit diagnostic criteria and structured interview schedules, psychiatric diagnosis was notoriously unreliable. This meant that the same patient would be diagnosed in different ways by different clinicians, resulting in many different diagnoses when treated over time in a variety of facilities or at different times in the same facility. Research studies now show that ratings can be made with high reliability if systematic structured interviews are carried out and multiple diagnoses are recorded. In this way, research investigations can be carried out so as to produce replicable results, although this can be difficult because of heterogeneity in comorbid disorders when research is focused on a primary diagnosis. However, the situation regarding reliability is much worse in clinical practice. In daily practice, clinicians often do not report all the comorbid diagnoses of a patient for many reasons. The reasons include: incomplete assessment of all possible diagnoses because the number of disorders in the classification is too extensive for routine work; disinterest in diagnoses not relevant to the chief complaints or available treatment being requested; enthusiasm for or prejudice against particular diagnoses; or consideration of insurance coverage and reimbursement.

Consider a patient who has a recurrent major depression and recurrent panic attacks in addition to a childhood history of extreme abuse, chronic dysthymia and somatization, and many features of borderline personality disorder. The treatment records of such patients often vary between primary diagnoses of major depression, panic disorder, post-traumatic stress disorder, dysthymic disorder, somatization disorder, and borderline personality disorder. In clinical practice, the choice of a primary diagnosis will depend on the interests and skills of the clinician, the chief complaint at the time of presentation, the treatment facilities available, and reimbursement policies of available insurance. Consequently, communication between clinicians does not have the reliability and specificity suggested by research results. Comorbidity allows clinicians now to be as unreliable in their choice of primary diagnoses as were clinicians before the introduction of current criteria. As a result of comorbidity, the classification of mental disorders does not appear to be any more reliable in clinical practice now than it was before the introduction of explicit criteria. In fact, modern records that I have reviewed often have less individualized and detailed description of cases than older records prior to introduction of explicit criteria. So, paradoxically, current classification methods may have actually impoverished case description without improving reliability in communication between practicing clinicians.

In summary, current classification methods appear to be reliable, but this is only illusory, because of comorbidity. Such inconsistency could be overcome by a system in which a practical number of criteria or quantitative parameters were always rated on every patient. It is not feasible for clinicians or researchers to rate all the criteria underlying diagnoses in current classifications. Classifications need to be comprehensive, but they also need to be parsimonious and efficient if they are to be used in a reliable manner in practice. Current classifications are not efficient and so they are not reliable in practice.

NEED FOR A FUNDAMENTAL SHIFT OF PERSPECTIVE

Comorbidity provides a major clue that the classification of mental disorders requires an integrative psychobiological approach. Comorbidity indicates that subdivision of patients with mental disorder into categories fails to produce mutually exclusive or discrete groups. This failure is the consequence of focusing on the components of an interactive system rather than functional aspects of the system as a whole. Consequently, it should be more useful to shift the focus of classification from narrowly defined categories to the self-organizing functions of the psychobiological system as an interactive whole.

Fortunately, there are examples with which we are all familiar of ways of describing a self-organizing complex adaptive system as a whole. The most enduring and informative metaphor compares mental self-government to political systems of government [34, 35]. More specifically, at an intellectual level of description, the functional properties of a complex adaptive system can be compared to the higher cognitive functions of the brain or dimensions of mental self-government. For example, human self-government can be characterized in terms of several properties that I will refer to as executive, legislative, emotional, judicial and integrative functions. Often a government is described as having only executive, legislative and judicial branches, but to describe human emotional and cognitive processing adequately we must add the emotional and integrative functions for a total of five aspects.

Executive functions are concerned with the implementation of plans, rules and procedures. Well-developed executive function is behaviorally characterized by purposefulness and resourcefulness, as in the character trait of self-directedness, which focuses on what an individual does intentionally [16]. Legislative functions are concerned with the formulation of laws and procedures. Well-developed legislative function is behaviorally characterized by being principled and helpful, as in the character trait of cooperativeness, which is concerned with the supervision of the relationships of people with one another in society [16]. No laws would be needed if each person was an isolate with no impact on anyone else; thus, we can see that the need for legislation is a consequence of the need to organize and regulate social interaction according to principles. Emotive functions are concerned with adaptive fluidity and coherence. Emotional functions are characterized by variation from happiness and harmony at one extreme to fear and insecurity at the other extreme. Judicial functions involve insight and judgement, such as knowing about the meaning of underlying facts or understanding whether a situation is an instance of a rule, as in the character trait of self-transcendence. Thus judicial function involves knowledge about the processes of thought, which is sometimes called meta-cognition. Integrative functions involve a sense of participation in wholeness or unity between what is apprehended as inside and outside oneself.

However, these five properties have usually been described in intellectual terms that do not fully capture the unique characteristics of human beings that are important in understanding mental disorders. That is, they do not recognize fundamental aspects of human psychobiological (i.e. mind–brain) correspondence. Human beings are distinguished from other primates by their capacity for such properties as creativity, freedom of will and spirituality [36–38]. These unique human characteristics are analogous to phenomena in quantum physics that have recently been rigorously documented as characterizing nature at the most fundamental levels that have been observed, as summarized in Table 4.1.

It is probably not surprising that the subtlest aspects of human cognition may be based on the subtlest aspects of laws known to physics. Mechanical deterministic views of human psychobiology are simply inadequate to

TABLE 4.1 Properties of human beings and analogous quantum phenomena

Property of human beings	Analogous quantum phenomenon
Creativity	Non-causality
Freedom of will	Uncertainty principle
Serenity/fluidity	Distributed coherence
Intuitive awareness	Non-locality
Sense of unity of being	Universality of Higgs field

account for the properties of the most sophisticated human abilities, such as subjectivity, creativity and intuition. The correspondence between uniquely human cognition and quantum processes, summarized in Table 4.1, is remarkable. Psychiatry has not kept pace with the revolutionary changes in physics, which inform us about the nature of reality. This is evidence of the inertia of human thought and the extent to which we can be bound by tradition. Intellectually we know that our traditional concepts are fundamentally flawed perspectives on reality and that those traditional concepts serve us poorly in the work we want to do. Psychiatry and psychobiology have failed during the past century to switch to an understanding of human behavior and cognition compatible with quantum physics, even though we know that these very quantum properties are what define our humanity.

First, let us consider the properties of human will. The psychological concepts of creative and free will are incompatible with classical Newtonian physics, which would require that nature behave as a machine whose function is necessarily determined by initial conditions [38]. Classical views of mechanics are inadequate to explain human personality development. The classical view of mechanics is also implicit in categorical classifications in which individuals are considered as separate objects with discrete boundaries and independent properties, rather than the quantum view of objects as inseparable condensations of interdependent activities within a universal field.

Creativity in humans involves more than clever application of what has been done before; it involves productions without precedent, which could not have been predicted from what had previously occurred. Such psychological creativity corresponds to non-algorithmic processes in quantum physics, such as non-causality. Non-causality is demonstrated by physical events that are unpredictable, under-determined, or under-constrained by all information about initial conditions.

Freedom of will is a closely related psychological phenomenon, corresponding to the uncertainty principle of Heisenberg: there is a finite limit to the precision with which events in space–time can be specified from initial conditions. In other words, there are aspects of the future that are unpredictable, under-constrained, or free because we can have only limited knowledge about their initial conditions. Furthermore, this freedom is somehow entangled with subjective awareness of the observer because there is a choice of the degree of constraint placed on different parameters [39].

Next, let us consider the properties of intuitive awareness and understanding. Certain states of awareness have been described as moments of optimal experience, peak performance, states of fluidity, or flow states, and are associated with creative insight, happiness, and fluid mental and physical performance [40]. Such awareness carries with it qualities of certainty and serenity. The understanding also inspires what to do like a spontaneously received gift without deliberation, tension or effort, and is regularly experienced by gifted children when they function intuitively [41]. These states of psychological fluidity are analogous to macroscopic quantum manifestations of distributed coherence similar to superfluidity.

The intuitive and subjective aspects of human awareness involve what Schrodinger [42] referred to ambiguously as the "singularity" of consciousness. This also corresponds to the integration at a conscious level of our awareness of the external world through our exteroceptive senses and our awareness of our interior milieu through our interoceptive senses mediated by the autonomic nervous system. This integration is accomplished through the reciprocal connections between the limbic system and the prefrontal cortex [43]. I will refer to our consciousness of our inner feelings and interior milieu as our interoceptive sensorium or intuition, as distinguished from our consciousness of the external world. A unique aspect of human evolution is the extent to which we are able to integrate our interoceptive and exteroceptive awareness at a conscious level as a result of the differentiation and development of connections between the mediodorsal thalamus and prefrontal cortex [43, 44]. Furthermore, ordinary states of human consciousness involve temporal "binding" so that past–present–future can all be experienced as a subjective interior continuity in a stream of consciousness, which is regarded as a unique capacity of modern human beings [36]. Such "binding" is crucial to the subjective sense of identity (i.e. self or ego), which should be distinguished from the general function of intuitive processing. The singularity of information in intuition is more analogous to the quantum phenomenon of non-locality (also called inseparability). The term non-locality is used because entangled quantum entities share information simultaneously regardless of distance, as if the same thing is in more than one place at the same time [39, 45].

Finally, in intuitive states of awareness, there is often a sense of participation in a unity of being. According to Quantum Field Theory, space is a universal field of infinite energy. In other words, space is a plenum of energy, which is the beginning and end of all physical phenomena in space–time or, more broadly, the unity of all being. This concept has been confirmed repeatedly by experimental high-energy physics, which regularly encounters phenomena that can only be explained by quanta emerging from space or returning into space. This movement in space–time indicates a direction of all physical developments to and from its source.

Physics is lacking a general theory of the nature of space and the space energy field. However, a consensus has emerged that a universal field, called a Higgs field, pervades all space. The Higgs field has been used to develop a unified field theory incorporating all the fundamental interactions of matter. Experimental support for the field has been indicated in recent particle discoveries, but not all predicted particles have yet been observed.

Such phenomena as non-causality and non-locality were so contrary to everyday experience that physicists, including Einstein, were forced to undergo a revolution in their thinking during the past century [39]. Now these phenomena are firmly established experimentally in physics [46–49]. Nevertheless, most psychologists, neuroscientists, and philosophers of mind continue to think in terms of classical physics [50]. Fortunately, other leaders in the same fields have begun to consider seriously quantum phenomena in relation to human cognition [36, 38, 51–53].

THE PSYCHOBIOLOGICAL STRUCTURE OF HUMAN THOUGHT

The problems of comorbidity and lack of discreteness in current classifications can be avoided by characterizing individuals in terms of a developmental matrix of variables, which involve stepwise increases in awareness of the processes of thought. That is, to increase the level of awareness means to apprehend more of what is given in experience. It is useful to distinguish five major levels of awareness. As illustrated in Table 4.2, these five levels can be described as a hierarchy of increasing sublimation of thought. At the lowest level (1), awareness is limited to aspects of our sexual drive, which is usually predominant in individuals with personality disorders. At the second level (2), labeled consumption, there is awareness of aspects of nutrition and growth. At the third level (3), there is awareness of the emotional attachments and aversions of oneself and others. At the fourth level (4), there is social communication and awareness of the processing and the formation of words as we try to understand experience by our individual intellect. The fifth level (5), integration, is the level of direct awareness or apperception of experience intuitively. Thus individual differences in maturity are understood as individual differences in the usual level of apprehension of reality, i.e. awareness of the processing of our thoughts.

Each level also has five sublevels, because each level has aspects of each of the other levels. For example, there are sexual, material (i.e. consummatory),

TABLE 4.2 Matrix of levels and sublevels of thought illustrating transcendence of temperament and sublimation of character: sublimation is lightening from level 1 to level 5, and transcendence is elevation within each level, going from sublevel A to sublevel E. There is increasing order or maturity in personality as thought rises from 1A to 5E

Sublevels of transcendence of thought	Levels of sublimation of thought				
	1 Sexuality	2 Consumption	3 Emotion	4 Intellect	5 Integrity
E (integration aspects)	discretion	generosity	humor	morality	integrity (unity)
D (intellectual aspects)	moderation	curiosity	sympathy	insight (self-transcendence)	wisdom (non-local)
C (emotional aspects)	validation	satisfaction	security	community	serenity (coherence)
B (consummatory aspects)	eroticism safety	consumption satiety	attachment aloofness	altruism egoism (cooperation)	love (free will)
A (sexual aspects)	sex (libido vs. harm avoidance)	aggression (novelty seeking)	insecurity (reward dependence)	Self-direction (persistence)	creativity (non-causal)

emotional, intellectual, and integrative aspects of sexuality. This progression involves an elevation or transcendence of the level. The forces from the body associated with each of the first four non-integrated levels are called temperaments. Each temperament dimension involves information processing in partly overlapping subdivisions of the limbic system, which are centrally integrated in the hypothalamus and supervised by neocortical association cortex according to extensive work on comparative neuroanatomy [54] and more recent brain imaging and neurophysiological research [28, 55]. The hypothalamus centrally integrates input from the limbic subdivisions and regulates the tonic opposition of sympathetic and parasympathetic branches of the autonomic nervous system. The autonomic nervous system maintains homeostasis by the opposition of its parasympathetic functions (such as sexual arousal, feeding, digestion and storage of nutrients, elimination, and sleep) and its sympathetic functions (such as sexual orgasm, preparation for fighting or flight, wakefulness). Accordingly, it is not surprising that each of the limbic subdivisions also regulates the tonic opposition of pairs of such psychodynamic drives, each of which has advantages and disadvantages depending on the context. In terms of functional neuroanatomy, there are opposing drives for sexuality vs. preservation of safety in the septal subdivision, feeding and aggression vs. satiety and satisfaction in the amygdaloid subdivision, social attachment vs. aloofness in the thalamo-cingulate subdivision, and industriousness vs. impersistence in the striato-thalamic subdivision.

In psychodynamic terms [56], the first level of sexuality involves the opposition of the outpouring of libidinal energy vs. preservation from harm (libido vs. harm avoidance). Harm avoidance is manifest as shyness and fatigability whereas libido is manifest as outgoing vigor and daring. When libido is not satisfied, anxiety develops, whereas sexual orgasm reduces anxiety. The second level of consumption involves the opposition of the drive for feeding vs. satiety (novelty seeking). When the drive for feeding is not satisfied, aggression develops, whereas feeding reduces irritability. Novelty seeking is manifest as impulsive aggression and consumption vs. stoicism and frugality with material possessions. The third level of emotionality involves the opposition of social aloofness and attachment (reward dependence). This reward dependence is manifest as strong social attachment, loyalty, and sympathy vs. social aloofness and distance. Separation or loss of attachments provokes insecurity, whereas inseparability facilitates sympathy and humor. The level of intellect initially involves the strengthening of ego-directedness or self-directedness by persistence. As intellect matures, there is reconciliation of the opposition of egoism with altruism, leading to increasing integration of character with increases in cooperativeness and self-transcendence. Unbridled egoism leads to conflict and delusion, whereas altruism leads to the insight and judgement underlying realistic and moral behavior. These opposing body forces are indicated by the two action tendencies (sublevel B) described for four material levels (sexuality, consumption, emotion and intellect) corresponding to the four temperaments in Table 4.2.

The transcendence of each level involves the elevation of each temperament by climbing up step by step from its sexual aspects to its integrated aspects until there is freedom from conflict or reconciliation of the opposing material forces in the integrative aspect of each level. For example, the opposition of eroticism and preservation from harm is transcended by discretion in the integrated sublevel of level 1 (lE). Likewise, the opposition of competitive consumption and possessive hoarding is reconciled and transcended in generosity to others in the spiritual sublevel of level 2 (2E). The opposition of social attachment and aloofness, manifest as social insecurity, is transcended in humor and merciful forgiveness of any offenses in the integrative sublevel of level 3 (3E). The opposition of egoism and altruism is reconciled by self-transcendence, which leads to morality in sublevel 4E, which is universally acceptable for all people. Thus transcendence involves elevation of each level by climbing up through four material sublevels to integrative reconciliation of opposed body forces.

In Table 4.2, transcendence of thought, which is elevation of thought within each level, is also distinguished from the sublimation of thought, which is maturation of thought across levels. For example, the sublevels of emotional transcendence range from insecurity (3A) to humor (3E). In contrast, sublimation involves thoughts lightening from level 1 (sexuality) to level 5 (integration). As seen in Table 4.2, this includes a combination of increasing self-directedness (particularly the sublimation of reproduction and sexuality), cooperativeness (particularly the sublimation of everyday activities related to nutrition and growth), and self-transcendence (particularly the sublimation of communication and intellectual activities).

The descriptors of emotional aspects of each of the levels are meant to indicate that there are multiple dimensions of positive emotionality or pleasurable stimulation. Gratification of sexuality, hunger or aggression, attachment needs, and intellectual judgement are distinguished here as validation, satisfaction, security, and community respectively. In contrast, some models of reinforcement which have dominated behavioral and clinical psychology for several decades are inadequate accounts of the neurobiological basis of motivated behavior, because they distinguish only dualities, such as reward and punishment, pleasure and distress, positive and negative emotionality, or behavioral inhibition and activation.

Using the descriptors in this matrix, it is possible to provide a qualitative or a quantitative account of variation in thought, including the average value and the range. This provides an idiographic description of each individual unlike nomothetic trait models; that is, it provides a description of variation in thought that is unique to each individual. If we consider thought as varying in level of energy, then these levels and sublevels are analogous to discrete energy levels, with the variation occurring in steps or energy quanta. In contrast, when we describe personality and psychopathology with traditional methods, we only measure reports about the way people are usually, but with this matrix of levels and sublevels it is possible to attend to idiographic patterns of variation in thought. Specifically, I have found it useful and efficient to distinguish the average or most frequent types of thoughts a person has, as well as their range (maximum and minimum) over specified periods of observation.

I have found this approach to observation and description of thought useful in both psychological assessment and therapy. It helps to make people aware of their processes of thought and how they can elevate and sublimate their thoughts. Table 4.3 summarizes strategies that facilitate personality maturation and sublimation of thought. This approach is called Coherence Therapy. It involves approaches that facilitate and sublimate increasing levels of self-directedness (letting go), cooperativeness (working at the service of others), and self-transcendence (awareness), as well as understanding the processes of thought (meta-cognition). Use of all of these approaches in concert appears to be synergistic. Overall, the emphasis of this approach is on progressing along a path of non-resistance. It is counter-therapeutic to strive to become something we are not, because this is effortful and intensifies conflicts and struggles that interfere with sublimation. It is natural for thought to be sublimated if we simply relax and stop struggling with our self and others. Sublimation simply means to enter into a state of lightness with intuitive awareness.

The reconciliation of opposing forces without tension or effort involves the use of paradoxical intention, as summarized in Table 4.3. Letting go of all struggles to change allows the spontaneous expression of creative change. Working to serve others leads to receiving love as well as giving it. Awareness without being judgemental allows insight and judgement to be wise. Knowledge of the processes of thought allows thought to become self-regulating without effort or tension.

My experience with Coherence Therapy suggests the hypothesis that fundamental character change only occurs when we are in a state of fluidity and freedom. In other words, we can only change when we are intuitively aware of our actual living being. In contrast, we do not change when we are thinking intellectually about images of our self because the images are dead things of the past and we are not sufficiently fluid for character change when we are emotionally tense or thinking judgementally.

Essentially then the matrix shown in Table 4.2 is a description of patterns of transition in thought as well as a description of the path of development of a person as a whole being. I will refer to this as a functional

TABLE 4.3   Principles of Coherence Therapy: the path of non-resistance

1. Letting go
   (a) no struggles with self or others
   (b) being what you are and following truth without any effort to become what you are not
   (c) hopeful calmness with anticipation that reality is unfolding in a way that is really good even if you cannot understand it
   (d) paradoxical intention to let go of struggles allows spontaneous expression of creativity

2. Working at service of others
   (a) spontaneous acts of kindness and cooperation
   (b) altruism, unconditional compassion
   (c) forgiveness of those who are aggressive
   (d) paradoxical intention to serve others results in receiving love as well as giving it

3. Awareness
   (a) simply being light and listening to our intuitive sensitivity
   (b) sublimation
   (c) intuitions have quality of certainty and clarity
   (d) paradoxical intention to be aware without judging allows integration of inner feelings and thought, leading to wisdom

4. Knowledge of the processes of thought
   (a) initial perspective is what makes us strong or weak
   (b) words of judgement can lead to untrue ideas
   (c) automatic reactions can amplify our errors of judgement

psychobiological matrix because it is a model of the functional psychobiology of human development that takes both neurobiology and psychodynamics into account on an equal footing. It is intended to describe mind–brain connections in terms that recognize the quantum-like properties of brain–mind duality, suggesting the possibility of a psychophysics corresponding to particle-wave duality. Actually Table 4.2 is only the matrix of thought. Corresponding matrices can be rated for other aspects of development, such as freedom of will or levels of insight and judgement (wisdom). Basically, rather than focusing on the content of thought, the rater can consider the extent to which the sublimation of thought through each sublevel is facilitated or resisted by different dynamic functions operating within each person under consideration. For example, is a person's freedom of will constrained by attachments to sexual objects, material possessions, emotional loyalties, intellectual theories, or concepts of the divine? This will be explained further in the next section, along with practical clinical descriptive indicators to clarify the clinical application of this approach. I will not attempt to give a complete description of this approach but only to illustrate how it provides a solution to the inadequacies of current classification methods.

APPLYING THE PSYCHOBIOLOGY OF COHERENCE TO CLASSIFICATION

In order to understand the clinical applicability of this novel way of understanding human nature, I will first discuss the findings from mental status examinations and psychiatric history that enable ratings of each of the basic parameters. Afterwards, I will provide a semi-quantitative overview of how individual differences in these psychobiological functions provide a basis for classification of mental health and disorders as dysfunction in this developmental matrix.

First, let us consider the clinical basis for rating the executive function parameter underlying the potential development of creativity (C). Creativity is related to intelligence and self-directedness, but it is more than these intellectual and character functions [57]. Individuals who are very low in executive function have impaired reality testing. In contrast, those who are high in executive function are highly purposeful, resourceful, and with full development of this function, inventive and creative [16, 57]. Thus creativity involves a realistic awareness of an ever-expanding reality to which we adapt our executive activities in an inventive manner in order to move with the flow of emerging opportunities that are truly novel. The degree of such creative awareness of reality can be rated qualitatively, quantitatively, or semi-quantitatively. Qualitatively, individuals who are psychotic are dominated by their basic urges for pleasure and safety, and these wishes distort the accuracy of their reality testing (lower part of level 1). In contrast, the average modern-day person, who is predominantly materialistic and has a classical mechanical view of the world, is preoccupied in their executive functions with competition for the acquisition of material goods (level 2). Higher levels of executive function are indicated by ease in dealing with the emotions of others in social interaction (level 3). Still higher levels of executive function involve intellectual analysis and communication, leading to high self-directedness, indicated by being purposeful and resourceful (level 4). Ultimately, the highest levels of executive function are manifest by creativity or inventiveness without tension (level 5).

In other words, both originality and adaptiveness must be considered in rating creativity [58, 59]. High creativity is the combination of originality with adaptation to reality. On the other hand, psychoticism or low creativity is the combination of original or divergent thinking with maladaptation to reality [59]. Intermediate or average creativity corresponds to the absence of originality. Thus, this emphasis on creativity as an adaptive executive function results in its corresponding to generation of products that are realistic and useful to society. Furthermore, the originality comes from recognizing and following the creative potential inherent in an ever-expanding reality.

For a fully quantitative approach, each level can be subdivided on a decimal scale. Level 1 (impaired reality testing dominated by sexuality and safety issues) varies from 1.0 to 1.9, level 2 (materialistic focus dominated by acquisition of goods, possessions, dependencies) from 2.0 to 2.9, level 3 (emotional focus dominated by issues of security and control versus sympathy and humor) from 3.0 to 3.9, level 4 (intellectual focus dominated by issues varying from rational egoism to ethical principles and morality) from 4.0 to 4.9, and level 5 (integration dominated by creativity, service to others, and spirituality) from 5.0 to 5.9. Poor reality testing varies from disorganized, borderline, or magical thinking (1.7 to 1.9 as in many severe personality disorders) to frank psychosis (1.0 to 1.6). These subdivisions within a level correspond to the sublevels. Because there are five sublevels of each level and 10 points in a decimal system, each sublevel involves two points in a decimal system. In other words, the first sublevel of level 1 (sex) can be rated 1.0 to 1.1, the second sublevel of 1 (eroticism) 1.2 to 1.3, the third sublevel of 1 (validation) 1.4 to 1.5, the fourth sublevel of 1 (moderation) 1.6 to 1.7, and the fifth sublevel of 1 (discretion) as 1.8 to 1.9. In executive planning, most people operate at intermediate levels near (i.e. above or below) 2.6, but are more often materialistic in their executive planning than they are concerned about social attachment issues. Only a small minority of people are directed by intellectual quest for truth and morality. Creative individuals are truly rare. Ratings are based on the cumulative total of a person's executive functioning for a period of time that the rater can specify (such as during a period of active illness or the month before onset or after remission).

For most purposes, a semi-quantitative approach is adequate. Each of the five levels can be divided into a lower and an upper half. Thus the five levels are divided into a total of 10 half-levels, which are then numbered in sequence 1 through 10. Accordingly, 1 corresponds to 1.0 to 1.4 (sex and eroticism), 2 to 1.5 to 1.9 (moderation and discretion), 3 to 2.0 to 2.4 (aggression and competition), etc., to 9 for 5.0 to 5.4 (creative and loving service to others) and ultimately 10 for 5.5 to 5.9 (wisdom and unity of being).

Second, let us consider what to measure in rating legislative function. Legislation refers to the ability to make laws and to operate according to rules or principles. However, life is constantly changing, so we must be flexible and free to make new rules as circumstances shift if we are to remain adaptive. Hence individuals who are low in legislative function are inflexible or low in freedom of will, as in patients with character disorder, which is characterized by inflexible maladaptive behavior. Other individuals with low free will include patients with impulse control disorders (like intermittent explosive disorder, kleptomania, pyromania), paraphilias (like fetishism, voyeurism, pedophilia), and factitious disorder. In contrast, individuals who are highly advanced in legislative function are those who are flexibly adaptive, that is, who have a high degree of freedom of will. Individuals who are dominated in their actions by need for immediate gratification, that is, who are stimulus and context bound in their actions, are inflexibly opportunistic and very low in freedom of will (level 1, 1.0 to 1.9). Those who are able to delay gratification but are dominated by acquisition of wealth or other dependency needs are at level 2 (2.0 to 2.9), and are usually described as self-centered, competitive, aggressive, prejudiced and intolerant. An individual whose will is dominated by emotional attachments and aversions is at level 3 (3.0 to 3.9), and is often described as highly empathic and compassionate. Those whose will is dominated by intellectual considerations are at level 4 (4.0 to 4.9), and are generally described as cooperative with well-developed principles, and certainly not as being opportunistic.

These descriptors of the degree of free will apply to the overall freedom of the individual across a wide variety of contexts. However, the nature of free will is most clearly seen when considering specific levels of function. People can vary in their degree of free will in relation to different situations. A person can have low free will with regard to specific stimuli, for example, sex, food, drugs, emotional attachments. Thus dependence on drugs or excessive eating indicates low free will in level 2, which involves the regulation of consumption versus satiety. This explains why indicators of physiological dependence on a drug do not predict the ability of a human being to quit. The prediction of success in quitting drug use is best explained by "self-efficacy", which is a way of describing the level of a person's free will and confidence in their ability to quit once they have decided to do so [60–62]. In contrast, degree of physiological dependence or severity of withdrawal does not predict success in drug cessation [62, 63].

Third, the emotional fluidity function involves the capacity to adapt to change without emotional insecurity or distress. Fluidity in adaptation is also called personality coherence [64] or psychological flow [40]. Individuals who are low in emotional fluidity are fearful, insecure and emotionally labile. In contrast, those who are high in emotional fluidity are described as serene, because they can adapt to adversity and misfortune without loss of their calmness and confidence. It is usually sufficient to measure a person's overall level of serenity but there are clearly particular areas in which different people vary in their sensitivity. However, low serenity is characteristic of most mental disorders, so is most helpful in distinguishing those with and without mental disorder.

Fourth, the judicial function of wisdom involves the degree of insight into the meaning or significance of what we know, as well as judgement about when something is an instance of a rule [35, 65]. Judgement is not something that can be taught [65] because it is intuitive, based on the ability to listen to one's inner feelings in response to possible intentions or external plans; e.g.

"Just the thought of doing that makes me feel unwell". In other words, wisdom involves the integration of our inner feelings and our plans for external action. Consequently, individuals who are moderately high in judicial function are described as high in self-transcendence; that is, they are judicious, insightful, intuitive and spiritual. Furthermore, such judicious people are also more cheerful than others, and individuals who are very high in judicial function are described as wise and serene. In contrast, those who are low in judicial function have poor insight and judgement, and often have depression and mood disorders. In fact, patients with mood disorders often have poor judicial function, even when they are euthymic and other parameters described here have normalized. Furthermore, individuals with mood and somatization disorders tend to be low in their judicial functions with regard to all aspects of their life (levels 1 through 5), whereas those who have anxiety disorders have poor insight and judgement primarily regarding sex, safety and possessions (i.e. levels 1 and 2).

The integrative function involves a sense of participation in the unity of all things. In other words, highly integrated people feel in touch with the world around them, which has sometimes been called the "common sense". Those who are very low in integration feel emptiness and separateness from the rest of society and nature, whereas those who are very high in integration feel completeness, participation in wholeness and integrity. For example, integrative function is very low in borderline personality disorder, which is marked by identity diffusion and splitting in which the same object is alternately viewed as all-good or all-bad. Splitting of objects is considered the most primitive psychodynamic defense. In splitting, objects that elicit ambivalent feelings in a person are compartmentalized into images that are all-good (idealized) or all-bad (devalued), so that images of self and others are not integrated. Patients with splitting of objects range from 1 to 2 on the semi-quantitative scale for integration, depending on the frequency and severity of their splitting. Likewise, integration is very low in factitious disorder (formerly called Munchhausen's syndrome), which is marked by dishonesty and deceptive simulation of a sick role for financial or emotional gain. Integration is frequently very low in people who have complaints of emptiness or alienation. Integration is also low in many patients who have disturbances of their self-image or ability to identify with others, such as many patients with eating disorders, dissociative disorders (like amnesia and multiple personality disorder) and schizophrenia. In contrast, in well-integrated individuals, their sense of integrity and completeness results in absence of conflict and the emergence of spiritual gifts, such as what are often called virtues. In other words, wholeness also is associated with holiness or a divine perspective that is concerned with the ongoing betterment of all things rather than individual separateness. These gifts can be understood in psychological terms as the emergence of the spontaneities of human nature, such as creativity, love, serenity, wisdom and integrity. In Table 4.2, these are the characteristics of the integrated level (e.g. wisdom) or integrated aspects of the other levels (e.g. discretion, generosity, humor, morality). Consequently, this dimension of human nature indicates both the extent of integration of the individual personality (internal mental order) and the degree of integration of the individual with society and nature as a whole. On the other hand, patients with borderline personality disorder are very low in both their internal mental order (splitting vs. integrity) and their sense of completeness (alienation, separateness, emptiness vs. participation, inseparability, wholeness). This indicates that health varies quantitatively by degrees and is more than the absence of disease, as is recognized in current ratings of global adaptive functioning in DSM-IV [66]. Rather, well-being involves the integration of all aspects of our being without resistance to the overall design inherent in the nature of reality as a whole, which is itself fluid and expanding in its evolution.

Another psychobiological parameter that is important for classification is the force of the self, which I will call ego. Ego refers to the binding function of consciousness, which provides continuity to the components of the individual self through time [36]. When it is too weak, as in dissociative disorders, there is loss of continuity of the stream of consciousness of self-awareness. When ego is too strong, as in conditions with pathological narcissism like delusional disorder, mania, eating and many adjustment disorders, there are ego struggles involving emotionality and intellectual tasks. Sublimation of thought is associated with self-assurance and confidence in the spontaneity of thought as a self-regulating process, rather than struggling for control. Accordingly, when adaptive function is high, the force of the individual self needs only a modest level of strength.

With these descriptions in mind, let us consider the characteristics of major groups of mental disorder in relation to these parameters. A semi-quantitative description of these relationships is summarized in Table 4.4, along with ratings of individuals with higher adaptive functioning that complete the range of values across all five levels described in Table 4.2. These ratings are based on my clinical work with this approach, including ratings of more than 2000 individuals from the general population and 1000 psychiatric inpatients and outpatients. Here I will only describe the pattern of results to illustrate the method as a clinical tool for classification.

The classifications in Table 4.4 are listed according to the average level of thought during active illness unless otherwise specified. The list begins with the highest levels of adaptive function, as seen in creative characters, and descends to the lowest level of disorganization, as observed in schizophrenics. Clearly, mental health is much more than the absence of disease, as shown by the intermediate levels of thought and other psychobiological parameters in individuals with no mental disorder.

TABLE 4.4 Average values of self-integrating functions and the classification of mental order and disorder using a semi-quantitative scale from 1 to 10, with 1 and 2 for lower and higher half of sexual level 1, 2 and 3 for consummatory level 2, and so on to 9 and 10 for lower and higher half of integrated level 5

Classification	Thought	Creativity	Free Will	Serenity	Wisdom	Integration	Ego
High adaptive function							
Top 0.1%	9	9	9	9	9	9	3
Top 5%	8	8	8	8	8	8	3
Top 10%	7	7	7	7	7	7	3
Top 20%	6	6	6	6	6	6	3
No mental disorder	5	5	5	5	5	5	3
Average	4	3	3	3	3	3	3
Mental disorders							
Eating disorders	3	3	3	3	3	1	5
Paraphilias	3	3	2	3	3	3	3
Substance dependence	3	3	2	3	3	3	4
Anxiety disorders	3	3	3	2	3	3	3
Delusional disorder	3	1	1	1	2	3	6
Major depression							
Euthymic	3	2	3	3	2	2	3
Non-psychotic	3	2	2	2	2	2	3
Psychotic	2	1	2	2	2	2	3
Bipolar disorder							
Euthymic	3	3	3	3	2	2	4
Manic	2	2	2	2	2	2	5
Depressed	2	2	2	2	2	2	3
Adjustment disorders							
In remission	3	3	3	3	3	3	4
Active disorder	2	3	3	3	3	3	4
Impulse control disorders	3	3	1	2	3	3	3
Factitious disorders	3	3	1	2	1	1	4
Dissociative disorders	2	2	2	2	2	1	2
Delirium	2	2	3	2	3	3	3
Personality disorders	2	3	2	3	3	3	4
Somatization disorders	1	2	2	2	2	2	4
Schizophrenia	1	1	1	1	1	1	3

Average levels of thought and psychobiological function are materialistic, as described in level 2 of Table 4.2 and rated semi-quantitatively by 3 for its lower half (aggression and competition) and 4 for its higher half (curiosity and generosity). Individuals with no mental disorder have average thought levels of 5 on our semi-quantitative scale, which means that they are usually instantaneously aware of the emotional aspects of their thought and behavior. A substantial minority shows high adaptive function, which is characterized by excellent intellectual insight and judgement. Individuals who are integrated to the extent that they are regarded by others as creative, loving, serene, wise, or holy occur only rarely.

Mental disorders are all associated with low average levels of thought and emotional serenity, which is appropriate since mind is sometimes defined as the emotional and intellectual aspects of our being. Differential diagnosis is possible using the psychobiological functions described earlier, so we gain by being able to account for many partly overlapping categories by a modest number of parameters that may help us understand better the neurodynamics and psychodynamics of the syndromes we observe. A more penetrating analysis is possible by making ratings of these parameters for each level rather than overall, but the present set of observations should be sufficient for illustrating the approach.

The milder mental disorders, with average thought levels of 3, include eating disorders, paraphilias, substance dependence and anxiety disorders. These differ from one another by particularly low scores in integration (eating disorders), free will (paraphilias, substance dependence) or serenity (anxiety disorders).

Observations on individuals with mood disorders reveal the value of this functional approach for understanding susceptibility and onset of episodes. Even when euthymic, patients with mood disorder are impaired in their judicial function (i.e. they are unwise in their insight and judgement). In other words, they do not listen to their heart, and consequently are vulnerable to their thoughts and mood falling. When this happens, their ego levels often increase as they struggle with themselves and others, and their thought falls leading to hopelessness and psychosis in severe cases (i.e. low creativity). Likewise, adjustment disorders appear to involve primarily a problem with ego struggling with undesired circumstances, leading thoughts to plummet acutely despite no major problems with other psychobiological parameters.

Problems with free will are predominant in patients with personality and impulse control disorders. Patients with factitious and dissociative disorders have more pervasive problems, including very low integration. The importance of the ego for the binding function of consciousness is shown by loss of recall of identity when ego levels fall below 3 on our semi-quantitative scale.

Average thought levels are very low in somatization disorder and schizophrenia. It is particularly interesting to compare delusional disorder and schizophrenia in terms of these psychobiological parameters. These conditions may appear very similar superficially, but they are fundamentally different psychobiologically. Both are psychotic disorders so the creativity function is very low in both. However, otherwise the disorders differ completely. In delusional disorder, thought remains coherent, and the decreases in reality testing (creativity), free will and serenity are proportional to the pathological elevation of the ego. In contrast, in schizophrenia there is pervasive dysfunction of all the psychobiological parameters except the ego.

It is possible to extend these descriptions to capture more details of information for differential diagnosis and treatment planning. For example, thought should be assessed in terms of average and range at each of the five levels depicted as columns in Table 4.2. Specifically, the average and range should be determined for thoughts about sexuality, everyday material concerns, emotions, intellectual communication, and integration or spirituality. Remember each of these levels has five sublevels, so each can be quantified on a 10-point scale, as we did for our semi-quantitative ratings overall. Likewise, it is useful and possible to obtain sufficient information to do this for free will (legislative function) and wisdom (judicial function).

CONCLUSIONS

Comorbidity and the absence of discrete boundaries between different mental disorders does not mean that classification is not useful or valid. It means that the categorical and molecular approaches to diagnosis are inappropriate. Neither brain-less categorical systems nor mind-less molecular systems can provide optimal accounts of phenomena that are complex adaptive systems with multiple dimensions of phenotypic variation, multifactorial in their origins, and non-linear in their development. We need a way to preserve information contained in syndromal descriptions but shift our perspective to their underlying psychobiological functional properties.

Complex adaptive systems can only be meaningfully classified using multiple parameters that describe the self-organizing functions of the system as a whole. Fortunately, sufficient information is known about the phylogeny and ontogeny of learning abilities that it has been possible here to describe a set of psychobiological parameters that provide a thorough description of both mental health and disease. This is an integration of both neurobiological and psychodynamic properties in a developmental matrix that is appropriate for the quantum-like properties of human consciousness. Perhaps the parameters described here are not optimal, but they serve to illustrate the general approach of functional psychobiology by describing the behavior of adaptive systems as a whole.

What then would classification be like if based on the functional psychobiology of coherence? Cases would be assessed at a clinical level in terms of multidimensional profiles of temperament and character, as well as recent changes in physical events and life events. Syndromes associated with this would be described, much as is done now, but without any illusion that the syndromes represent discrete diseases. These steps are not very different from what we like to do now, except that many psychiatrists now do not elicit accounts of temperament and character in much detail.

Next this information would be formulated and interpreted in terms of both functional neuroanatomy and psychodynamics. This requires assessment of the psychobiological functions described in Table 4.2 and applied in Table 4.4. These formulations should eventually be testable by psychophysiological tests and functional brain imaging, which are currently revealing strong relations between specific brain circuits and personality traits closely related to the psychobiological parameters described here [67, 68]. Pharmacotherapy and psychotherapy would then be planned with this functional psychobiology as its basis.

Practically, then, the classification of mental disorders is truly a medical or neuropsychological specialty, in which expertise is needed in both neurodynamics and psychodynamics. Functional psychobiology, as envisioned here, is intended to take psychodynamics from an intellectual or emotional level to an even more integrated level of awareness with quantum-like characteristics. Such functional psychobiology should help to improve the effectiveness of classification and treatment. It would also help to re-emphasize the importance of medical and psychiatric training in the diagnosis and treatment of mental disorders. We cannot expect others to recognize the complexity of mental disorders when we rely on outdated systems of classification and approach treatment as a diagnosis-dependent cookbook. Furthermore, we cannot expect classification of mental disorders to be reliable and valid when our system of classification depends on so many redundant categories that clinicians and researchers find it impractical to do comprehensive assessments. Fortunately, functional psychobiology can be assessed in a way that is at once comprehensive, efficient and practical.

REFERENCES

1. Cloninger C.R., Martin R.L., Guze S.B., Clayton P.J. (1985) Diagnosis and prognosis in schizophrenia. *Arch. Gen. Psychiatry*, **42**: 15–25.
2. Millon T., Klerman G.L. (1986) *Contemporary Directions in Psychopathology: Toward the DSM-IV*. Guilford, New York.
3. Goodwin D.W., Guze S.B. (1996) *Psychiatric Diagnosis*, 5th edn. Oxford University Press, New York.
4. Robins E., Guze S.B. (1970) Establishment of diagnostic validity in psychiatric illness: its application to schizophrenia. *Am. J. Psychiatry*, **126**: 983–987.
5. Woodruff R.A. Jr., Reich T., Croughan J.L. (1977) Strategies of patient management in the presence of diagnostic uncertainty. *Compr. Psychiatry*, **18**: 443–448.
6. Feighner J.P., Robins E., Guze S.B., Woodruff R.A., Jr., Winokur G., Munoz R. (1972) Diagnostic criteria for use in psychiatric research. *Arch. Gen. Psychiatry*, **26**: 57–63.
7. Boyd J.H., Burke J.D., Gruenberg E., Holzer L.E. III, Rae D.S., George L.K., Karno M., Stoltzman T., McEvoy L., Nestadt G. (1984) Exclusion criteria for DSM-III: a

study of co-occurrence of hierarchy free syndromes. *Arch. Gen. Psychiatry*, **41**: 983–989.

8. Kessler R.C., McGonagle K.A., Zhao S., Nelson C.B., Hughes M., Eshleman S., Wittchen H.U., Kendler K.S. (1994) Lifetime and 12-month prevalence of DSM-III-R psychiatric disorders in the United States: results from the National Comorbidity Survey. *Arch. Gen. Psychiatry*, **51**: 8–19.

9. Wu L.T., Kouzis A.C., Leaf P.J. (1999) Influence of comorbid alcohol and psychiatric disorders on the utilization of mental health services in the National Comorbidity Survey. *Am. J. Psychiatry*, **156**: 1230–1236.

10. Andrews G., Henderson S., Hall W. (2001) Prevalence, comorbidity, disability and service utilisation: overview of the Australian National Mental Health Survey. *Br. J. Psychiatry*, **178**: 145–153.

11. McElvoy S.L., Altshuler L.L., Suppes T., Keck P.E. Jr., Frye M.A., Denicoff K.D., Nolen W.A., Kupka R.W., Leverich G.S., Rochussen J.R., Rush A.J., Post R.M. (2001) Axis I comorbidity and its relationship to historical illness variables in 288 patients with bipolar disorder. *Am. J. Psychiatry*, **158**: 420–426.

12. Kendell R.E. (1982) The choice of diagnostic criteria for biological research. *Arch. Gen. Psychiatry*, **39**: 1334–1339.

13. Eysenck H.J. (1986) A critique of contemporary classification and diagnosis. In *Contemporary Directions in Psychopathology* (Eds T. Millon, G.L. Klerman), pp. 73–98. Guilford, New York.

14. Sigvardsson S., Bohman M., von Knorring A.L., Cloninger C.R. (1986) Symptom patterns and causes of somatization in men. *Genet. Epidemiol.*, **3**: 153–169.

15. Cloninger C.R. (1987) A systematic method for clinical description and classification of personality variants: a proposal. *Arch. Gen. Psychiatry*, **44**: 573–587.

16. Cloninger C.R., Svrakic D.M., Przybeck T.R. (1993) A psychobiological model of temperament and character. *Arch. Gen. Psychiatry*, **50**: 975–990.

17. Cloninger C.R., Svrakic D.M. (2000) Personality disorders. In *Comprehensive Textbook of Psychiatry*, 7th edn (Eds B.J. Sadock, V.A. Sadock), pp. 1723–1764. Lippincott Williams & Wilkins, New York.

18. Moldin S.O. (1997) The maddening hunt for madness genes. *Nature Genet.*, **17**: 127–129.

19. Comings D.E., Gade-Andavolu R., Gonzalez N., Wu S., Muhleman D., Blake H., Mann M.B., Dietz G., Saucier G., MacMurray J.P. (2000) A multivariate analysis of 59 candidate genes in personality traits: the temperament and character inventory. *Clin. Genet.*, **58**: 375–385.

20. Cloninger C.R., Martin R.L., Guze S.B., Clayton P.J. (1990) The empirical structure of psychiatric comorbidity and its theoretical significance. In *Comorbidity of Mood and Anxiety Disorders* (Eds J.D. Maser, C.R. Cloninger), pp. 439–498. American Psychiatric Press, New York.

21. Battaglia M., Przybeck T.R., Bellodi L., Cloninger C.R. (1996) Temperament dimensions explain the comorbidity of psychiatric disorders. *Compr. Psychiatry*, **37**: 292–298.

22. Cloninger C.R., Przybeck T.R., Svrakic D.M., Wetzel R.D. (1994) *The Temperament and Character Inventory (TCI): A Guide to its Development and Use*. Washington University Center for Psychobiology of Personality, St. Louis.

23. Cloninger C.R., Bayon C., Svrakic D.M. (1998) Measurement of temperament and character in mood disorders: a model of fundamental states as personality types. *J. Affect. Disord.*, **51**: 21–32.

24. Cloninger C.R. (1999) *Personality and Psychopathology*. American Psychiatric Press, Washington.

25. Cloninger C.R., Svrakic N.M., Svrakic D.M. (1997) Role of personality self-organization in development of mental order and disorder. *Develop. Psychopathol.*, **9**: 681–906.
26. Maser J.D., Cloninger C.R. (1990) *Comorbidity of Mood and Anxiety Disorders.* American Psychiatric Press, Washington.
27. Bloom F. (1993) The neurobiology of addiction: an integrative view. In *Biological Basis of Substance Abuse* (Eds S.G. Korenman, J.D. Barchas), pp. 3–18. Oxford University Press, New York.
28. Cloninger C.R. (2000) Biology of personality dimensions. *Curr. Opin. Psychiatry*, **13**: 611–616.
29. Stewart I., Stewart A. (1997) *Life's Other Secret: The New Mathematics of the Living World.* Wiley, New York.
30. Eisenberg L. (1995) The social construction of the human brain. *Am. J. Psychiatry*, **152**: 1563–1575.
31. Eisenberg L. (2000) Is psychiatry more mindful or brainier than it was a decade ago? *Br. J. Psychiatry*, **176**: 1–5.
32. Plomin R., Owen M.J., McGuffin P. (1994) The genetic basis of complex human behaviors. *Science*, **264**: 1733–1739.
33. Baltes P.B. (1997) On the incomplete architecture of human ontogeny: selection, optimization, and compensation as foundation of developmental theory. *Am. Psychol.*, **52**: 366–380.
34. Plato (c. 400 BC/1977) *The Republic of Plato.* Oxford University Press, New York.
35. Sternberg R.J. (1990) *Wisdom: Its Nature, Origins, and Development.* Cambridge University Press, New York.
36. Eccles J. (1989) *Evolution of the Brain: Creation of the Self.* Routledge, London.
37. Mithen S. (1996) *The Prehistory of the Mind: The Cognitive Origins of Art, Religion, and Science.* Thames & Hudson, London.
38. Walker E.H. (2000) *The Physics of Consciousness: Quantum Minds and the Meaning of Life.* Perseus Books, Cambridge.
39. Bell J.S. (1993) *Speakable and Unspeakable in Quantum Mechanics.* Cambridge University Press, New York.
40. Csikszentmihalyi M. (1990) *Flow: The Psychology of Optimal Experience.* Harper Collins, New York.
41. Winner E. (1996) *Gifted Children: Myths and Realities.* Basic Books, New York.
42. Schrodinger E. (1967) *What is Life?* Cambridge University Press, New York.
43. Nauta W.J.H. (1971) The problem of the frontal lobe: A reinterpretation. *J. Psychiatr. Res.*, **8**: 167–187.
44. Reep R. (1984) *Relationship between Prefrontal and Limbic Cortex: A Comparative Anatomical Review.* Karger, Basel.
45. Bohm D. (1980) *Wholeness and the Implicate Order.* Routledge, London.
46. Tittel W., Brendel J., Zbinden H., Gisen N. (1998) Violation of Bell inequalities by photons more than 10 km apart. *Phys. Rev. Lett.*, **81**: 3563–3566.
47. Weihs G., Jennewein T., Simon C., Weinfurter H., Zeilinger A. (1998) *Violation of Bell's inequality under strict Einstein locality conditions. Phys. Rev. Lett.*, **81**: 5039–5043.
48. Bouwmeester D., Pan J.W., Mattle K., Eibl M., Weinfurter H., Zeilinger A. (1997) Experimental quantum teleportation. *Nature*, **390**: 575–579.
49. Zeilinger A. (2000) Quantum teleportation. *Scientific American*, **282**: 50–59.
50. Rey G. (1997) *Contemporary Philosophy of Mind.* Blackwell, Oxford.
51. Penrose R. (1989) *The Emperor's New Mind: Concerning Computers, Minds, and the Laws of Physics.* Oxford University Press, New York.

52. Chalmers D.J. (1996) *The Conscious Mind: In Search of a Fundamental Theory.* Oxford University Press, New York.
53. Stapp H. (1999) Attention, intention, and will in quantum physics. *Journal of Conscious Studies: The Volitional Brain*, 6: 143–164.
54. MacLean P.D. (1990) *The Triune Brain in Evolution: Role in Paleocerebral Functions.* Plenum Press, New York.
55. Cloninger C.R. (1998) The genetics and psychobiology of the seven factor model of personality. In *The Biology of Personality Disorders* (Ed. K.R. Silk), pp. 63–84. American Psychiatric Press, Washington.
56. Freud S. (1938) *A General Introduction to Psychoanalysis.* Garden City Publishing Co., Garden City.
57. Sternberg R.J. (1988) *The Nature of Creativity: Contemporary Psychological Perspectives.* Cambridge University Press, New York.
58. Simonton D.K. (1999) Creativity and genius. In *Handbook of Personality*, 2nd edn (Eds L.A. Pervin, O.P. John), pp. 629–653. Guilford, New York.
59. Eysenck H.J. (1995) *Genius: The Natural History of Creativity.* Cambridge University Press, Cambridge.
60. DiClemente C.C., Prochaska J.O., Gibertini M. (1985) Self-efficacy and the stages of self-change of smoking. *Cogn. Ther. Res.*, 9: 181–200.
61. Kavanagh D.J., Pierce J., Lo S.K., Shelley J. (1993) Self-efficacy and social support as predictors of smoking after a quit attempt. *Psychol. Health*, 8: 231–242.
62. Kenford S.L., Fiore M.C., Jorenby D.E., Smith S.S., Wetter D., Baker T.B. (1994) Predicting smoking cessation: who will quit with and without the nicotine patch. *JAMA*, **271**: 589–594.
63. Robins L.N., Helzer J.E., Davis D.H. (1975) Narcotic use in southeast Asia and afterward. An interview study of 898 Vietnam returnees. *Arch. Gen. Psychiatry*, **32**: 955–961.
64. Cervone D., Shoda Y. (1999) *The Coherence of Personality: Social-Cognitive Bases of Consistency, Variability, and Organisation.* Guilford, New York.
65. Kant I. (1798) *Anthropology from a Pragmatic Point of View.* Martinus Nijhoff, The Hague.
66. American Psychiatric Association (1994) *Diagnostic and Statistical Manual of Mental Disorders*, 4th edn. American Psychiatric Association, Washington.
67. Sugiura M., Kawashima R., Nakagawa M., Okada K., Sato T., Goto R., Sato K., Ono S., Schormann T., Zilles K., Fukuda H. (2000) Correlation between human personality and neural activity in cerebral cortex. *NeuroImage*, **11**: 541–546.
68. Vedeniapin A.B., Anokhin A.A., Sirevaag E., Rohrbaugh J.W., Cloninger C.R. (2001) Visual P300 and the self-directedness scale of the temperament–character inventory. *Psychiatry Res.*, **101**: 145–156.

5

Evolutionary Theory, Culture and Psychiatric Diagnosis

Horacio Fabrega Jr.

Department of Psychiatry, University of Pittsburgh, Pittsburgh, PA, USA

INTRODUCTION

Psychopathology is universal, found in all societies regardless of their ancestry, size, organization, political economy, and culture. The conditions for it are products of the inherited biology of *Homo sapiens*. However, societies differ in terms of such things as language, beliefs, world-views, notions of personhood and emotion, and rules and standards regarding social behavior. These cultural factors affect the content of psychopathology. Moreover, since culture is internalized and enters into the very construction of human psychology and the experience of bodily functions, it significantly influences the structure of psychopathology.

This gives rise to two seemingly opposed views about the character of psychopathology. The first is a culture-free conceptualization based on generic, biologically rooted mechanisms; the other, cultural relativism based on historical, national and ideological differences. My goal in this chapter is to review the two perspectives, compare them using three clinical examples, and critically discuss their strengths and limitations. Based on suppositions about the future interplay between psychiatry and society, I will discuss briefly why evolutionary and cultural tenets need to be incorporated in a system of psychiatric diagnosis.

ON THE GENEALOGY OF PSYCHIATRIC DIAGNOSIS AND CLASSIFICATION

All of the traditions of medicine associated with ancient civilizations that have been studied have developed approaches to the understanding of

Psychiatric Diagnosis and Classification. Edited by Mario Maj, Wolfgang Gaebel, Juan José López-Ibor and Norman Sartorius. © 2002 John Wiley & Sons, Ltd.

problems of behavior and sickness that today are classified as psychiatric. The civilizations of India and China each developed a naturalistic conception of disease and mental illness which to this day retains a measure of identity and viability in the respective societies [1, 2]. The contemporary perspective about psychiatric diagnosis and classification is a product of the social history of mental illness and of the discipline and profession of psychiatry in European and Anglo-American societies. Its roots extend into the medicine of the Greco-Roman period of antiquity exemplified by the writings of Hippocrates and Galen. Descriptions of symptoms in these writings (formulated in terms of the four humors) referred to abnormal forms of experience and behavior that pre-figure descriptions of contemporary psychiatric disturbances. During the medieval period, academic scholarly medicine continued its emphasis on humors, but was also strongly influenced by Christianity. Conceptions about and approaches to psychiatric problems as madness and insanity became associated with notions of spirituality, sin and punishment. The early modern period witnessed the eclipse of humoral theory and growth of iatrochemical and mechanical points of view. This involved a heightening of secular, naturalistic tenets. Eventually, diseases came to be formulated as separate entities having their own identity, history or course, and treatment. The central task of medicine became that of identifying, describing, and understanding these natural objects or disease entities. The evolving "modern" theory of disease eventually was applied to psychopathology.

In association with scientific developments in the theory and understanding of disease, changes in society during the early modern and then modern era came to shape the care of the mentally ill and eventually the evolution of the profession of psychiatry [3]. These changes are complex and wide-ranging. From a sociological standpoint, they involved increases in population, urbanization and migration, political changes affecting the growth of liberalism and democracy, and the growth of industrial capitalism. The changes affected the prevalence and visibility of mental illness, attitudes about its victims, and changes in social policy.

Starting in the seventeenth century in France and later spreading to other nations, marginal, impoverished, and dependent segments of the populations came to pose a major problem in large communities, especially in cities throughout Europe. Problem populations were placed in institutions and, with time, victims of mental illness were set apart from the larger class of disabled, diseased, dependent, and marginal. Eventually, special asylums were established for their care, while more affluent establishments provided a "private trade in lunacy". Later, during the reform era, the deplorable conditions existing in public institutions became the concern of municipal regulatory bodies. Inquiries into conditions of asylums with attempts at reform culminated in the establishment of more humane conditions of care and treatment of mental illness. In some societies, the central government played an influential role in spearheading treatment, education, and research; in others, universities and faculties of medicine; and in still others, local municipalities.

The evolution of actual knowledge of clinical psychiatry is largely a product of developments during the nineteenth century. It involved two empirically interconnected trends that can be separated only analytically. One development culminated in the refinement of a system of concepts about and terms referring to disturbances of human psychology and behavior along with the criteria and principles pertaining to how this descriptive system was to be used. The other one involved the creation of a science about the many psychiatric disorders that came to be named and described, disorders that were delineated by means of the descriptive system and which came to be studied by means of the new science of medicine prevalent in the nineteenth century, involving diagnosis and explanation pertaining to causes, lesions, and natural history. The former development involved the evolution of a science of *descriptive psychopathology* and the latter the scientific knowledge linked to the *historiography of clinical psychiatry* [4, 5].

In summary, it was in groups of physicians involved in the study and care of mentally ill patients, in both private and public institutions, that the modern approach to mental illness evolved. Different national conceptualizations about psychopathology evolved reflecting linguistic, cultural, and societal experiences and traditions. However, to improve communication and promote research, there arose a need for the discernment of commonalities. A conviction grew that the various syndromes, disorders, and illnesses that had emerged in national classification systems exhibited common features and conformed to a smaller set of conditions that transcended national boundaries and cultural experience. The members of this class of disorders are assumed to be amenable to careful scientific definition and description in a general language of psychopathology. The traditional view holds that human populations show different vulnerabilities to disease linked to differences in geography, social ecology, and culture, but it does not undermine the official position about universals in the pathology and clinical presentation that underpin the international approach to psychiatric diagnosis and classification.

An emphasis on the development of psychiatric knowledge and mental health services in European and Anglo-American societies is important to emphasize, because it gained international eminence and now claims allegiance across the world. The imperialism and colonialism of the nineteenth and twentieth centuries had many obvious political and economic repercussions. One of them was the exportation of biomedical knowledge that initially came to be applied to improve general public health. As the modern conception of disease became ascendant and with this understandings of mechanism and control embodied in the biological sciences, biomedicine attained a major colonizing influence in developing societies. In relation to this social movement, modern European and Anglo-American knowledge about psychiatric disorders has attained world significance and along with this principles of diagnosis and practice that increasingly have come to be formulated in a common language of nosology.

EVOLUTIONARY THEORY AS A BASIS FOR PSYCHIATRIC THEORY AND NOSOLOGY

General Remarks

Many psychiatric disorders have a genetic basis. Their prevalence is substantially higher than average mutation rates. These facts are held to imply that the responsible genes may have been positively selected during human biological evolution. Many genes underlying psychopathology may have benefits in other areas of functioning and their role in psychopathology may simply reflect a cost incurred as a result of trade-offs. In the case of psychological mechanisms or personality traits that are due to multiple genes, instances of psychopathology may simply reflect heavy loading of genes that in lower amounts or degree of penetrance happen to be adaptive. Not all psychiatric disorders are the direct expression of genetic coding but are related indirectly to evolutionary factors nonetheless [6].

Evolutionary Theory, Human Behavior, and Psychopathology

Social relations play a central role in evolutionary theory. Natural selection did not produce "logically consistent" routines of behavior, "good solutions" to problems and conflicts, or "pleasant" emotions. Instead, inherited behavior routines, termed psychological adaptations or algorithms, are responsible for aspects of human behavior. These are the product of a long history of constraints in the design of hardware (e.g. the brain) that occurred early in evolution and of a myriad of trade-offs and balances that were required over hundreds of thousands of years and that were aimed at solving recurring biological problems that tracked changes in ancestral environments.

The emotions play an important role in evolutionary accounts of psychopathology. They are behavioral indicators that reflect naturally designed mechanisms that have a bearing on or relationship to important biological functions. When the mechanisms are exaggerated or inappropriately elicited, psychopathology may result. Positive emotions (e.g. satisfaction, pleasure) reflect mechanisms and behavior exchanges that in past environments were associated with fitness and survival, while negative ones (e.g. anxiety, sadness, anger) are signals of threats and challenges to fitness. Like adaptations, emotions are *evolutionary residuals*: the "leftovers" of mechanisms of social behavior that were naturally designed during evolution in relation to happenings in ancestral environments. Negative emotions are not "bad" things, but rather "good", inherited signals that operate to inform (though not consciously and willfully) the individual as to the current status or functioning of adaptive patterns of behavior and about needed choices, avoidances, and strategies.

Psychiatric Disorders as Harmful Dysfunctions

Evolutionary theory has been used in the study of disease and the general medical care of patients [7]. A *disorder* has been defined as a harmful dysfunction (HD); namely, a failure or breakdown of an internal mechanism to perform its natural function [8]. Harmfulness is a condition that is painful and/or detrimental to an individual's well-being and functioning. Harmful conditions have many causes, being based on environmental happenings that conflict with biological imperative; however, only dysfunctions of *natural mechanisms* are applicable to the evolutionary argument of disorder.

The HD slant on a disorder is compelling. On the one hand, it has general resonance: a "natural function" and a "failure" of it are, from a conceptual standpoint, what persons ordinarily intuitively mean when they think of disease or disorder involving something that has gone wrong or is not working properly. On the other hand, it also has a seeming rigor. It rests on the classical theory of categories (see below) and invokes a scientific epistemology (i.e. a failure of a naturally designed function). While the HD approach has general medical implications (e.g. diabetes, hypertension, kidney failure), it has been systematically applied to psychopathology. The psychological adaptations singled out by evolutionary psychologists were naturally designed to solve recurring biological problems during evolution and hence are examples of "natural functions". The HD analysis holds that true or "scientifically valid" psychiatric disorders are based on harmful dysfunctions of such adaptations. The HD analysis of a psychiatric disorder reinforces the link between psychiatry and general medicine [9, 10].

An evolutionary conception of psychiatric disorder is an essentialist or classical approach to the definition of a concept. The definition of HD stipulates two individually necessary and jointly sufficient defining features of "psychiatric disorder". The HD analysis has been the target of critical analysis by both psychiatrists and social scientists. Whether the concept of (psychiatric) disorder is "Roschian" and conforms to the prototype theory of concept formation (i.e. any one condition qualifying as a disorder because it approximates or resembles an ideal or prototype) has constituted one line of attack [11, 12]. In addition, emphasis has been given to its disregard of cultural influences, social values, and sheer practical exigencies [6]. Further critiques of the HD perspective are taken up later in the chapter.

THE THEORY OF CULTURE AS A BASIS FOR PSYCHIATRIC THEORY AND NOSOLOGY

General Remarks

Culture theory argues for the influence of social symbols and their meanings on a person's general psychology, outlook and tenor of life, including psychopathology. There are two ways in which the ideas of culture and cultural differences have been used in the study of psychiatric disorders. First, as a marker for a group, like age, gender, social class, religion, or ethnicity. This *demographic view* is then used to compare group differences in psychopathology. A contrast is the *psychological view* that stresses determinative and constitutive aspects of a person's sense of reality, personal identity, and behavior.

Psychiatric Disorders as Culturally Constituted Human Conditions

The cultural theory position stipulates that culture cannot easily be separated out of the material basis of psychiatric disorders [13]. While disorders are universal, conditioned if not produced by human biological evolution (i.e. having a phylogeny), they also are cultural and hence variable. This position holds human psychology is an essential locus of psychopathology. The traditional history of psychiatry informs that conditions of interest involve the "psyche". The latter includes cognition, emotion, and motivation, on the one hand, and social, symbolic behavior, on the other. Together they constitute essential characteristics of psychopathology (as well as psyche), however it may be formulated. Culture theory emphasizes and complements the social mandate that gave rise to the discipline and profession of psychiatry and that underlies the efforts of all societies to cope with mental illness. The second conception of culture reviewed above implies that cultural psychology is a proper locus of psychopathology. It stresses that language, culture and cognition, realized in world-views, conceptions of persons and behavior, and ways of understanding self, other, and the outside, behavioral environment, in their integration, "make up" psycho-pathology.

The vaunted properties of *Homo sapiens* (e.g. language, cognition, culture) are assumed to result from a slow process of natural selection during biological (i.e. genetic) evolution [6]. Rather than subscribing to the view that these properties are mere by-products of brain size and comparatively recent in origin, a Rubicon crossing that happened "once and for all" during the transition to the Upper Paleolithic era, they are assumed to have a much longer ancestry. Not 50 000 or so years ago but hundreds of thousands of years mark the gradual, progressive march towards the human symbolic capacity [14–16]. Coincident with this pattern of slow evolution of symbolization in the hominid line, behavior problems became better differentiated and began to be accorded a corresponding social and cultural significance. Varieties of psychopathology, then, were "natural" to hominid populations well before the transition to the Upper Paleolithic [6].

DEPRESSION: CASE NO. 1 IN THE EVOLUTIONARY AND CULTURAL STUDY OF PSYCHOPATHOLOGY

General Remarks

Disorders associated with the mood of depression are firmly placed in the history of psychiatric nosology and systems of classification [17]. They have a complex etiology, pathogenesis, set of manifestations, and natural history. Many contemporary conditions (e.g. chronic anxiety, somatoform disorders, fibromyalgia, irritable bowel) resemble or overlap with depression. The medical authenticity of depression is beyond reproach: it enjoys a universal prevalence in human societies and presence in medical traditions of the world [1].

Evolutionary Theory Considerations

Evolutionary psychiatrists have made depression an object of analysis. Its genetic basis and high frequency have implied positive selection and raised the question of it constituting an actual adaptation. For example, its emotional manifestations have suggested a warning function that the victim's current strategies are failing; its physiological signs of slowing, withdrawal, and seeming conservation as prompting that the individual shift to more profitable environments and enterprises; and its external, behavior/demeanor characteristic signs as communications designed to elicit others' help. However, several factors about depression have argued against a strict adaptationist interpretation. Its protean character is one and another is the possibility that each of its sets of manifestations has diverse origins and functions—some maladaptive [18]. That the depression spectrum or "phenotype" seems to constitute a "common final pathway", the resultant of many causes, and a variable course (e.g. remitting spontaneously or responding only to some medications) has suggested that it is not unitary and homogeneous and thus unlikely to constitute an adaptation *per se*. Some hold that depression is the result of disruption of a maturation program [18, 19].

The *social competition hypothesis* is the most systematic evolutionary formulation of depression [20, 21]. It posits that humans share with their primitive ancestors an involuntary strategy of subordination, a mechanism for yielding in situations of competition. The theory draws on ideas from ethology and the social biology of behavior about how individuals compete for rank. The functions of the strategy are to inhibit aggression towards rivals and superiors by creating a subjective sense of incapacity, to communicate a lack of threat and a yielding, and to facilitate function by putting the individual into a "giving up" frame of mind that encourages acceptance and voluntary yielding. The features of depression and the situations and circumstances surrounding its victims are all explained in terms of ethological notions of group dynamics and rituals of behavior.

Nesse [22] has recently offered a critical analysis of the idea that the depression spectrum constitutes an adaptation. Based on much earlier work involving the evolutionary function of emotions and the biological basis of responses linked to general medical disease, he offers a summary of the possible functions of low mood (states in the common range of normal experience) and depression (severe states of negative affect, usually pathological). He sees these as pleas for help, the elicitation of help from group mates, and also as a communication designed to manipulate others to provide resources and then conserve them. Depression is part of a motivational package to plan and reassess a course of action with a possible view to change or alter goals. Even some conditions of frank clinical depression, Nesse implies, can be explained as serving evolutionary functions. However, his analysis and experience lead him away from explaining depression in terms of one function and instead to view the spectrum as states shaped to cope with a number of unpropitious situations.

Culture Theory Considerations

While the universal prevalence of depression constitutes an indisputable generalization in psychiatric epidemiology, that these conditions are brought on, shaped, expressed, and interpreted in culturally specific terms constitutes an axiom of cultural psychiatry that is also beyond dispute. Nowhere is this better illustrated than with respect to China. There is much evidence, as well as controversy about, the presentation of depression in China. It has been claimed that in China depression manifests in a "somatized" as compared to a "psychologized" way [23]. Many explanations have been invoked, including innate patterns of physiological response, culturally shaped processes in brain/behavior, linguistic conventions pertaining to self and emotion, social attitudes about emotional expression, and political strictures affecting how one should explain and communicate hardship. The idea that in some countries like China mental disorders take a somatized form as compared to a psychologized one has also been attributed to sheer educational factors and to the possibility that the attitudes of the doctor ("accepting" or "rejecting" psychological complaints from patients) are determinant of the form of presentation of distressing experiences. Of course, as indicated above, some conventions regarding self-expression through language favor the use of examples ("I feel as bad as . . . ") whereas others do not and this may be a consideration as well. All of these factors, it has been stated, shape, color, and configure the depression in a distinctly Chinese pattern.

The complex association between culture and the depression spectrum is illustrated by the findings, and subsequent responses to their dissemination, of the study by Kleinman [24] of neurasthenia and depression in China. He studied 100 patients there who were diagnosed as showing neurasthenia. This is a "condition" coined by *American* neurologist George Beard to denote "exhaustion of the nervous system". It consisted of a mixture of fatigue, weakness, impaired concentration and memory, headaches, poor appetite, and any number of variegated "physical" symptoms. It is interesting to note that the concept of neurasthenia appears to have been introduced into China via the training of psychiatrists in the former Soviet Union and the model of neurasthenia as presented in the former Soviet Union was different from that of European countries and the United States. The eventual translation of neurasthenia into Chinese (as *shenjing shuairuo*) is significant, since it drew on important local concepts of vitality, cognitive activity or "energy", and motivation (*shen*), and the traditional medical knowledge of meridians or channels of the body (*jing*) which carried "vital energy" (*qi*) and "blood" (*xue*). "Conceptually, *shen* and *jing* are treated by Chinese people as one term (*shenjing*), that means 'nerve' or 'nervous system'. When *shenjing* becomes *shuai* (degenerate) and *ruo* (weak) following undue nervous excitement, a variety of psychic and somatic symptoms may reasonably ensue" [25]. The Chinese interpretation of neurasthenia encapsulates in a succinct way a whole tradition and theory about self, experience, sickness, bodily experience, and psychopathology that is integral to its native systems of medicine.

Not surprisingly, then, because the diagnosis of neurasthenia as *shenjing shuairuo* is connected in vital ways with deeply rooted, traditional notions and idioms of well-being, it consequently "caught on" in Chinese medicine soon after it spread there during the nineteenth century. What Kleinman showed was that 87% of neurasthenic patients met criteria for depression and moreover on follow-up appeared to respond to antidepressant medication. Not all who were biomedically improved, however, necessarily defined themselves as not sick, a fact that underscored the political economic embedment of sickness including depression in China as well as its "natural" fit with Chinese cultural psychology. Personal and culturally rooted political economic factors, it would appear, strongly influence whether a diagnosis pertaining to the depression spectrum embodies a condition of sickness and maladaptation as the individual, at any rate, defines this.

One obvious implication of Kleinman's study was to demonstrate that local conventions of meaning and traditions pertaining to body, emotion, self, and situation profoundly determine how aspects of the depression spectrum play out in relation to culture and society. A complex amalgam of factors, which include biology, culture and local experience, shape how the depression spectrum is configured and enacted. The influence of cultural factors in the depression spectrum has been studied in other social groups. Manson *et al.* [26] studied the links between depression and several indigenously defined conditions of sickness among members of the Hopi Nation of American Indians. The similarities and differences between scientific definitions of depression and those representative of the residents of the region were discussed. Manson makes clear that general characteristics of the various sickness conditions differ as a function of culture, but so do also the phenomenology, putative cause, duration, and circumstances surrounding actual episodes. An argument can be made that among the Hopi people, no less than among the Chinese, the depression spectrum is configured and enacted differently. Kinzie *et al.* [27] have developed and validated a Vietnamese-language depression rating scale precisely because among refugees the disorder has a different configuration. There exist numerous other approaches to the cultural study of depression [28].

SOCIAL PHOBIA: CASE NO. 2 IN THE EVOLUTIONARY AND CULTURAL STUDY OF PSYCHOPATHOLOGY

General Remarks

Few human conditions embody as much face validity for a form of social maladaptation as do those marked by worry, fearfulness, psychic pain, somatic experiences of autonomic hyperactivity, and associated social avoidance. The distress, misery, and social disruption that anxiety can cause extend beyond psychiatry to encompass religion and philosophy. Because of its wide prevalence, anxiety has received attention from evolutionary and cultural psychiatrists. The anxiety that seems concentrated in social relations and interactions has evolutionary importance because of the hominid trait of sociality and it has cultural relevance because in personal experience and human activity one finds concentrated the meanings of any culture.

Evolutionary Theory Considerations

Anxiety, like fear, pain, and fever, is a natural defensive response, one of the body's protective mechanisms [7, 29, 30]. The process of natural selection in the environment of evolutionary adaptedness (EEA) designed the regulatory mechanisms that underlie anxiety so as to enable individuals to avoid threats and promote survival and reproduction. Anxiety, in other words, is a "good thing". Whenever a threat or the likelihood of harm occurs, anxiety can be expected to result and its degree will bear a relationship to the magnitude of harm/threat. However, even if the cost is low, the defense will be expressed in anxious behavior when the mechanism is operating normally, much like a smoke detector may be triggered even in the absence of a real fire. It is assumed that hominid ancestors existed in environments that had a wide range of levels of danger that were recurrent. Genes that shaped the anxiety response continued to be adaptive for a very long time and have left a residue of low threshold for the generation of protective responses to situations of potential harm and danger.

Many varieties of phobias have been the object of evolutionary analysis and each one has been explained as the outcome of "the smoke detector principle" in response to an evoking situation that had fitness implications in EEA. In the case of social phobia, threats to reputation and status have been singled out as important. Drawing on principles from ethology and evolutionary biology, Stevens and Price [20] emphasize the importance of contests and tournaments as a way of establishing social rank, something individuals persist in striving to maintain or improve upon. Success in such tournaments earns individuals a measure of value and power, termed resource holding power (RHP). During evolution, hedonic as compared to strictly agonistic modes of social interaction became increasingly important. This involved competition not by intimidation but by attraction, with competitors disarming rivals and attracting mates and also achieving status and rank in the group. This gave rise to a new capacity for self-assessment, termed social attention holding power (SAHP). According to Stevens and Price [20], anxiety generally and social anxiety in particular is commonly released in situations that are perceived to constitute a threat to the individual's RHP or SAHP.

Social phobia may thus be regarded as a psychiatric disorder that conforms to the harmful dysfunction model proposed by evolutionary psychologists and reviewed earlier. Psychological mechanisms and algorithms serve the natural function of maintaining an individual's sense of competence and ranking in a group. Through such mechanisms individuals are able to project and protect their social resources, establish their credibility, compete, attract mates, and assure the maintenance of their offspring. When a perturbation of this mechanism takes place, a disorder of behavior results. Social phobia is assumed to correspond to a dysfunction of mechanisms promoting social competence in a group setting and in face-to-face relationships. Its presence and definition in international systems of diagnosis attest to its presumed universal, pan-cultural characteristics.

Culture Theory Considerations

While the international and evolutionary viewpoints about social phobia suggest universality, research work from Japan argues the case for cultural specificity. Kirmayer [31] reviewed characteristics of *Taijin Kyofusho* (TKS), a common disorder in Japan featured by fear of offending others through one's social awkwardness or because of an imagined social defect. In Japanese psychiatry TKS comprises a spectrum of disorders. While symptoms consistent with social phobia are predominant in all its varieties, their characteristics in Japan differ significantly. Moreover, while TKS involves a Japanese set of disorders marked by a unitary and distinctively Japanese content and meaning, it includes varieties that in the relatively culture fair nosology of international psychiatry suggest several different disorders.

Social relationships in Japan are systematically shaped into and calibrated on the basis of emphasis on one's effect on an immediate audience. Parties to a relationship strive to reduce psychological distance by intuiting what others are thinking and feeling. Indirect, implicit communication is valued, the obverse is considered blunt and insensitive. An assumption prevails that a socially competent person can understand others without having to resort to words. Even eye contact is regarded as bold and potentially offensive and averting one's gaze is enjoined, creating a normative basis for concern and fear of injuring others with one's gaze. It goes without saying that the expression of negative emotions is restricted and that attributes of the self and indeed of the body, such as appearance, skin blemishes, and odor are regarded as potentially offensive to others and the possibility that this may prevail is a source of obsessive worry if not preoccupation. Cognitive factors are associated with these interpersonal characteristics; for example, an emphasis on consciousness of self in social situations, of being on a social stage, and of having to act appropriately in front of others. Rules of etiquette include elaborate forms of respect language, awareness of posture, and self-presentation with respect to management of facial expressions and the masking of emotions.

In Japan, then, a distinctive social psychological calculus shapes how selves should behave in public settings. There exists a dictum that one must search and scan facial expressions so as to anticipate what best to say and how to "come across" so as not to offend. It is no surprise that pathological deviations of this social language of communication and of interpersonal relations influence not only the origins of social anxiety and phobia but also color its manifestations in a significant way. Child rearing and patterns of social interaction all appear to function so as to create vulnerabilities to varieties of social anxiety.

TKS is extremely common in Japan and since the 1960s has been regarded by Japanese psychiatrists as a unique form of psychological disorder. Many patients fulfill DSM criteria of social phobia. However, fear of eye-to-eye contact, of physical deformity, and of emitting an unpleasant body odor as well as of blushing are among the commonest symptoms of TKS, yet were not especially emphasized in DSM-III [31]. The fear that one has a deformed body constitutes a subtype of TKS in Japan, yet in DSM-III-R such a dysmorphophobia was classified as a separate condition, namely, as a form of somatoform disorder. The conviction that one may harm others either by appearance, behavior, body odor, or physical deformity often appears to reach delusional proportions, yet this symptom is judged to fall squarely within the TKS spectrum and is not regarded as a psychosis. It should be noted that the German introduction of the terms ereuthophobia and erithophobia was known in Japan and found to be useful; however, the fear of others did not appear to be extremely common. Moreover, the concept of dysmorphophobia in its original definition was characterized by the delusional conviction that one's body is deformed; however, the clarity of that experience did not fall into the rubric of fear that an organ of the body might be deformed.

The TKS spectrum, then, illustrates rather vividly the role of culture not only in influencing the origins of social phobia but also its content and constitution. Socialization and enculturation create expectancies regarding emotions and personal expression in social relations that predispose individuals to this variety of anxiety. The semantic content that provides meaning to what is expected of the self and how feelings and actions should be shaped in social relations create the normative conventions on the basis of which deviations that constitute the spectrum are calibrated. This endows those deviations in behavior with a blend of concerns that shape and give a distinctive meaning to the syndrome in Japanese culture. Its cultural psychology, as it were, shapes social anxiety into a Japanese disorder.

PSYCHOPATHY: CASE NO. 3 IN THE EVOLUTIONARY AND CULTURAL STUDY OF PSYCHOPATHOLOGY

General Remarks

Antisocial personality traits and behavior constitute a challenge for a nosology of psychiatry. Studies in cultural anthropology suggest that a construct or cognitive category about antisocial behavior is a human universal [32, 33]. Murphy [34] used antisocial personality as an example of universalism in her study that argued against the view that psychiatric disorders were culturally variable and relative. These generalizations about views on antisocial behavior and personality are consistent with the history of psychiatric thinking. Since the very late eighteenth century, when the American Benjamin Rush and the Frenchman Philippe Pinel published their respective dissertations, the antisocial constellation and construct has fallen within the perimeter of psychiatric attention [35]. Currently, it is represented in the two international systems but defined somewhat differently: DSM-IV emphasizing antisocial behaviors and ICD-10 personality factors.

The history of psychiatry embodies tensions with respect to behavior and mental illness. As a medical discipline, psychiatry is concerned to develop and use a system of knowledge so as to diagnose, treat and prevent illness. Its social functions, on the other hand, are various and they overlap: as a social medical institution with a distinctive social mandate (i.e. public health functions), psychiatry seeks to control and regulate social problems associated with mental illness; as part of the social welfare system, it validates if not justifies the disbursement of social security and disability payments to victims of mental illness; and as a sanctioning, disciplining body of the criminal justice system, its decisions about mental illness appear to absolve, punish, stigmatize, and/or medicalize.

How antisocial behavior has fared within psychiatry illustrates the quandary presented by psychiatry's dual functions and the goals of its nosology. While including a disorder whose indicators are socially divisive, contravene social norms, and can include patterns of delinquent and criminal activity, psychiatry has been accused of mitigating or condoning the behaviors of individuals diagnosed as antisocial personality disorder or psychopathic [36]. The relationship between psychiatry and antisocial behavior and personality thus raises a fundamental challenge to the medical as compared to the social functions of psychiatry. It is thus important that one distinguish analytically between the antisocial constellation and construct (a recurring, universal presence in society), its social interpretation (generally negative, but can lead to positive traits and also fascination), the species of behavior involving misdemeanors and crimes which the legal system adjudicates, and what properly belongs in a nosology of psychiatry considered as a medical discipline or institution.

Evolutionary Theory Considerations

A disturbance of behavior that is relatively discrete, consists of circum-scribed signs/symptoms, and can result in social breakdowns, for example, anxiety and phobia, paranoia, mood related problems, and even schizophre-nia, would seem to present a "cleaner" case for an evolutionary conception of psychiatric disorder [37, 38]. The abnormal personality constellations do not readily conform to intuitive notions of disorder and disease. Rather, they comprise complex programs of behavior, encompass traits and behav-iors that appear ego-syntonic and by definition presuppose inferred, unob-servable features of persons.

There are two different and seemingly contradictory ways in which evolu-tionary theory has approached antisocial behavior. A harmful dysfunction (HD) formulation would presumably rest on the "natural function" of soci-ality, including competition and mutualism or altruism. A defect of this function undermines an individual's pursuit of biological goals and causes "harm", thus qualifying as a disorder according to the HD formulation. Problems associated with this perspective are covered later.

The second way in which evolutionary theory has been applied to "anti-social" strays away from the HD disorder conceptualization and views the antisocial constellation as a lifelong social strategy. It was one of any number of strategies naturally selected for in the ancestral environment and can, depending on the circumstances facing an individual early in development, be adaptive even in the contemporary environment. This formulation draws on a complex synthesis and interpretation of knowledge from the fields of biological anthropology, developmental psychology, per-sonality theory, sociobiology, criminology, and evolutionary ecology [39, 40]. It holds that ecological stimuli or "clues" that suggest uncertainty and risk (e.g. parents' inability or unwillingness to offer support, resources, and stability) cause patterns of attachment behavior that trigger or elicit (during early childhood) a social strategy designed to maximize reproduction in conformance with life history theory. This involves the differential alloca-tion of resources (e.g. pertaining to survival, growth, repair, reproduction) throughout the life cycle, affecting the onset of sexuality, the timing of mating and reproduction, the quality of mating relationships, and the qual-ity of parenting. This social strategy, by definition, promotes long-term goals, but in the short run and in some environments can encompass many of the personality, emotional, and social behavior traits associated with the antisocial constellation.

Culture Theory Considerations

The cross-cultural validity of virtually any psychiatric disorder presents conceptual and methodological problems, but the personality disorders are more knotty ones since they involve more style of behavior and less psychological distress and social impairment [38]. Antisocial personality disorder adds to this a consideration of social norms, rules, and social practices involved in the definition of deviance and criminality. Many questions have been raised about its cultural validity [41]; for example, whether its essential properties are culturally invariant or merely reflect Anglo-European standards of behavior, its relationship to concepts of personhood like ego-centricity or social-centricity (as seen in individualistic as compared to collectivistic societies, respectively), and tensions between an underlying trait or construct compared to sociological and cultural parameters that may hinder or favor its expression as per self-disclosure (e.g. whether the processes of socialization and enculturation promote or suppress personality and behavior tendencies suggesting antisocial personality).

The prevalence and characteristics of psychopathic personality in Scottish compared to North American samples of psychiatric, forensic and criminal populations have been studied recently [41–43]. These authors relied on the Psychopathy Checklist-Revised (PCL-R) developed by Hare [44], which consists of two factors that measure personality factors and antisocial behavior. Cooke and co-workers employed the item response theory approach in the measurement of antisocial personality disorder, a strategy that copes successfully with many of the problems of cross-cultural measurement [43]. In particular, item response theory allows establishing whether the same trait or phenotype is being measured and by means of the same metric in two populations, in this case, two cultures.

Results revealed a statistically significant and substantially higher prevalence of psychopathy (i.e. based on cut-off scores and mean scores) in North America compared to Scotland. Even when cut-off points were adjusted so as to conform to the differences in overall measures, substantially more psychopaths were found in the North American sample. This parallels findings that have been obtained in Scandinavian and British samples, suggesting that enculturation and socialization lead to suppression or exaggeration of traits of psychopathy cross-culturally. With respect to North American and Scottish samples, the slope parameters of the measures obtained did not differ significantly cross-culturally, suggesting that the disorder is defined by the same characteristics in the two cultures. A number of items produced significantly different measures in the two cultures, but most showed cross-cultural equivalence of measurement.

Many of the features of the disorder apparently do not become apparent among Scottish prisoners until high levels of the trait are present. This suggests that cultural factors dampen, inhibit, or suppress their expression in Scotland. For example, the level of the underlying traits of glibness, lack of remorse, and pathological lying at which the characteristics of the disorder become apparent differed in the two cultures: in Scotland those who show these traits have a higher measure of the underlying trait of psychopathy. Cooke and Michie explain the difference observed as resulting from cultural differences in pressure for psychopathic behavior. The importance of differences between levels of individualism in the two societies and cultures, a factor that has been invoked to explain cultural variability in the expression and manifestations of psychopathy, was considered as a possibility but could not be verified. Classically, individualism compared to sociocentrism is a parameter that has been observed in Anglo-European as compared to Asian societies.

CRITIQUE OF THE TWO APPROACHES TO DIAGNOSIS AND CLASSIFICATION

The Evolutionary Conception of Psychiatric Disorder

Many harmful dysfunctions of psychological mechanisms, disorders in the evolutionary sense, are treatable conditions, but the latter need not constitute disorders [45]. From an evolutionary standpoint, conditions of potential psychiatric relevance involve a behavior condition, its evaluation, someone who evaluates, and an evaluation context. The condition can be positive or negative; the evaluator can be the subject, an observer, or a reference group; the evaluation involves whether the condition results from a naturally designed mechanism that is or is not "doing its job" (i.e. is evolutionarily functional or dysfunctional) or is simply a by-product of a mechanism; and finally, the environment in which a condition is situated can vary (i.e. the ancestral or the present one). In this light, a treatable condition is the product of a decision based on values and conventions, either that of the individual, significant other, or reference group in society. Some treatable conditions may arise because a function naturally designed in an ancestral environment and operating "naturally" in the current one nevertheless causes impairment or suffering (sexual jealousy or predation). The converse is also true: natural functions may be dysfunctional (e.g. repeated sensation seeking and dangerous risk taking) yet produce behavior in contemporary environments that is satisfying and not impairing (e.g. bold personalities, rock climbing). Finally, many treatable conditions may have no relationship to a natural function but are simply by-products of such, or due to simple human variation [1].

Echoing a treatable condition perspective, Kirmayer and Young [46] point out that the HD analysis is not fully impersonal and objective, but depends on implicit positions of value, totally disregarding social and cultural conventions. Sadler [47] has emphasized that the HD position started out as a prescriptive formula validating what a disorder constituted. Its exponents seem now to be concerned mainly with descriptive questions (why and how generally held psychiatric disorders conform to a HD analysis) and less so with prescriptive ones that clarify what and why a condition (e.g. hyperactivity, premenstrual syndrome) should or should not constitute a disorder. It is clear that in the debate about prescriptive questions regarding a particular condition, one can point to fuzzy concepts about what constitute natural functions and, thus, whether the condition constitutes a disorder. Sadler, like Kirmayer and Young, then, makes clear that despite the seeming rigor of the HD formulation, its application can entail messy questions of politics, values, and conventions and standards about normality, deviance, adaptation, and natural functions.

There are several additional reasons why a HD prescription cannot be expected to neatly serve the needs of diagnostic systems, at least in the foreseeable future. Most diagnoses that have emerged in psychiatry do not conform in point-for-point way with failures or breakdowns of a natural function. Entities like depression, schizophrenia, anxiety, and somatization disorder embrace many levels and layers of social and psychological function, and there is little evidence that they can be reduced to or equated with failures of one or even a few adaptations or mechanisms [9, 10]. Most embody complex behavior phenomena that are the outcome of failures of several natural functions and mechanisms. Furthermore, many of the functions or mechanisms governing pathological behavior involve the interplay of hierarchically arranged levels of functions. Perturbations and dysfunctions in one level can be propagated up and down the hierarchy and at different levels may be subject to positive or negative feedback. If a systems view is used to conceptualize individual functioning and what constitutes a disorder, the elegant solutions that a HD analysis promises become opaque and fuzzy.

Many so-called psychological adaptations are really descriptions of domains of biologically significant but highly complex social behavior. They may have promoted the solution of biological problems, for example, mate selection, acquisition of rank, and social competition; however, they do not readily map on to well-demarcated spheres of behavior (other than tautologically) nor can they be equated with conditions or "disorders" as classified in psychiatry. Other adaptations, while certainly fundamental in promoting fitness and adaptation, really refer to rather narrowly defined (i.e. content specific) cognitive/perceptual functions that serve or contribute to the solution of many biological functions. For example, mate selection, achievement of high social rank, solution of subsistence problems, and/or ability to avoid predators in the hominid environment of evolution required adaptive functions in many areas of perception, cognition, recognition of emotion, linguistic and/or emotional communication. Some of the evolutionary arguments that have been developed for psychiatric disorders (depression, schizophrenia) embody whole packages of maladaptive behavior that can be reduced or fitted into a HD analysis only with great difficulty.

Problems in the evolutionary conception can be illustrated by considering psychopathy. It obviously incorporates many so-called psychological mechanisms and does not easily or neatly profile a disorder as per the HD analysis. Mechanisms pertaining to care giving, mating, social commitment, and social responsibility come to mind and these can apply to kin, non-kin group mates, competitors, strangers, and/or potential mates. Where and on what basis does one place the antisocial in this array of behavior and experience? Moreover, there is in evolutionary biology a well-established "theory" about the complexities of social relationships. Emphasis is placed on the intricacies of competition and trade-offs which of necessity must take place across different spheres of relationships and behaviors, for example, between giving and taking, between differences in what it is adaptive for parents to "invest in" or "hold back from" offspring compared to the unlimited demands that the latter make, and between the obvious residuals of sexual selection that involve sharply divergent mating strategies of males (i.e. impregnate and if necessary coerce many) and females (i.e. select few on the basis of their resources and commitment). Finally, there is the quandary raised by the trait not only of selfishness/competition but also of social cunningness and dissimulation in the service of personal goals, aptly termed Machiavelianism. Behavior meriting this qualification has been described for primates attesting to its presumed adaptive, selective basis. Thus, while on first impression the HD formulation of disorder appears relevant and valid to the antisocial constellation and construct, closer analysis reveals problems. There is a great deal of complexity and ambiguity regarding what is "social" and altruistic/responsible compared to "unsocial" or selfish/expedient. Consequently, where and on what basis the calibration of antisocial fits within the domain of social activity is problematic. Unambiguously disentangling what is evolutionarily prudent from what is antisocial, and from whose standpoint will the latter be calibrated, all would seem to present problems to the HD formulation of the antisocial constellation/construct.

In summary, there are reasons to be cautious with respect to the proposed evolutionary conception of psychiatric disorder generally and on the HD formulation in particular. While the classic theory of categories that support the HD formulation is theoretically compelling and aesthetically pleasing, its use for deciding whether any one condition of psychiatric relevance is, is not, or should be defined as a disorder raises numerous problems. Nevertheless, evolutionary biology and psychology generally, and the HD analysis of disorder more specifically, embody insights that should be included in a science of psychiatric diagnosis and classification.

The Cultural Conception of Psychiatric Disorder

It can be argued that evolution provided conditions for the emergence of culture but the latter was not naturally selected. Mechanical and physical changes affecting the brain (e.g. size and/or structure) and/or an exaptation and not an adaptation [48] may explain the behavioral plasticity that makes culture possible. Behavioral traditions and systems of communication observed in higher primates, likely features of hominids and earlier varieties of species *Homo*, can be regarded as qualitatively different from human language, cognition, and culture. These traits may constitute, on the one hand, either a singular, unique development of the final phase of human biological evolution, integral to what brought about the emergence of *Homo sapiens* and the move out of Africa some time after 100 000 or so years ago; or, on the other hand, merely a set of traits that were conditioned by social ecological exigencies. Thus, culture may merely add surface manifestations to behavior and psychopathology, constituting mere epiphenomena rather than essential features. One could argue that a vulnerable Japanese subject raised in America is not "prepared" to develop manifestations resembling *Taijin Kyofusho* but is instead vulnerable to whatever variety of social phobia is present in the local culture.

In summary, one can argue that essential behavioral properties of *Homo sapiens* (including their vulnerability to suffer from psychopathology) may reside in psychological mechanisms (or algorithms) but that characteristics linked to culture are largely evoked, learned, and/or acquired. The HD position, for example, underscores natural functions that are culture free. Essential aspects of "cultural psychology" that shape a culturally specific psychopathology may not be part of an ensemble that in any way was naturally selected for and genetically based. Whether human language, cognition, and culture constitute capacities that were naturally selected gradually or merely a by-product of a unique event or "explosion" of comparatively recent origin, is highly contested and cannot be discussed further here [6]. However, even if human language, cognition, and culture do not constitute naturally selected and genetically based traits, one can still claim that they constitute essential features of *Homo sapiens* and are necessarily implicated in psychopathology.

Psychiatry seeks a universal science about the functioning of the "psyche" and its disturbances. However, how the mind works involves an amalgam of two sets of factors: conceptual models and reasoning principles, on the one hand, and features of language and culture, on the other. The two are very difficult if not impossible to untangle [49–53]. Anthropologists and linguists agree that through an amalgam of meaning-creating systems individuals fashion their personal experience, sense of reality, social behavior, and the requirements for social order. According to culture theory, systems of meaning are crucial. It does not posit an opposition or exclusivity between the domains of brain function and cultural meaning systems. Both together form an integral whole and are products of the evolutionary process.

Psychopathology, then, arises only in a symbolically determined setting of behavior. There are good reasons to presume that even were psychiatric disorders to be conceptualized in purely neurobiological terms, cultural factors have to in some way be taken into account in making sense of them. The three test cases discussed earlier illustrate that social conventions and cultural meanings about behavior and deviance of necessity come into play in decisions regarding how psychopathology is configured, enacted, and accorded significance in a society. Elsewhere I have argued on general grounds that what constitutes a psychiatric disorder, who should be treated, and what constitutes the proper domain of a medical psychology, all require taking into consideration cultural conventions [6, 54].

Another criticism of the cultural conception of psychiatric disorder is that it may rely on a view of culture that is losing ground and eventually may become outdated. The importance of cultural psychologies in the constitution of psychopathology is best visualized for members of monolithic cultures that contrast sharply with one another. The examples discussed earlier involved Japan and China and to this could be added India, societies of the African continent, and of course members of isolated, non-industrial societies. It is among people holding traditions and conceptions that articulate self-contained and integrated world-views that differ sharply from society to society and that speak different languages that one finds contrasts in cultural psychologies that, in turn, would configure different constitutions of psychopathology. In the modern world, a global, capitalist culture holds sway, communication of traditions is widespread, and migration very prominent. This criticism, then, stipulates that modernity melts away cultural heterogeneity and that, in the long run, truly contrastive constructions of cultural psychologies and psychopathology will lessen. However, this argument does not contravene the importance of culture: while suggesting the possible erasure of cultural differences, it actually reinforces the importance of symbols and meaning (see below).

That a system of psychiatric diagnosis and classification is first and foremost a practical enterprise designed to facilitate international communication and comparability of clinical practice and research is another argument that challenges the cultural conception. A practical argument for universality weakens the position that cultural differences should be accorded primacy. This is consistent with the point mentioned earlier; namely, that in the modern world science, secularism and rationalism have become so integral to the idiom of contemporary societies and of medicine more generally that these developments undermine monolithic cultural differences, homogenize world-views, and create internationalist cultures and human psychologies that a science of descriptive psychopathology has evolved to cope with [4, 5]. In this view of the matter, holding on to the reality and importance of cultural variability becomes an impediment and distraction. All of this would appear to demand a common language of psychopathology and undermine the cultural conception.

IMPLICATIONS FOR THE FUTURE OF PSYCHIATRIC DIAGNOSIS AND CLASSIFICATION

Theoretical Perspective

Psychopathology is one of the social problems that societies cope with. Institutions for this are diverse and include social welfare, religion, medicine, and the systems of social control that embrace ethics, morality and criminal adjudication. Depending on context, any particular variety of psychopathology can be interpreted as a condition of disadvantage requiring support and assistance, a condition of wickedness and impiety requiring spiritual and religious counseling, a type of sickness requiring medical treatment, a special category of sickness as per psychiatry, or a moral transgression and offense that needs control, correction and/or incarceration. Provided it takes into consideration culture and language, a science of diagnosis seeks to address universal characteristics. It allows determining exactly where in the social spaces and institutions of any society conditions of psychopathology are situated, keying in on essential characteristics. A culturally sensitive science of diagnosis allows claims that some members of devotional sects of ancient India or medieval Islam may have been victims of psychopathology whereas many dissidents labeled as schizophrenic in the former Soviet Union decades ago were not. Such claims are possible because the system would handle specific disorders as tokens of types defined on the basis of a theory or nosology that incorporates biology, neurobiology, language, and culture.

Generalizations About the Character of Psychopathology

Evolutionary conceptions of psychopathology can be nothing if not elaborate, complex, and also variable. At other times, they are direct, trim, and uncomplicated; sometimes, they seem like "as if" stories. Nevertheless, such conceptions cannot be ignored and should be represented in a diagnostic system; either prescriptively, stipulating which complex of behavior should be included in the system (e.g. those that constitute breakdowns of a natural function) or at least descriptively, illustrating why a treatable condition is a disorder. Ideally, evolutionarily conceived biological goals that a psychiatric disorder undermines should be represented as criteria in a psychiatric nosology.

The theory of culture authorizes equally compelling claims about psychiatric disorders. It certainly challenges the notion that their phenomenology, interpretation, and social effects are universal and pan-cultural. The fact of cultural differences also renders problematic the very enterprise of diagnosis by emphasizing how aspects of personal experience and behavior that shape a clinical condition are based on culturally constituted world-views. This is clearly the case with depression and social phobia. Yet, even the make-up of psychopathy is in some ways different in Scotland and America, two "cultures" that share many traditions. One cannot but expect that in societies with more divergent histories and cultural traditions differences in psychopathy would be greater. It would seem to follow that culture theory, like evolutionary theory, makes claims about psychiatric disorders that a system of diagnosis should incorporate.

Generalizations About the Future of Human Societies

Given the apparent trends in migration and immigration and the possible future weakening of totalitarian/autocratic governmental controls as a function of the spread of modern ideas of individualism and liberalism, one would argue that human populations are likely to manifest greater genetic mixing and assimilation in the long run. Since evolutionary biology points to the innate bases for human psychology, it can safely be assumed that a view about the universality or essentialism of psychopathology will continue to be relevant. Furthermore, given modern developments in transportation and communication, one may assume the continued spread of an internationalist political economy and associated values of capitalism. In the long run, this should lessen cultural boundaries and distinctions, contributing however slowly to the homogenization of human beliefs, values, traditions, and outlooks. Barring major collisions among large and small national powers, with consequent time-limited reactions of insularity and isolationism, the pace of social and cultural change in the direction of a common global culture can be expected to continue. Events in recent history both support and challenge these generalizations [55, 56].

Prospects of future social change may be anticipated. The role of cultural factors in critically influencing political economic developments in

Western and non-Western societies has been emphasized [57]. Social crises undermine traditional institutions of social control and legitimate structures of authority, with consequent loosening of psychological controls and the hold of traditional systems of morality and conscience [58–60]. Modern societies show waxing and waning of the hold of traditional values, grudging tolerance of social deviance seen in juxtaposition to racial hatreds and divisive competition, openness to differences in lifestyle and religion yet increased distrust, and suspicion; they resort to adversative modes of conflict resolution, and a heightening of narcissism. Modernity tends to increase interpersonal self-disclosure along with an awareness and openness to cultural differences, sometimes including sexual experience and behavior.

One can assume that such features of culture will not only continue to influence the character of personal experience and social behavior, but will also sharply influence interpersonal conflicts in circumscribed communities. Migration and cultural pluralism will likely increase and this implies not only a clash between "old" traditions and the "new" narcissism and internationalism of the culture of capitalism, differences between host and parent country, but also clashes between competing traditions, values, and sects in large urban "melting pots". In other words, individuals come to be influenced by global, secular trends and migrate to foreign soils where they then interact with other immigrant, minority populations.

Here it is important to keep in mind the distinction between the two conceptions of culture mentioned earlier. While the demographic (demarcating) view of culture may diminish in importance because of the assimilation of modernity, culture as lived reality shaped by diverse and even competing tenets and feelings (and different in emphasis from that of other citizens) will continue to be important. Even if one agrees that a brain-based model of rationality and belief formation is an innate property of *Homo sapiens*, ascertaining its workings necessarily enmeshes the diagnostician in a complex exegesis that requires knowledge of his/her and client's language and culture. How items of information are labeled, confirmed, disconfirmed, and incorporated into meaningful social discourse constitutes the essence of culture and language and of higher cortical functions. Consequently, while cultural differences across societies may lessen in importance, intra-societal differences between an individual in work and institutional settings, including psychiatrist/patient dialogues, are likely to increase in societies of the future. It is thus to be expected that symbols, meanings, and world-views will continue to be influential in shaping personal experience and behavior, constituting aspects of social reality that systems of psychiatric diagnosis should contend with in the future, if such systems are to realistically incorporate important characteristics of the individual.

Incorporating Evolutionary Theory in a Psychiatric Nosology

Although the HD formulation may not serve as the ultimate "scientific" criterion for the definition of a psychiatric disorder, this by no means implies tenets of evolutionary theory should not be represented in a system of psychiatric diagnosis. The history of psychiatry and empirical research underscore the importance that disorders (e.g. Axis I of DSM-IV) will likely continue to play in future systems of diagnosis. Because of the high prevalence of comorbidity and the difficulty of establishing clear boundaries between disorders [61–63], it seems prudent to hold that individuals in need of psychiatric care embody a clinical condition made up of one or several disorders. Moreover, the condition more than the disorders is what limits an individual's capacity and ability to function [64].

This means that the basic functional capacities to execute behavior as authorized by evolutionary theory constitute important "facts" about a psychiatric condition of an individual. McGuire and Troisi [19] have provided a comprehensive listing of these including their behavior components. Such functional capacities constitute human universals that could be incorporated by means of separate axes or numerical coding schemes in a system of diagnosis. Many of the directives of evolutionary psychiatrists are highly consistent with basic psychosocial, behavioral, and psychotherapeutic approaches in psychiatry.

Incorporating Culture Theory in a Psychiatric Nosology

At least for the foreseeable future, settings of evaluation, especially in large Western cities, will involve individuals from non-Western, less developed societies. Proficiency in the language of the host country is likely to be low. The social backgrounds and cultural orientations of potential patients are likely to: (a) contrast with that of the host country and especially with basic conceptions about self, experience, and behavior that are integral to scientific medicine and psychiatry; (b) emphasize more somatic as compared to psychological factors in health and disease; (c) manifest a more social centered as compared to a person centered orientation regarding the meaning, purpose, and calibration of behavior; and (d) include a more spiritual emphasis on experience, purpose, obligation, and personal accounting. The concept of what is private and hence closed to inquiry will differ as well. Ease of self-disclosure and openness to questions regarding social, interpersonal, and spiritual matters are likely to differ from what is regarded as relevant to the ordinary, typical psychiatric history. The lay conception of a "mental illness" will not coincide with that of psychiatry, and the way personal symptoms and impairments are explained (i.e. explanatory models) will likewise differ as well. Finally, all of the parameters of social and biological functions mentioned earlier will require formulation in an idiom that realistically takes into account the cultural perspective of the patient.

A psychiatric diagnosis should serve to identify and describe a person's clinical condition in a way that accurately represents his or her disorder or disorders. It should optimize formulation of an effective treatment plan that accurately measures the person's condition and merges or translates between the person's conception of his/her condition with that of the provider of mental health services. Diagnosis should also facilitate communication among professionals, staff, patients, and families of patients. Factors listed above constitute some of the rubrics of information and domains of experience that psychiatric diagnosis should encompass. The requirements for reaching a valid psychiatric diagnosis and the functions served by a system of diagnosis and classification imply that culture will continue to be important in how psychopathology is assessed and how information about it is used in a clinically effective and prudent way.

REFERENCES

1. Fabrega H. Jr. (1997) *Evolution of Sickness and Healing*. University of California Press, Berkeley.
2. Fabrega H. Jr. (2001) Mental health and illness in traditional India and China. In: *Cultural Psychiatry: International Perspectives* (Eds J.E. Mezzich, H. Fabrega Jr.). Harcourt Brace, Orlando, in press.
3. Fabrega H. Jr. (1989) An ethnomedical perspective of Anglo-American psychiatry. *Am. J. Psychiatry*, **146**: 588–596.
4. Berrios G., Porter R. (1995) *A History of Clinical Psychiatry: The Origin and History of Psychiatric Disorders*. Athlone Press, London.
5. Berrios G.E. (1996) *The History of Mental Symptoms: Descriptive Psychopathology Since the Nineteenth Century*. Cambridge University Press, Cambridge.
6. Fabrega H. Jr. (2001) *Origins of Psychopathology: The Phylogenetic and Cultural Basis of Mental Illness*. Rutgers University Press, Piscataway.
7. Nesse R.M., Williams G.C. (1994) *Why We Get Sick: The New Science of Darwinian Medicine*. Random House, Times Books, New York.
8. Wakefield J.C. (1999). Evolutionary versus prototype analyses of the concept of disorder. *J. Abnorm. Psychol.*, **108**: 374–399.
9. Klein D.F. (1978) A proposed definition of mental illness. In *Critical Issues in Psychiatric Diagnosis* (Eds R. Spitzer, D.F. Klein), pp. 41–71. Raven Press, New York.
10. Klein D.F. (1999) Harmful dysfunction, disorder, disease, illness and evolution. *J. Abnorm. Psychol.*, **108**: 421–429.
11. Lilienfeld S.O., Marino L. (1995) Mental disorder as a Roschian concept: a critique of Wakefield's "harmful disfunction" analysis. *J. Abnorm. Psychol.*, **104**: 411–420.
12. Lilienfeld S.O., Marino L. (1999) Essentialism revisited: evolutionary theory and the concept of mental disorder. *J. Abnorm. Psychol.* **108**: 400–411.

13. Fabrega H. Jr. (2000) Culture, spirituality and psychiatry. *Curr. Opin. Psychiatry,* **13**: 525–530.
14. Donald M. (1991) *Origins of the Modern Mind: Three Stages in the Evolution of Culture and Cognition.* Harvard University Press, Cambridge.
15. Deacon D.W. (1997) *The Symbolic Species.* W.W. Norton, New York.
16. Hayden B. (1993) The cultural capacities of Neanderthals: a review and re-evaluation. *J. Human Evolution,* **24**: 113–146.
17. Jackson S.W. (1986) *Melancholia and Depression: From Hippocratic Times to Modern Times.* Yale University Press, New Haven.
18. McGuire M., Troisi A., Raleigh M. (1997) Depression in evolutionary context. In *The Maladapted Mind: Classic Readings in Evolutionary Psychopathology* (Ed. S. Baron-Cohen) pp. 255–282. Psychology Press, East Sussex.
19. McGuire M., Troisi A. (1998) *Darwinian Psychiatry.* Oxford University Press, New York.
20. Stevens A., Price J. (1996) *Evolutionary Psychiatry: A New Beginning.* Routledge, New York.
21. Price J., Sloman L., Gardner R., Jr., Gilbert P., Rohde P. (1994). The social competition hypothesis of depression. *Br. J. Psychiatry,* **164**: 309–315.
22. Nesse R.M. (2000) Is depression an adaptation? *Arch. Gen. Psychiatry,* **57**: 14–20.
23. Kirmayer L.J. (1984) Culture, affect and somatization. *Transcult. Psychiatr. Res. Rev.,* **23**: 159–188.
24. Kleinman A. (1986) *Social Origins of Distress and Disease: Depression, Neurasthenia, and Pain in Modern China.* Yale University Press, New Haven.
25. Lee S. (1999) Diagnosis postponed: Shenjing Shuairuo and the transformation of psychiatry in post-Mao China. *Cult. Med. Psychiatry,* **23**: 349–380.
26. Manson M., Shore J.H., Bloom J.D. (1985) The depressive experience in American Indian communities: a challenge for psychiatric theory and diagnosis. In *Culture and Depression: Studies in the Anthropology and Cross-Cultural Psychiatry of Affect and Disorder* (Eds A. Kleinman, B. Good), pp. 331–368. University of California Press, Berkeley.
27. Kinzie J.D., Manson S.M., Vinh D.T., Tolan N.T., Anh B., Pho Y.N. (1982) Validation of the Vietnamese Depression Scale. *Am. J. Psychiatry,* **139**: 1276–1281.
28. Kleinman A., Good B. (1985) *Culture and Depression: Studies in the Anthropology and Cross-cultural Psychiatry of Affect and Disorder.* University of California Press, Berkeley.
29. Marks I.M. (1987) *Fears, Phobias, and Rituals: Panic, Anxiety, and Their Disorders.* Oxford University Press, New York.
30. Nesse R. (1998) Emotional disorders in evolutionary perspective. *Br. J. Med. Psychol.,* **71**: 397–415.
31. Kirmayer L.J. (1991) The place of culture in psychiatric nosology: Taijin Kyofusho and DSM-III-R. *J. Nerv. Ment. Dis.,* **179**: 19–28.
32. White G.M. (1980) Conceptual universals in interpersonal language. *Am. Anthropol.,* **82**: 759–781.
33. D'Andrade R.G. (1984) Cultural meaning systems. In *Culture Theory: Essays on Mind, Self and Emotion* (Eds R.A. Shweder, R.A. Levine), pp. 89–108. Cambridge University Press, Cambridge.
34. Murphy J.M. (1976) Psychiatric labeling in cross-cultural perspective. *Science,* **191**: 1019–1028.
35. Werlinder H. (1978) *Psychopathy: A History of Concepts.* Almqvist and Wiksell International, Uppsala.

36. Kittrie N.N. (1971) *The Right to Be Different*. Johns Hopkins Press, Baltimore.
37. Fabrega H., Jr. (1989) The self and schizophrenia: a cultural perspective. *Schizophr. Bull.*, **15**: 277–290.
38. Fabrega H., Jr. (1994) Personality disorders as medical entities: a cultural interpretation. *J. Personal. Disord.*, **8**: 149–167.
39. Mealey L. (1995) The sociobiology of sociopathy: an integrated evolutionary model. *Behav. Brain Sci.*, **18**: 523–599.
40. Chisholm J.S. (1999) *Death, Hope and Sex: Steps toward an Evolutionary Ecology of Mind and Morality*. Cambridge University Press, Cambridge.
41. Cooke D.J. (1998) Cross cultural aspects of psychopathy. In *Psychopathy: Theory, Research and Implications for Society* (Eds D.J. Cooke, A.E. Forth, R.D. Hare), pp. 13–45. Kluwer, Dordrecht.
42. Cooke D.J. (1996) Psychopathic personality in different cultures. *J. Personal. Disord.*, **10**: 23–40.
43. Cooke D.J., Michie C. (1999) Psychopathy across culture: North America and Scotland compared. *J. Abnorm. Psychol.*, **108**: 58–68.
44. Hare R.D. (1991) *The Hare Psychopathy Check List, Revised*. Multi Health Systems, Toronto.
45. Cosmides L., Tooby J. (1999) Toward an evolutionary taxonomy of treatable conditions. *J. Abnorm. Psychol.*, **108**: 453–464.
46. Kirmayer L.J., Young A. (1999) Culture and context in the evolutionary concept of mental disorder. *J. Abnorm. Psychol.*, **108**: 446–452.
47. Sadler J.Z. (1999) Horsefeathers: a commentary on "Evolutionary versus prototype analyses of the concept of disorder". *J. Abnorm. Psychol.*, **108**: 433–437.
48. Gould S.J. (1991) Exaptation: a crucial tool for an evolutionary psychology. *J. Soc. Issues*, **47**: 43–65.
49. Lakoff G. (1987) *Wonder, Fire and Dangerous Things: What Categories Reveal about the Mind*. University of Chicago Press, Chicago.
50. Lakoff G., Johnson M. (1980) *Metaphors We Live By*. University of Chicago Press, Chicago.
51. Holland D., Quinn N. (1987) *Cultural Models in Language and Thought*. Cambridge University Press, Cambridge.
52. Lucy J.A. (1992) *Language Diversity and Thought*. Cambridge University Press, Cambridge.
53. Ingold T. (Ed.) (1996) *Key Debates in Anthropology*. Routledge, London.
54. Fabrega H., Jr. (1994) International systems of diagnosis in psychiatry. *J. Nerv. Ment. Dis.*, **182**: 256–263.
55. Mittelman J.H. (2000) *The Globalization Syndrome*. Princeton University Press, Princeton.
56. Micklethwait J., Wooldridge A. (2000) *A Future Perfect: The Challenge and Hidden Promise of Globalization*. Crown Publishers, Random House, New York.
57. Lal D. (1998) *Unintended Consequences: The Impact of Factor Endowments, Culture, and Politics on Long-Run Economic Performance*. MIT Press, Cambridge.
58. Sanchez L. (1986) Social crises and psychopathy. In *Antisocial Personality and Related Syndromes* (Eds W.H. Reid, D. Door, J.I. Walker, J.W. Bonner III), pp. 78–97. Norton, New York.
59. Fromm E. (1941) *Escape from Freedom*. Avon Books, New York.
60. Lasch C. (1991) *The Culture of Narcissism*. Norton, New York.
61. Jablensky A. (1988) Methodological issues in psychiatric classification. *Br. J. Psychiatry*, **152** (Suppl. 1): 15–20.

62. Kendell R.E. (1989) Clinical validity. *Psychol. Med.*, **19**: 45–55.
63. Millon T. (1991) Classification in psychopathology: rationale, alternatives and standards. *J. Abnorm. Psychol.*, **100**: 245–261.
64. Fabrega H., Jr., Mezzich J., Ulrich R.F. (1989) Interpreting the structure of diagnosis in intake settings. *J. Psychiatr. Res.*, **23**: 169–186.

6

The Role of Phenomenology in Psychiatric Diagnosis and Classification

Josef Parnas[1] and Dan Zahavi[2]

[1]*Department of Psychiatry, Hvidovre Hospital, Hvidovre, Denmark*
[2]*Danish Institute for Advanced Studies in the Humanities, Copenhagen, Denmark*

INTRODUCTION

As with most classifications, psychiatric classification has essentially a pragmatic purpose, that is to delimit entities useful for the choice of treatment, prevention and prediction of outcome. Moreover, classifications create important constraints for aetiological and pathogenetic research, because they dictate, more or less explicitly and authoritatively, the boundaries of what is declared as relevant fields of research. According to the medical model, psychiatric classification should be ultimately based on aetiological knowledge, and any other approach, be it symptomatic, syndromatic or even more complexly descriptive (like the multiaxial) is considered as provisional. Validity of psychiatric diagnosis is considered as a problem of matching clinical entities with "real" processes of nature [1]. In the case of most psychiatric disorders, however, hoping for a segmentation of "real" processes of nature into neat "real kind" categories is perhaps overoptimistic or even expressive of a certain epistemological naïveté. In any case, the majority of current diagnostic categories are based on *typologies of human experience and behavior*, and in all likelihood this state of affairs will continue to prevail in a foreseeable future. Therefore, a search for a faithful *description of experience* must be considered as a necessary first step in any taxonomic effort, including attempts of reducing abnormal experience to its potential biological substrate. This prerequisite, articulated in psychopathology by Karl Jaspers in 1923 [2], has been more recently expressed by Thomas Nagel [3] in the context of consciousness research: "a necessary requirement for any coherent reductionism is that the entity to be reduced is properly understood". But the

Psychiatric Diagnosis and Classification. Edited by Mario Maj, Wolfgang Gaebel, Juan José López-Ibor and Norman Sartorius. © 2002 John Wiley & Sons, Ltd.

search for a coherent taxonomy in psychiatry is caught in a sort of *rationalist–empiricist* dilemma: either we know in advance *what* (and how) to describe, in other words we have some, however dim, *a priori* knowledge of the entities to be described, or, assuming a thoroughly atheoretical stance (as it is programmatically stated in the DSM-IV [4]), we do not know at all what to look for and are therefore doomed to an endless process of accumulation of disconnected atomistic observations with no obvious prospect of eventual, finite synthesis into useful categories (which is well illustrated by the contemporary proliferation of comorbidity studies). The rationalist tendency is usually regarded as a sort of sinful transgression, only to be overcome by empirical data collection untainted by any theoretical preference. The real problem, however, in our view, is not to choose between a theoretical approach and an atheoretical stance but rather between an adequate and inadequate theoretical approach.

Phenomenology, as it will be argued, is in a unique position to contribute to the issues of classification and diagnosis, because it involves *a step-by-step account of how abstractions are derived from everyday clinical experiences and encounters* [5]. It articulates the essential features of experience and so clarifies the typification processes involved in its classification. The claim of this chapter is that continental phenomenology, i.e. as originally outlined by Edmund Husserl and his followers, is at the present moment an essential tool for any further progress in psychiatric classification, and that familiarity with its basic tenets should be included in the psychiatric training curriculum. A scientific interest in studying the nature of consciousness and experience has dramatically exploded during recent decades, and phenomenology is increasingly being seen as a crucial component in research in cognitive science and the neurosciences [6–11]; oddly enough, a position that hardly has been heard of in psychiatry [12].

We will first chart the conceptual puzzles inherent in the contemporary psychiatric classification, placing it in a general epistemological context. We will describe aspects of phenomenology pertinent to psychiatry and then draft the basic structures of human consciousness that should serve as a departure for classificatory efforts. We will finally try to articulate the basic steps through which phenomenology may contribute to a taxonomic progress.

THE PROBLEM OF DESCRIPTION IN CONTEMPORARY PSYCHIATRY

The realm of human subjectivity or conscious experience has been a taboo for operational psychiatry as well as for other so-called "behavioral sciences" [10], and until recently for the neurosciences as well [13].

Notwithstanding the claim of the authors of modern psychiatric classifica-tory systems that the latter are "phenomenologically descriptive" [14], it is more appropriate to characterize them as *behavioral*. Neither is the claim of an atheoretical stance in the current classifications true; theory is simply concealed and rarely made explicit and reflected upon [15].

The epistemological underpinnings and historical and sociological aspects of the contemporary psychiatric classification have been described in detail elsewhere [16, 17]; here we will only sketch the main line of thinking behind operationalism as a contrastive background to the phenom-enological approach. Operationalism in psychiatry stems from the ideals of logical positivism (logical empiricism), a philosophical position inaugurated in Austria and Germany in the beginning of the twentieth century (the so-called "Vienna Circle") and imported into academic psychiatry, partly due to a strong influence of the positivist philosopher Carl Hempel, in the 1960s. Logical positivism claims that sensory experience is the only valid source of knowledge about reality. Although in its original anti-metaphysical attitude it refrained from ontological claims, it gradually slipped into a position which in its contemporary version is usually desig-nated as materialistic (naturalistic) *objectivism* and *physicalism*: reality is as it is, independently of any human perspective (objectivism), and the nature of reality is wholly physical (physicalism). Whatever exists, is (at least in principle and in the future) reducible to the subatomic particles and their interactions governed by eternal physical laws. It follows from these prem-ises that science must be unified both in method and in goal, the latter being a reduction of complex realities into simpler forms, and ultimately express-ible in the form of mathematical equations. Logical positivism was strongly preoccupied by the issue of how theories, stated in human language, might correspond to reality and this preoccupation came to mark decisively modern psychiatric classifications. In the early years of logical empiricism, it was hoped that "reality" might be faithfully linguistically reproduced by means of very simple, atomistic, theory-free "observational" sentences (*Beobachtungssätze*) or "record" statements (*Protokollsätze*). However, it soon became clear that language is never theory-free, nor can a statement be protected from the impurities inflicted upon it by a human speaker. Conse-quently, a concept of *operational definition*, assuring an "objective" link between a concept and its "real" referent in nature, was presented to the psychiatric community by Carl Hempel in his famous address to the Ameri-can Psychiatric Association: "An operational definition of a term is con-ceived as a rule to the effect that the term is to apply to a particular case if the performance of a specified operation in that case yields a certain char-acteristic result" [18].

For example, we could operationally define the term "ice" as some volume of water, which changes into solid state if it is brought to a specified measurable temperature under a specified measurable barometric pressure. Unfortunately, this type of definition is not practically applicable for psychiatric terms (e.g. what kind of *operation* might be envisaged to decide whether a statement is delusional). Moreover, Hempel considered operational definitions as *provisional* tools only. Ultimately, and in accordance with the ideal of unity of science, a scientific understanding of a term must be based on its nomological dependence on the laws of nature. Thus, Hempel believed that *mental terms* would be replaced *with time* by appropriate vocabulary of physical science and their reality asserted by lawfully predictable regularities. A more radical, contemporary version of this view is known as materialistic *eliminativism*: mental terms (e.g. hoping, wishing, etc.) are mere illusions with no referent in nature and should be replaced by neuroscientific terms about brain events [19].

Upon this sketch it is now possible to summarize what are the central problems of psychiatric taxonomy and diagnosis as it has been instantiated from the DSM-III [20] onwards:

1. There is a reliance on a mixture of simple and technical language in the hope that such an approach may compensate for a lack of truly operational definitions (e.g. "affect is to mood as weather is to climate" [4]). Yet, it is widely accepted that even ordinary language is replete with historically handed-down tacit metaphysics [21].

2. There is an unwarranted claim that diagnostic systems are atheoretical, yet numerous crucial defining terms (e.g. delusions, hallucinations, dysfunction, mental, behavioral, etc.) are either loaded with metaphysical assumptions (e.g. implicit opposition between non-organic and organic disorders) or are tainted by references to hypothetical extra-clinical, sub-personal processes (e.g. a notion of "incorrect inference" in the definition of delusion).

3. There is a systematic underemphasizing of the patient's subjective experience [5, 22, 23]. In fact, no account of human subjectivity and inter-subjectivity is to be found in the contemporary psychiatric manuals, not even in the textbooks specifically dedicated to the nature of psychiatric interviewing.

4. Correspondingly, there is an emphasis on behavioral terms, in the hope of better reliability (e.g. the so-called "negative" symptoms), without any inquiry or reflection into the relationships between experience, its modes and contents on the one hand and expression on the other hand.

The systematic neglect of subjective experience is simply a consequence of a pervasive lack of a suitable theoretical psychopathological framework to address human *experience* or, in more general terms, human *subjectivity*.

Spitzer [24] summarized the empiricist predicament in contemporary psychopathology in the following way:

> The impossibility of pure description brings with it a corollary, that might be even more important: if everything that we have so far regarded as "pure" data is a result of certain steps of interpretation, these steps should be the subject of thorough reasoning. So any attempt to get better descriptions and a better understanding of (disturbed) perception, thought, and the experiencing I can only consist in reflections on the theories we have and use, i.e.: in philosophical reasoning.

In practice, these fundamental conceptual problems in the operationalist psychopathology entail manifold and serious deleterious practical consequences. Vast domains of human experience (e.g. notions of self, self-identity, varieties of delusional experience, subtle perceptual and cognitive experiences) have been deleted from the diagnostic manuals because they are not suitable for descriptions in a simplistic lay vocabulary, disconnected from any comprehensive account of human subjectivity. Similarly, any reflection on possible links between different symptoms and their expression is systematically and strongly discouraged because it is perceived as an unacceptable transgression of the dominant empiricist dogma. Moreover, such reflection cannot be intersubjectively articulated because of the unavailability of a systematic descriptive framework for human consciousness. Psychiatrists are increasingly trained solely on the basis of official manuals, with a drastic impoverishment of the knowledge of abnormal phenomena. In most psychiatric handbooks, the clinical descriptions of mental disorders hardly occupy more than 10% of the text and are being increasingly simplified to a reproduction of the operational diagnostic criteria.

VARIETIES OF PHENOMENOLOGY

The term "phenomenology" is so heavily polysemic that in order to clarify our position it is necessary to briefly address the semantics of this term. In its most loose, colloquial usage, the term phenomenology is simply synonymous with the notion of description; e.g. one may speak of phenomenology of social exchanges. In the contemporary Anglo-Saxon psychiatric use, the term refers to a description of signs and symptoms of mental disorders, a description relying on a commonsensical view of how things seem to be at a perceptual or introspective glance. It is tacitly assumed that we all know *and* can articulate what we are talking about: e.g. that we are all familiar with, say, the essential *experiential differences* between a remembered event and a remembered fantasy. This way of addressing experience is tacitly permeated by metaphysical assumptions stemming from common sense and the "natural attitude". In this framework, consciousness and subjective experience are treated on a par with spatio-temporal objects of the natural world, as "things" amenable to the same descriptive approach, which we could use in describing a stone or a waterfall. A recent version of such a commonsensical approach is known as *heterophenomenology*; a method proposed by the philosopher Daniel Dennett [25]. It recommends a collection and *averaging* of "third person" descriptive data and subjective reports ("second-person" data) followed by inferential construction of explanatory scientific models. Dennett's data collector is never really situated and, faithful to his behavioristic–empiristic heritage, he relies on "external traces" of subjectivity for his model construction.

A more restrictive use of the term phenomenology was proposed by Karl Jaspers [2]: phenomenology is a *study of inner experience*. The psychiatrist is obliged to recreate or capture the patient's experience in his own mind through a process of imaginative variation. The patient's *spontaneous* statements or written materials are particularly invaluable for a "phenomenological analysis", because they are undistorted by questioning and thus faithfully reflect the patient's experiencing. Jaspers's magnum opus, *General Psychopathology*, substantially revised in 1923, provided a first systematic description of anomalous mental phenomena (usually presented upon the corresponding descriptive background of normal experience; e.g. the discussion of delusions followed the exposition of a sense of reality) as well as a thorough exposition of basic philosophical and other theoretical concepts relevant for psychiatry. Jaspers believed that familiarity with the methods and viewpoints of philosophy and other fields in the human sciences had a special value for psychiatry and abnormal psychology. He hoped it would foster a curious and sophisticated attitude of mind, one allergic not only to scientism but also to "platitudinous speculation, dogmatic theorizing, and absolutism in every form". The impact of *General Psychopathology* remained quite limited outside Germany (its first English translation appeared only in 1963), and its potential as a basis for creating a unified discourse, relevant for the taxonomic efforts, was never fully exploited.

Jaspers must be credited with an explicit realization and emphasis on the fact that studying anomalous subjective experience has no analogue in the somatic medicine and therefore requires a suitable method, a phenomenology. However, as aptly pointed out by Spitzer [24], Jaspers never really solved the problem of description. In order to describe the processes of experience, says Jaspers, we need a conceptual framework, a vocabulary suitable for description. In other words we need to isolate, characterize and conceptually determine the investigated phenomena ("knowledge only consists in psychological determinations"). We cannot get the concepts from descriptions, because the former are the tools for performing the latter. For this reason, Jaspers speaks of a "phenomenological analysis". Unfortunately, however, he is never explicit in explaining what this phenomeno-logical analysis is actually about. As emphasized by Spitzer [24], Jaspers

> speaks of "phenomenological analysis" with reference to single cases, thus presupposing the existence of a conceptual framework which can be used for description...Jaspers refers to single cases when he speaks of his method in general and refers to his general method when he discusses single cases. What is left is his emphasis on detailed descriptions of single cases and on the necessity to clarify concepts. How this should be done—in other words: what the science of psychopathology consists in—he does not say.

The term phenomenology that we employ differs both from the Anglo-Saxon use, denoting descriptive psychopathology, and from the more re-strictive concept of Jaspers. We refer by this term to an endeavor inspired by phenomenological philosophy [26–28], a tradition specifically *aiming at grasping the essential structures of human experience and existence*, and for this reason highly significant for psychiatry.

The epistemology of phenomenology, especially in the work of Heidegger and Merleau-Ponty, represents a radical critique of the Cartesian subject–object dualism and overcomes the problems inherent in both the rationalis-tic over-reliance on the "subjective *a priori*" and in the empiricistic unilateral emphasis on purely sensory sources of knowledge. The subject does have *a priori* capacities, but these capacities only emerge on the background of his pre-linguistic tacit understanding of and embeddedness in the world. The subject does not *create* the world but contributes actively to its articulation and significance. As pointed out by Merleau-Ponty [28]:

> The world is inseparable from the subject, but from a subject which is nothing but a project of the world, and the subject is inseparable from the world, but from a world which the subject itself projects. The subject is a being-in-the-world and the world remains "subjective" since its texture and articulations are traced out by the subject's movement of transcendence.

One fundamental issue addressed by phenomenology is how to approach consciousness. Is it just as straightforward to investigate consciousness as it is to examine the chemical structure of gasoline, or estimate the number of cod in the Baltic Sea, or is it rather the case that consciousness as object of investigation has a quite peculiar status which our choice of methodology must reflect? According to phenomenology, consciousness is *not* just one object among others. Consciousness differs from everything else by being that which is in possession of comprehension, by being that which relates itself comprehendingly to both self and world. It should therefore be obvious that an investigation of consciousness has the highest priority and significance. Any other investigation (including the two mentioned above) necessarily presupposes the epistemic and cognitive contribution of consciousness, that is, any investigation *whatsoever* has consciousness as its pivot and condition.

Phenomenology calls attention to the fact that it is possible to investigate consciousness in several ways. It is not only possible to consider it as an empirical object somehow endowed with mental properties, as a causally determined object in the world, but also as the subject of intentional direct-edness to the world, i.e. as the subject for the world, as—to paraphrase Wittgenstein—*the limit of the world* [29]. And as long as consciousness is only considered as an empirical object, which is the predominant case in contemporary materialism, the truly significant aspect of consciousness, the fact that it is the dimension that allows the world to manifest itself, will be overlooked.

The term *phenomeno-logy* literally means an account or knowledge of a phenomenon. *Phenomenon* is that which shows itself, that which manifests itself, an appearance. Consciousness enables or *is a condition of such manifest-ation*; it is a dative of all appearing (phenomenality). Phenomenology does not distinguish between the inaccessible noumenon (thing-in-itself) and its "outer" appearance (phenomenon in the Kantian sense): for phenomen-ology the phenomenon is always a manifestation of the thing itself. This way of discussing consciousness, as the *constitutive* dimension that allows for identification and manifestation, as the "place" "in" which the world can reveal and articulate itself, is radically different from any attempt to treat it as merely yet another object in the world.

PHENOMENOLOGICAL ACCOUNT OF THE FUNDAMENTAL FEATURES OF CONSCIOUSNESS

We will now present some of those central features of consciousness that phenomenology has elucidated in numerous analyses. Such an account is, as it has been argued above, a necessary first step in any scientific explana-tory account and in any classification of pathological experience. The very notion of anomalous experience is a *contrastive* concept, i.e. it can only be articulated against the background of the normal experience. It is therefore our contention that this brief exposition will not only familiarize the reader more closely with the ways in which phenomenology performs its analyses; it will also provide a much needed introduction to the essential structures of human subjectivity, a comprehension of which is indispensable for a sophisticated and faithful description of anomalous experience. To mention just a few examples: to identify the essential differences between, say, obsessions, pseudo-obsessions, and episodes of thought interference in the incipient schizophrenia, it is necessary to grasp different possible ways of being self-aware; to differentiate between the non-psychotic and the psychotic somatic complaints, it is important to comprehend the notions of the body-subject and the body-object; to distinguish between an identity disturbance in the borderline personality disorder and in the schizophrenia spectrum condition one has to realize that identity operates at different and hierarchically ordered levels of experiential complexity.

Phenomenal Consciousness and Self-awareness

To undergo an experience is to be in a conscious state with a certain quality, often designated as "qualia" in contemporary literature. Experiences have a subjective "feel" to them, i.e. a certain (phenomenal) quality of "what it is like" or what it "feels like" to have them. This is obviously true of bodily sensations like pain or nausea. But it is also the case for perceptual experiences, desires, feelings and moods. There is something it is like to touch an ice cube, to crave chocolate, to feel envious, nervous, depressed, or happy. However, *the phenomenal dimension of experience* is not limited to *sensory* or *emotional* states alone. There is also something "it is like" to entertain abstract beliefs; there is an experiential difference between hoping and fearing that justice will prevail, and between accepting and denying theoretical propositions. But we need to elucidate this experiential quality in further detail. Whereas the object of my perceptual experience is intersubjectively accessible in the sense that it can in principle be given to others in the same way that it is given to me, my perceptual experience itself is only given directly to me. Whereas you and I can both perceive the numerically identical same cherry, each of us has our own distinct perception of it, and can share these just as little as we can share each other's pain. You might certainly realize that I am in pain, you might even empathize with me, but you cannot actually feel my pain the same way I do. We can formulate this by saying that you have no access to the *first-personal givenness* of my experience. We can therefore distinguish between at least three levels of self-awareness: (a) the immediate, prereflective level; (b) the level of "I-consciousness"; and (c) the level of personhood or narrative self-awareness. This sequence reflects a hierarchical structure from the most founding or basic to the most founded or complex.

When one is *directly* and non-inferentially conscious of one's own occurrent thoughts, perceptions or pains, they are characterized by a first-personal givenness, that immediately reveals them as one's own. This first-personal givenness of experiential phenomena is not something quite incidental to their being, a mere varnish that the experiences could lack without ceasing to be experiences. On the contrary, it is this first-personal givenness that makes the experiences *subjective*. To put it differently, their first-personal givenness entails a built-in self-reference, a primitive experiential self-referentiality. When I am aware of an occurrent pain, perception, or thought from the first-person perspective, the experience in question is given immediately, non-inferentially as *mine*, i.e. I do not first scrutinize a specific perception or feeling of pain, and subsequently identify it as mine. Phenomenologically speaking, we are never conscious of an object as such, but always of the object as appearing in a certain way (as judged, seen, feared, remembered, smelled, anticipated, tasted, etc.). The object is given *through the experience*, and if there is no awareness of the experience, the object does not appear at all. This dimension of self-awareness, its first-personal givenness, is therefore a medium in which specific modes of experience are articulated. Following these analyses, self-awareness cannot be equated with reflective (thematic, conceptual, mediated) self-awareness. On the contrary, reflective self-awareness presupposes a prereflective (unthematic, tacit, non-conceptual, immediate) self-awareness. Self-awareness is not something that only comes about the moment *I* realize that *I* am perceiving the Empire State Building, or realize that *I* am the bearer of private mental states, or refer to myself using the first person pronoun. On the contrary, it is legitimate to speak of a more primitive type of self-awareness whenever I am conscious of my feeling of joy, or my burning thirst, or my perception of the Empire State Building. If the experience is given in a first-personal mode of presentation to me, it is (at least tacitly) given as *my* experience, and therefore counts as a case of self-awareness. The first-personal givenness of an experience, its very self-manifestation, is the most basic form of selfhood, usually called *ipseity* [30–32]. To be aware of one*self* is not to apprehend a pure self apart from the experience, but to be acquainted with an experience in its first-personal mode of presentation, that is, from "within". That is, the subject or self referred to is not something standing opposed to, or apart from or beyond experience, but rather a feature or function of its givenness.

Given these considerations, it is obvious that all phenomenal consciousness is a basic form of self-awareness. Whenever I am acquainted with an experience in its first-personal mode of givenness, whenever I live it through, that is whenever there is a "what it is like" involved with its inherent "quality" of *myness*, we are dealing with a form of self-awareness: "...all subjective experience is self-conscious in the weak sense that there is something it is like for the subject to have that experience. This involves a sense that the experience is the subject's experience, that it happens to her, occurs in her stream" [33]. More recently, Antonio Damasio has also defended a comparable thesis: "If 'self-consciousness' is taken to mean 'consciousness with a sense of self', then all human consciousness is necessarily covered by the term—there is just no other kind of consciousness as far as I can see" [34].

This primitive and fundamental notion of self must be contrasted to what might be called explicit "I-consciousness"; an awareness of oneself as a source, agent and centre of experience and action. Though exceedingly difficult to define, the I-consciousness appears to involve, on the experiential plane, some kind of self-coinciding that confers a sense of coherence to the field of experience. Other features of the I-experience comprise its synchronic singularity, linked to the unity of the stream of consciousness and the diachronic identity or persistence of the self. This is the invariant singularity of the "I" in the midst of its changing experiential contents. But *what is*, precisely, the "I", the entity which is endowed with such possessing powers? Phenomenology emphasizes that this "I" is not *just* a formal construct or a logical subject (i.e. a subject whose existence can be logically deduced from the unity of consciousness). *Neither* is it an object in the usual sense of the term; it *is* possible to grasp it reflectively, not as a "content" or a "mental object", but as *a pole or focus of experience*. The "I" polarizes the flux of consciousness into its intentional subject–object relational structure.

At the most sophisticated level, we can speak of a narrative self, a constructed unity. This type of self-reference points to the *person*. The person as a carrier of self-reference is phenomenologically complex, involving multiple aspects such as subjective experience, "external" behavior, dispositions–habits (historical sediments) and embodiment. Self-identity at the level of person emerges in a narrative-mediated (and therefore linked to *history* and to linguistic competence and practice) and intersubjectively embedded *dialectic* between indexicality of mutable, yet persisting sameness (*idem*-identity) and a constancy of the experiential self-hood (*ipse*-identity) [35]. Idem-identity refers to the *what* of a person and is expressible as a cluster of intrinsic and extrinsic predicates, e.g. personality-type; ipse-identity refers to the *who* of a person: the focus or source of experience (see I-consciousness above). These two aspects only make sense in conjunction with each other. The notions of social self, personal identity, self-esteem, self-image and "persona", are all concepts that can be construed at this level of description. The construction of narrative identity starts in early childhood, it continues the rest of our life, and is a product of complex social interactions that in crucial ways depend on language. It should be clear, however, that the notion of a narrative self is not only far more complex than but also logically dependent upon what we might call the experiential selfhood. Only a being with a first-person perspective could make sense of the ancient dictum "know thyself", only a being with a first-person perspective could consider her own aims, ideals and aspirations *as* her own, and tell a story about it [32].

Temporality

It is customary to speak of the stream of consciousness, that is the stream of changing, even saccadic, yet unified experiences. How must this process be structured if something like identity over time is to be possible? Not only are we able to perceive enduring and temporally extended objects, but we are also able to recollect on an earlier experience, and recognize it as *our own*. Our experience of a temporal object (as well as our experience of change and succession) would be impossible if we were only conscious of that which is given in a punctual now, and if the stream of consciousness would consequently consist in a series of isolated now-points, like a line of pearls.

The phenomenological approach is to insist on the *width of the presence*. The basic unit of perceived time is not a "knife-edge" present, but a "duration-block", i.e. a temporal field that contains all three temporal modes, present, past and future. Let us imagine that we are hearing a triad consisting of the tones C, D and E. If we focus on the last part of this perception, the one that occurs when the tone E sounds, we do not find a consciousness which is exclusively conscious of the tone E, but a consciousness which is still conscious of the two former notes D and C. And not only that, we find a consciousness which still *hears* the two first notes (it neither imagines nor remembers them). This does not mean that there is no difference between our consciousness of the present tone E, and our consciousness of the tones D and C. D and C are not simultaneous with E, on the contrary we are experiencing a temporal succession. D and C are tones which have been, but they are *perceived* as *past*, and it is only for that reason that we can experience the triad in its temporal duration, and not simply as isolated tones which replace each other abruptly. We can perceive temporal objects because consciousness is not caught in the now, because we do not merely perceive the now-phase of the triad, but also its past and future phases.

There are three *technical terms* to describe this case. First, there is a moment of the experience which is narrowly directed towards the now-phase of the object, and which is called the *primal impression*. By itself this cannot provide us with a perception of a temporal object, and it is in fact merely an abstract component of the experience that never appears in isolation. The primal impression is situated in a temporal horizon; it is accompanied by a *retention* which is the name for the intention which provides us with a consciousness of the phase of the object which has just been, and by a *protention*, which in a more or less indefinite manner intends the phase of the object about to occur: we always anticipate in an implicit and unreflected manner that which is about to happen. That this anticipation is an actual part of our experience can be illustrated by the fact that we would be *surprised* if the wax-figure suddenly moved, or if the door we opened hid a stonewall. It only makes sense to speak of a surprise in the light of certain anticipation, and since we can always be surprised, we always have a horizon of anticipation. The concrete and full structure of all lived experience is primal impression–retention–protention. It is "immediately" given as a unity, and it is not a gradual, progressive process of self-unfolding.

Both retention and protention have to be distinguished from the proper (thematic) *recollection* and *expectation*. There is an obvious difference between retaining and protending the tones that have just sounded and are just about to sound, and to remember a past holiday, or look forward to the next vacation. Whereas the two latter experiences *presuppose* the work of the retention and the protention, the protention and retention are intrinsic moments of any occurrent experience I might be having. They provide us with consciousness of the temporal horizon of the present object, they are the *a priori* structures of our consciousness, structures which are the very condition of temporal experience. They are *passive* or automatic processes that take place without our active contribution.

Comprehending the structure of time-consciousness proves crucial if we for instance wish to understand the important *syntheses of identity*: if I move around a tree in order to obtain a more exhaustive presentation of it, then the different profiles of the tree, its front, sides and back, do not present themselves as disjointed fragments, but are perceived as synthetically integrated moments. This synthetic process is temporal in nature. Ultimately, time-consciousness must be regarded as the formal condition of possibility for the constitution of any objects [36, 37].

Intentionality

An intrinsic, fundamental feature of consciousness is its object-directedness or *intentionality*. One does not merely love, fear, see or judge; one loves, fears, sees or judges *something*. In short, it characterizes many of our experiences, that they are exactly conscious *of* something. Regardless of whether we are talking of a perception, a thought, a judgement, a fantasy, a doubt, an expectation, a recollection, etc., all of these diverse forms of consciousness are characterized by intending objects, and they cannot be analyzed properly without a look at their objective correlate, i.e. the perceived, doubted, expected object. Likewise, affectivity discloses also intentional structure: whereas feelings are about the objects of feelings, moods exhibit a global intentionality of horizons of being by coloring the world and so expand, restrict or modify our existential possibilities.

The decisive question is how to account for this intentionality. One common suggestion is to reduce intentionality to causality. According to this view consciousness can be likened to a container. In itself it has no relation to the world; only if it is *causally influenced* by an external object can such a relation occur. That this model is severely inadequate is easy to show. The real existing spatial objects in my immediate physical surrounding only constitute a minority of that of which I can be conscious. When I am thinking about *absent* objects, *impossible* objects, *non-existing* objects, *future* objects, or *ideal* objects, my directedness towards these objects is obviously not brought about because I am causally influenced by the objects in question.

Thus, an important aspect of intentionality is exactly its *existence-independency*. In short, our mind does not become intentional through an external influence, and it does not lose its intentionality, if its object ceases to exist. Intentionality is not an accidental feature of consciousness that only comes about the moment consciousness is causally influenced in the right way by an object, but is on the contrary a feature belonging to consciousness as such. That is, we do not need to add anything to consciousness for it to become intentional and world-directed. It is already from the very start embedded in the world.

How do we intend an object? By *meaning* something about it. It is sense that provides consciousness with its object-directedness and establishes the objectual reference. More specifically, sense does not only determine which object is intended, but also *as* what the object is apprehended or conceived. Thus, it is customary to speak of intentional "relations" as being perspectival or aspectual. One is never simply conscious of an object, one is always conscious of an object in a particular way; to be intentionally directed at something is to intend something *as* something. One intends (perceives, judges, imagines) an object *as* something, i.e. under a certain conception, description or from a certain perspective. To think about the capital of Denmark or about the native town of Niels Bohr, to think of Hillary Clinton's husband or of the last US president in the twentieth century, to think about the sum of $2 + 4$ or about the sum of $5 + 1$, or to see a Swiss cottage from below or above, in each of the four cases one is thinking of the same object, but under different descriptions, conceptions or perspectives, that is with different senses.

The phenomenological take on intentionality can be further clarified by contrasting it with what is known as the *representational model*. According to this model, consciousness cannot on its own reach all the way to the objects themselves, and we therefore need to introduce some kind of interface between the mind and the world, namely *mental representations*. On this view, the mind has of itself no relation to the world. It is like a closed container, and the experiences composing it are all subjective happenings with no immediate bearing on the world outside. The crucial problem for such a theory is of course to explain why the mental representation, which per definition *is different* from the object, should nevertheless lead us to the object. That something represents something different (that X represents Y) *is not a natural property of the object in question*. An object is not representative in the same way that it is red, extended or metallic. Two copies of the same book may look alike, but that does not make one into a representation of the other; and *whereas resemblance is a reciprocal relation, this is not the case for representation*. On the contrary, if X is to represent Y, X needs to be *interpreted* as being a representation of Y. It is exactly the interpretation, i.e. a particular form of intentionality, which confers X with its representative reference. In short, representative reference is parasitic and ultimately faces the problem of an infinite regress of interpreters (the regress of homunculi). The object which is interpreted *as* a representation must first be perceived. But in this case, the representative theory of perception must obviously be rejected, since the claim of this theory was that perception itself is made possible through representation. If representation presupposes perception, and more generally, intentionality, it cannot explain it. Thus, phenomenology argues that we do in fact experience the external world directly, and that we should stop conceiving of perceptual experience as some kind of internal movie screen that confronts us with mental representations. Instead, perceptual experience should be understood as (in successful cases) an acquaintance with the genuine properties of external objects, not mediated by any "intra-mental images". The so-called qualitative character of experience, the taste of a lemon, the smell of coffee, are not at all qualities belonging to some spurious mental objects, but qualities of the presented objects. Rather than saying that we experience *representations*, we might say that our experiences are *presentational*, and that they *present* the world as having certain features.

One of the significant distinctions introduced by phenomenology is the distinction between signitive (linguistic), imaginative (pictorial), and perceptual intentions: I can talk about a withering oak, I can see a detailed drawing *of* the oak, and I can perceive the oak myself. These different ways to intend an object are not unrelated. On the contrary, there is a strict hierarchical relation between them, in the sense that the modes can be ranked according to their ability to give us the object as directly, originally and optimally (more or less *present*) as possible. It is only *perception* that gives us the object directly; it is only that type of intention that presents us with the object itself in its bodily presence.

Embodiment

Consciousness has always an experiential bodily background (embodiment/corporeality). It is quite trivial to say that we can perceive our body as a physical object, e.g. visually inspect our hands. It is however less obvious to realize that our subjectivity is incarnated in a more fundamental way. The phenomenological approach to the role of the body is closely linked to the analysis of perception. An important point here is the *partial givenness* of the perceptual (spatio-temporal) object. The object is never given in its totality, but always appears from a certain perspective. That which appears perspectivally always appears *oriented*. Since it also presents itself from a certain angle and at a certain distance from the observer, the point is obvious: there is no *pure* point of view and there is no view from nowhere, *there is only an embodied point of view*. A subject can only perceive objects and use utensils if it is embodied. A coffee mill is obviously not of much use to a disincarnated spirit, and to listen to a string quartet by Schubert is to enjoy it from a certain perspective and standpoint, be it from the street, in the gallery or on the first row. Every perspectival appearance presupposes that the experiencing subject has itself a relation to space, and since the subject only possesses a spatial location due to its embodiment, it follows that spatial objects can only appear for and be constituted by embodied subjects.

These reflections are radicalized the moment it is realized how intrinsically intertwined *perception* and *action* are. Not only does action presuppose perception, but perception is not a matter of passive reception but of active exploration. The body does not merely function as a stable center of orientation. Its *mobility* contributes decisively to the constitution of perceptual reality. We see with mobile eyes set in a head that can turn and is attached to a body that can move from place to place; a stationary point of view is only the limiting case of a mobile point of view [38]. In a similar way, it is important to recognize the importance of bodily movements (the movement of the eyes, the touch of the hand, the step of the body, etc.) for the experience of space and spatial objects. Ultimately, perception is correlated to and accompanied by the self-sensing or self-affection of the moving body. Every visual or tactile appearance is given in correlation to a *kinaesthesis* or *kinaesthetic experiencing*. When I touch the surface of an apple, the apple is given in conjunction with a sensing of finger-movement. When I watch the flight of a bird, the moving bird is given in conjunction with the sensing of eye-movement.

The thesis is not simply that the subject can perceive objects and use utensils only if it *has* a body, but that it can perceive and use objects only if it *is* a body, that is if we are dealing with an embodied subjectivity. Let us assume that I am sitting in a restaurant. I wish to begin to eat, and so I pick up the fork. In order to pick up the fork, I need to know its position in relation to *myself*. That is, my perception of the object must contain some information about myself, otherwise I would not be able to act on it. On the dinner table, the perceived fork is to the left (of me), the perceived knife is to the right (of me), and the perceived plate and wineglass in front (of me). Every perspectival appearance implies that the embodied perceiver is himself *co-given* as the zero point, the absolute indexical "here" in relation to which every appearing object is oriented. As an experiencing, embodied subject I am the point of reference in relation to which each and every one of my perceptual objects are uniquely related. I am the center around which and in relation to which (egocentric) space unfolds itself. This bodily self-awareness is a condition of possibility for the constitution of spatial objects, and conditions every worldly experience [26]. When I experience the world, the body is co-given in the midst of the world as the unperceived (i.e. pre-reflectively experienced) relatum that all objects are turning their front towards [28]. We may speak of space as "hodological", that is a space structured by *references of use*, where the position and orientation of the objects are connected to a *practical* subject. That the knife is lying there on the table means that I can reach and grasp it. The body is thus present in every project and in every perception. It is our "point de vue" and "point de départ" [39]. The body is not a medium between me and the world, but our primary being-in-the-world. A concept frequently used to describe this constituting function of embodiment is the notion of the *body schema*, which is an active corporeal dimension of our subjectivity, making perceptual experience not only possible but also structured or articulated in accordance with our bodily potentialities. This concept is distinct from the notion of the *body image*, which simply signifies an objectivated representation of our physical/spatial body [40].

Insofar as the body functions as the zero-point that permits a perceptual view on the world, the body itself is not perceived. My body is my perspective on the world. It is not among the objects that I have a perspective on. My *original* body-awareness is not a type of object-consciousness, is *not* a perception of the body as an object. Quite the contrary, the objective body or the body-object is, like every other perceptual experience, dependent upon and made possible by the pre-reflectively functioning body-awareness. The lived body precedes the perceived body-object. Originally, I do not have any consciousness *of* my body. I am not perceiving it, *I am it*. Originally, my body is experienced as a unified field of activity and affectivity, as a volitional structure, as a potentiality of mobility, as an "I do" and "I can". This is the most fundamental aspect of the thesis that consciousness has always an experiential bodily background (embodiment).

Thus a full account of our bodily experience reveals the body's double or ambiguous experiential status: both as a "lived body" (*Leib*), *identical or superposable with the subject*, and as a physically spatial, objective body (*Körper*) [26]. An incessant oscillation and interplay between these bodily modes constitute a fluid and hardly noticed foundation for all experiencing [28].

Intersubjectivity, "Other Minds", and Objectivity

In many traditions, including contemporary cognitive science, the problem of intersubjectivity has been equaled with the "problem of other minds", and a classical attempt to come to grip with this problem is known as the *argument from analogy*. It runs as follows: The only mind I have direct access to is my own. My access to the mind of another is always mediated by his bodily behavior. But how can the perception of another person's body provide me with information about his mind? Starting from my own mind and linking it to the way in which my body is given to me, I then pass to the other's body and, by noticing the analogy that exists between this body and my own body, I *infer* that the foreign body is probably also linked in a similar manner to a foreign mind. In my own case, screaming is often associated with pain; when I observe others scream, I infer that it is likely that they are also feeling pain. Although this inference does not provide me with indubitable knowledge about others, and although it does not allow me to actually experience other minds, at least it gives me some reason to believe in their existence.

This way of posing and tackling the problem of intersubjectivity is quite problematic from a phenomenological point of view. First of all, one could question the claim that my own self-experience is of a purely mental, self-enclosed nature, and that it takes place in isolation from and precedes the experience of others. Secondly, the argument from analogy assumes that we never *experience* the thoughts or feelings of another person, but that we can only *infer* their likely existence on the basis of that which is actually given to us, namely a physical body. But, on the one hand, this assumption seems to imply a far too intellectualistic account—after all, both animals and infants seem to share the belief in other minds but in their case it is hardly the result of a process of inference—and, on the other hand, it seems to presuppose a highly problematic dichotomy between inner and outer, between experience and behavior. Thus, a solution to the problem of other minds must start with a correct understanding of the relation between mind and body. In some sense, experiences are not internal, they are not hidden in the head, but rather expressed in bodily gestures and actions. When I see a foreign face, I *see* it as friendly or angry, etc., that is, the very face expresses these emotions. Moreover, bodily behavior is meaningful, it is intentional, and as such it is neither internal nor external, but rather beyond this artificial distinction. On the basis of considerations like these, it has been argued that we do not first perceive a physical body in order then to infer in a subsequent move the existence of a foreign subjectivity. On the contrary, in the face-to-face encounter, we are neither confronted with a mere body, nor with a hidden psyche, but with a *unified whole*. We see the anger of the other, we feel his sorrow, *we do not infer* their existence. Thus, it has been claimed that we will never be able to solve the problem of other minds unless we understand that the body of the other differs radically from inanimate objects, and that our perception of this body is quite unlike our ordinary perception of objects. The relation between self and other is not first established by way of an analogical inference; on the contrary, it must be realized that there exists a distinctive mode of consciousness, often called *empathy* or simply "Fremderfahrung", that allows us to experience the feelings, desires, and beliefs of others in a more or less direct manner. To be more specific, empathy has typically been taken to constitute a unique form of intentionality, and one of the phenomenological tasks has consequently been to clarify its precise structure and to spell out the difference between it and other forms of intentionality, such as perception, imagination and recollection.

A number of investigations have also been concerned with the way in which the very intentional relation between subjectivity and world might be influenced by intersubjectivity. It has been argued that a fundamental feature of those objects we first and foremost encounter in our daily life, namely artefacts, all contain references to other persons. Be it because they are produced by others, or because the work we are trying to accomplish with them is destined for others. Thus, in our daily life *we are constantly embedded in an intersubjective framework* regardless of whether or not there are *de facto* any others persons present. In fact, the very world we live in is from the very start given to us as already explored and structured by others. We typically understand the world (and ourselves) through a traditional conventionality. We participate in a communal tradition, which through a chain of generations stretches back into a dim past: "I am what I am as an heir" [41]. In short, the world we are living in is a public and communal world, not a private one. Subjectivity and world are internally related, and since the structure of this world contains essential references to others, subjectivity cannot be understood except as inhabiting a world that it necessarily shares with others. Moreover, this world is experienced as objective, and the notion of objectivity is intimately linked with the notion of intersubjectivity. That which in principle is incapable of being experienced by others cannot be ascribed reality and objectivity. To put it differently, the *objectivity of the world is intersubjectively constituted*, and my experience of the world as objective is mediated by my experience of and interaction with other world-engaged subjects. Only insofar as I experience that others experience the same objects as myself, do I really experience these objects as objective and real.

PHENOMENOLOGICAL CONTRIBUTION TO CLASSIFICATION

Phenomenology, through its specific interest in consciousness, is particularly suitable for reconstructing the patient's subjective experience. Phenomenology does not consider consciousness as a spatial object; in fact the fundamental feature of conscious experience is its intrinsically non-spatial nature. Consciousness is not a physical object but *a dimension of phenomenality*. Consciousness does not consist of separable, *substantial* ("thing-like") components, exerting a mechanical–efficient causality on each other. Rather, the phenomenological concept of consciousness implies a meaningful network of interdependent *moments* (i.e. non-independent parts), a network founded on intertwining, motivation and mutual implication [42], encompassing and framed by an intersubjective matrix. These views have important implications for psychopathological taxonomic endeavor.

First, examination of single cases, as already pointed out by Jaspers, is very important. Reports from few patients, able to describe their experiences in detail, may be more informative of the nature of the disorder than big N studies performed in a crude, simplified way. Subjective experience or first-person perspective, by its very nature, *cannot be averaged*, except at the cost of heavy informational loss. In other words, in-depth study of anomalous experience should serve as a complement to strictly empirical designs. But even the latter may be dramatically improved, if the psychopathological examinations are phenomenologically informed.

Second, a psychiatrist, in his diagnostic efforts, is always engaged in what is called a "typification" process [43, 44]. At the most elementary level, typification simply implies "seeing as", the fact that we *always* perceive the world perspectivally, i.e. we always see objects, situations and events as *certain types* of objects, situations and events (e.g. when we see a bus driving away from a bus-stop and a man running in the same direction, we will tend to perceive the man as trying to catch a bus that he had missed) [45]. The most frequent type of typification is the pre-reflective and automatic one, linked to the corporeal awareness, and this holds for the diagnostic encounter as well. We *sense* the patients as withdrawn, hostile, sympathetic, eccentric, etc., and such typifications depend on our knowledge and experience, and will be perhaps modified upon further interactions with the patient. But we can also engage in reflective attitudes in order to make our typifications more explicit.

The notion of typicality or of a prototype is crucial here: it is a notion important in all cognitive research [46–48]. *Prototypes* are central exemplars of a category in question: e.g. a sparrow is more typical of the category "birds" than is a penguin, which cannot fly and does not seem to have wings. Most cognitive and epistemic categories are founded upon a "family resemblance", a network of criss-crossing analogies between the individual members of a category [29], with very characteristic cases occupying central position, and less typical cases forming a continuum towards the border of the category, where the latter eventually blends into other, neighboring categories. Prototype can be empirically established by examining the co-occurrence of its various features; this happens tacitly in the formation of a diagnostic skill, due to pre-reflective sedimentations of experiences and acquisition of theoretical knowledge. This is also explicitly the case in the statistical detections of syndromatic entities. However, phenomenology would argue that the psychiatric typifications sedimented through encounters with patients are not only a matter of *simple averaging* over time of the accumulated atomistic sensory experiences, but are also motivated by a quest for *meaningful* interrelations between the observed phenomenal features. A concept of "ideal type" [49] or *essence* [26] plays here an important role. Ideal type exemplifies the *ideal and necessary* connections between its composing features. Ideal type transcends what is given in experience: e.g. all my possible drawings of a straight line will be somehow deficient (for instance if examined through a microscope) compared to the very (ideal) concept of a straight line.

Phenomenological approach to anomalous experience is precisely concerned with bringing forth the typical, and ideally necessary features of such experience. This is the aim of the *eidetic reduction*: to disclose the essential structure of the experience under investigation by means of an imaginative variation. This variation should be understood as a kind of conceptual analysis where we attempt to imagine the phenomenon as being different from how it currently is. This process of imaginative variation will lead us to certain borders that cannot be varied, i.e. changed and transgressed, without making the phenomenon cease to be the kind of phenomenon it is. The variation consequently allows us to distinguish between the accidental properties, i.e. the properties that *could* have been different, and the essential properties, i.e. the invariant structures that make the phenomenon be of the type it is. It is important not to confuse this claim with the claim that we can obtain infallible insights into the essence of every object whatsoever by means of some passive gaze. On the contrary, the eidetic variation is a demanding conceptual analysis that in many cases is defeasible.

The aim of psychopathological phenomenological analysis will be to disclose the essential, invariant properties of abnormal phenomena (e.g. a difference between obsession and thought interference). The same will be the case at the level of *diagnostic entities*: these are seen by phenomenology as certain typical modes of human experience and existence, possessing a meaningful whole reflected in their invariant phenomenological structures (e.g. the concept of "trouble générateur" by Minkowski [50]). Delimitation of diagnostic entities is supported by a concept of a *whole* or an organizing Gestalt (*Ganzheitsschau*) [51]. *Phenomena* exhibit such wholeness. For example, the schizophrenic autism is not a symptom, i.e. a sign referring to some underlying modular abnormality. As a phenomenon autism manifests *itself*, it expresses a certain fundamentally altered mode of existence and experience [52–53], which may serve to delimit schizophrenia as a disease concept.

Phenomenological psychopathology is more interested in the *form* than in the *content* of experience, a point already emphasized by Jaspers. It is likely that the altered form of experience is, pathogenetically speaking, closer to its natural/biological substrate; the content is always contingent and idiosyncratic because it is mainly, but not only, biographically determined. Therefore, formal alterations of experience will be of a more direct taxonomic interest.

It is on this point that phenomenology offers a method called *phenomenological reduction*, that is a specific kind of reflection enabling our access to the structures of subjectivity. It is a procedure that involves a shift of attitude, the shift from a natural attitude to a phenomenological attitude. In the natural attitude, that is *pre-philosophically*, we take it for granted that there exists a mind-, experience-, and theory-independent reality. But reality is not simply a brute fact, but a system of validity and meaning that *needs subjectivity*, i.e. epistemic and cognitive perspectives, if it is to manifest and articulate itself. Thus, a phenomenological analysis of the object *qua* its appearing necessarily also takes subjectivity into account. Insofar as we are confronted with the appearance of an object, that is with an object as presented, perceived, judged, evaluated, etc., we are led to the experiential structures, to the intentionality that these modes of appearance are correlated with. We are led to the acts of presentation, perception, judgement and valuation, and thereby to the subject that the object as appearing must necessarily be understood in relation to. We do not simply focus on the phenomenon exactly as it is given, we also focus on the subjective side of consciousness, and thereby become aware of the formal structures of subjectivity that are at play in order for the phenomenon to appear as it does. The subjective structures we thereby encounter are the structures that are the condition of possibility for appearance as such. A subjectivity which remains hidden as long as we are absorbed in the commonsensical natural attitude, where we live in self-oblivion among the objects, but which the phenomenological reduction is capable of revealing.

Formal configuration of experience includes modes and structures of intentionality, spatial aspects of experience, temporality, embodiment, modes of altered self-awareness, etc. However, as we have already argued, in order to address these formal or structural aspects of anomalous experience, the psychiatrist must be familiar with the basic organization of phenomenal awareness. Otherwise he would only have a superficial, commonsensical take on experience at his disposal. That would force him to focus only on the content of experience, because he would be unable to address its structural alterations. A good example here is the notion of "bizarre delusion", regarded today as being a diagnostic indicator of schizophrenia and defined by its "physically impossible content". Yet, as it has been argued, a true diagnostic significance of such delusions only emerges if the content of delusion reflects a profoundly altered (solipsistic and transitivistic) self-experience of the patient [54, 55].

CONCLUSIONS

Psychopathology is currently in a state of crisis which, if not ameliorated, will seriously impede any further pathogenetic and taxonomic progress [12, 15, 56]. Very simply stated, psychiatry, as an academic discipline, is at risk of quick disappearance, if the tendency will continue to reduce psychopathology to a list of commonsensically derived and crudely simplified operational features, and if any reflection on the relations between phenomenal aspects of mental disorders is systematically discouraged by a combination of editorial, teaching and funding policies. There is an urgent need to re-potentiate and re-emphasize clinical skills and sophistication. Continental phenomenology with its detailed descriptions of the structures of consciousness (and its ongoing integration with analytic philosophy of mind and cognitive science [10, 12, 57]) is ideally suited as a conceptual framework for such a psychopathological reappraisal. It enables a precise description and classification of single anomalous experience in relation to its more encompassing intentional structures (e.g. recent attempts to describe anomalous self-experience in early schizophrenia [58–62]) and helps to define mental disorders on the basis of their experiential structural features, linking apparently disconnected phenomena together (59, 63–65). The problem of reliability, often raised against the phenomenological approach, is not unsolvable; it is a matter of intense relearning and a profound transformation of psychiatric culture. High reliability of the current operational criteria is seldom achieved; if so, then only at the precious cost of validity. Even if we continue with the polythetic operational diagnostic systems, we will still need a prototypical, phenomenologically informed hierarchy of disorders in order to improve our diagnostic practices and taxonomic research.

REFERENCES

1. Robins L., Barrett J. (1989) Preface. In *The Validity of Psychiatric Diagnosis* (Eds L. Robbins, J. Barrett). Raven Press, New York.
2. Jaspers K. (1923) *Allgemeine Psychopathologie*, 3rd edn. Springer, Berlin.
3. Nagel T. (1974) What is it like to be a bat? *Philosoph. Rev.*, 83: 435–450.
4. American Psychiatric Association (1994) *Diagnostic and Statistical Manual of Mental Disorders*, 4th edn, revised (DSM-IV). American Psychiatric Association, Washington.
5. Mishara A. (1994) A phenomenological critique of commonsensensical assumptions in DSM-III-R: the avoidance of the patient's subjectivity. In *Philosophical*

Perspectives on Psychiatric Diagnostic Classification (Eds J.Z. Sadler, O.P. Wiggins, M.A. Schwartz), pp. 129–147. Johns Hopkins University Press, London.
6. Bermudez J.L.E., Marcel A.J.E., Eilan N.E. (1995) *The Body and the Self*. MIT Press, Cambridge.
7. Bermudez J.L. (1998) *The Paradox of Self-Consciousness*. MIT Press, Cambridge.
8. Eilan N.E., McCarthy R.A.E., Brewer B.E. (1993) *Spatial Representation: Problems in Philosophy and Psychology*. Blackwell, Oxford.
9. Gallagher S.E., Shear J.E. (1999) *Models of the Self*. Imprint Academic, Thorverton.
10. Petitot J., Varela F., Pachoud B., Roy J.-M. (1999) *Naturalizing Phenomenology: Issues in Contemporary Phenomenology and Cognitive Science*. Stanford University Press, Stanford.
11. Gallagher S. (1997) Mutual enlightenment: recent phenomenology in cognitive science. *J. Consciousness Studies*, **4**: 195–214.
12. Parnas J., Zahavi D. (2000) The link: philosophy–psychopathology–phenomenology. In *Exploring the Self* (Ed. D. Zahavi), pp. 1–16. John Benjamins Publishing Company, Amsterdam.
13. Varela F. (1996) Neurophenomenology: a methodological remedy for the hard problem. *J. Consciousness Studies*, **3**: 330–350.
14. Webb L., DiClemente C., Johnstone E., Sanders J., Perley R. (1981) *DSM-III Training Guide for Use with the American Psychiatric Association's Diagnostic and Statistical Manual of Mental Disorders*, 3rd edn. Brunner/Mazel, New York.
15. Parnas J., Bovet P. (1995) Research in psychopathology: epistemologic issues. *Compr. Psychiatry*, **36**: 167–181.
16. Parnas J. (1996) Epistemological issues in psychiatric research. In *Psychopathology. The Evolving Science of Mental Disorder* (Eds S. Mathysse, D.L. Levy, J. Kapan, F.M. Benes), pp. 511–538, Cambridge University Press, Cambridge.
17. Sadler J.Z., Wiggins O.P., Schwartz M.A. (1994) *Philosophical Perspectives on Psychiatric Diagnostic Classification*. Johns Hopkins University Press, Baltimore.
18. Hempel C.G. (1965) *Aspects of Scientific Explanation and Other Essays in the Philosophy of Science*. Free Press, New York.
19. Churchland P.S. (1986) *Neurophilosophy: Toward a Unified Science of the Mind/Brain*. MIT Press, Cambridge.
20. American Psychiatric Association (1980) *Diagnostic and Statistical Manual of Mental Disorders*, 3rd edn. American Psychiatric Association, Washington.
21. Putnam H. (1987) *The Many Faces of Realism*. Open Court, LaSalle.
22. van Praag H.M. (1992) Reconquest of the subjective. Against the waning of psychiatric diagnosing. *Br. J. Psychiatry*, **160**: 266–271.
23. Maj M. (1998) Critique of the DSM-IV operational diagnostic criteria for schizophrenia. *Br. J. Psychiatry*, **172**: 458–460.
24. Spitzer M. (1988) Psychiatry, philosophy, and the problem of description. In *Psychopathology and Philosophy* (Eds M. Spitzer, F.A. Uehlein, G. Oepen), pp. 3–18. Springer, Berlin.
25. Dennett D.C. (1991) *Consciousness Explained*. Little Brown, New York.
26. Husserl E. (1952) *Ideen zu Einer Reinen Phänomenologie und Phänomenologischen Philosophie II. Husserliana IV*. Martinus Nijhoff, Den Haag.
27. Heidegger M. (1962) *Being and Time*. Translated by J. MacQuarrie, E. Robinson. Harper & Row, New York.
28. Merleau-Ponty M. (1945) *Phénoménologie de la Perception*. Gallimard, Paris.
29. Wittgenstein L. (1961) *Tractatus Logico-Philosophicus*. Routledge and Kegan Paul, London.

30. Zahavi D., Parnas J. (1998) Phenomenal consciousness and self-awareness. A phenomenological critique of representational theory. *J. Consciousness Studies*, **5**: 687–705.
31. Henry M. (2000) *Incarnation. Une philosophie de la chair*. Seuil, Paris.
32. Zahavi D. (1999) *Self-Awareness and Alterity. A Phenomenological Investigation*. Northwestern University Press, Evanstone.
33. Flanagan O. (1992) *Consciousness Reconsidered*. MIT Press, Cambridge.
34. Damasio A. (1999) *The Feeling of What Happens*. Harcourt, San Diego.
35. Ricoeur P. (1990) *Soi-même comme un autre*. Seuil, Paris.
36. Husserl E. (1966) *Analysen zur Passiven Synthesis. Husserliana XI*. Martinus Nijhoff, The Hague.
37. Husserl E. (1966) *Zur Phänomenologie des Inneren Zeitbewußtseins (1893–1917). Husserliana X*. Martinus Nijhoff, The Hague.
38. Gibson J.J. (1979) *The Ecological Approach to Visual Perception*. Lawrence Erlbaum, Hillsdale.
39. Sartre J.-P. (1976) *L'Être et le Néant*. Gallimard, Paris.
40. Gallagher S. (1986) Body image and body schema: a conceptual clarification. *J. Mind Behav.*, **7**: 541–554.
41. Husserl E. (1973) *Zur Phänomenologie der Intersubjektivität II. Husserliana XIV*. Martinus Nijhoff, The Hague.
42. Marbach E. (1993) *Mental Representation and Consciousness. Towards a Phenomenological Theory of Representation and Reference*. Kluwer, Dordrecht.
43. Cantor N, Smith E.E., French R. (1980) Psychiatric diagnosis as prototype categorization. *J. Abnorm. Psychol.*, **89**: 181–193.
44. Schwartz M.A., Wiggins O.P. (1987) Diagnosis and ideal types: a contribution to psychiatric classification. *Compr. Psychiatry*, **28**: 277–291.
45. Hanson N.R. (1965) *The Patterns of Discovery: An Inquiry into the Conceptual Foundations of Science*. Cambridge University Press, Cambridge.
46. Rosch E. (1973) Natural categories. *Cogn. Psychol.*, **8**: 328–350.
47. Rosch E. (1999) Reclaiming concepts. In *Reclaiming Cognition. The Primacy of Action, Intention and Emotion* (Eds R. Nunez, W.J. Freeman), pp. 61–78, Imprint Academic, Thorverton.
48. Lakoff G. (1987) *Women, Fire, and Dangerous Things: What Categories Reveal About the Mind*. University of Chicago Press, Chicago.
49. Weber M. (1949) *The Methodology of Social Sciences*. Free Press, New York.
50. Minkowski E. (1997) *Au-delà du Rationalisme Morbide*. L'Harmattan, Paris.
51. Kraus A. (1994) Phenomenological and criteriological diagnosis: different or complementary? In *Philosophical Perspectives on Psychiatric Diagnostic Classification* (Eds J.Z. Sadler, O.P. Wiggins, M.A. Schwartz), pp. 148–162. Johns Hopkins University Press, Baltimore.
52. Parnas J., Bovet P. (1991) Autism in schizophrenia revisited. *Compr Psychiatry*, **32**: 7–21.
53. Tatossian A. (1979) *Phénoménologie des Psychoses*. Masson, Paris.
54. Bovet P., Parnas J. (1993) Schizophrenic delusions. A phenomenological approach. *Schizophr. Bull.*, **19**: 579–597.
55. Sass L.A. (1994) *The Paradoxes of Delusion: Wittgenstein, Schreber, and the Schizophrenic Mind*. Cornell University Press, Ithaca.
56. Parnas J. (2000) Genetics and psychopathology of spectrum phenotypes. *Acta Psychiatr. Scand.*, **101**: 413–415.

57. Mishara A., Parnas J., Naudin J. (1998) Forging the links between phenomenology, cognitive neuroscience, and psychopathology: the emergence of a new discipline. *Curr. Opin. Psychiatry*, **11**: 567–573.
58. Parnas J., Jansson L., Sass L.A., Handest P. (1998) Self-experience in the prodromal phases of schizophrenia. *Neurol. Psychiatry Brain Res.*, **6**: 97–106.
59. Parnas J. (2000) The Self and intentionality in the pre-psychotic stages of schizophrenia. A phenomenological study. In *Exploring the Self* (Ed. D. Zahavi), pp. 115–147. John Benjamins Publishing Company, Amsterdam.
60. Møller P., Husby R. (2000) The initial prodrome in schizophrenia: searching for naturalistic core dimensions of experience and behavior. *Schizophr. Bull.*, **26**: 217–232.
61. Gallagher S. (2000) Self-reference and schizophrenia: a cognitive model of immunity to error through misidentification. In *Exploring the Self* (Ed. D. Zahavi), pp. 203–242. John Benjamins Publishing Company, Amsterdam.
62. Parnas J. (2002) Anomalous self-experience in early schizophrenia: a clinical perspective. In *Self and Schizophrenia: A Neuropsychological Perspective* (Eds T. Kircher, A. David). Cambridge University Press, Cambridge, in press.
63. Parnas J. (1999) On defining schizophrenia. In *Schizophrenia* (Eds M. Maj, N. Sartorius), pp. 43–45. Wiley, Chichester.
64. Parnas J. (1999) From predisposition to psychosis: progression of symptoms in schizophrenia. *Acta Psychiatr. Scand.*, **100** (Suppl. 395): 20–29.
65. Parnas J. (1999) The boundaries of the schizotypal disorders and schizophrenia. In: *One World, One Language. Paving the Way to Better Perspectives for Mental Health* (Eds J. Lopez-Ibor, F. Lieh-Mak, H.M. Visotsky, M. Maj), pp. 164–169. Hogrefe & Huber, Göttingen.

Multiaxial Diagnosis in Psychiatry

Juan E. Mezzich[1], Aleksandar Janca[2] and Marianne C. Kastrup[3]

[1]*Division of Psychiatric Epidemiology and International Center for Mental Health, Mount Sinai School of Medicine of New York University, New York, NY, USA*
[2]*Department of Psychiatry and Behavioural Science, University of Western Australia, Perth, Australia*
[3]*International Rehabilitation and Research Center for Torture Victims, Copenhagen, Denmark*

INTRODUCTION

Diagnosis, as a central concept and activity in psychiatry and general medicine, is aimed at providing the basis for effective clinical care. To fulfil this fundamental role, a diagnostic statement must be adequately informative about the patient's condition.

Conventional approaches have aimed at identifying the main disorder of the patient (the single label model). This model has been considered insufficient in many circles [1, 2], which have pointed out its limitations in addressing the complexity of clinical conditions. These considerations have led to the proposal of more comprehensive diagnostic models, with the hope of providing a more complete and informative delineation of the patient's pathology and its contextualization.

The comprehensive diagnostic model that has received most attention over the past few decades has been the multiaxial diagnostic approach. It can be defined as the approach aimed at describing the patient's overall clinical condition through the systematic assessment and formulation of highly informative clinical axes or domains. In contrast to general narrative statements of comprehensive content, the multiaxial model ensures that all key domains are covered and that they are assessed and formulated in a structured manner [3].

A main purpose of the multiaxial diagnostic formulation is to create the basis for a comprehensive treatment plan as well as to facilitate and optimize the longitudinal reassessment of the patient's condition and contribute

Psychiatric Diagnosis and Classification. Edited by Mario Maj, Wolfgang Gaebel, Juan José López-Ibor and Norman Sartorius. © 2002 John Wiley & Sons, Ltd.

to a refinement of the validity of clinical diagnosis. The assumption is that, by providing a more detailed holistic picture of the patient's current condition, there is a better ground for planning treatment and determining prognosis. While the development of multiaxial systems continues, more encompassing comprehensive diagnostic models are emerging. They include multiaxial schemas supplemented by narrative statements focused on cultural framework or the uniqueness of the person of the patient.

This chapter presents an examination of the development of the multiaxial model, of experience obtained with established multiaxial diagnostic schemas, as well as of some of the newest comprehensive approaches.

EARLY USE OF MULTIAXIAL DIAGNOSIS

The first published attempts to introduce a systematic, multiaspect approach to psychiatric classification were made by Essen-Möller and Wohlfahrt in Sweden [4] and Lecomte *et al.* in France [5], who proposed an innovative model for the classification of mental disorders involving the separation of the description of psychiatric syndromes from their aetiology. These pioneering biaxial schemas were shortly followed by triaxial ones (psychiatric syndromes, personality conditions, and biopsychosocial aetiopathogenic constellations) published by Bilikiewicz in Poland [6] and Leme Lopes in Brazil [7]. These schemas served as a basis for the development of numerous other multiaspectual approaches suitable for providing more systematic and comprehensive characterization of different and separately assessed domains of the psychiatric patient's clinical condition.

The above-mentioned early proposals stimulated two decades later considerable creative interest in multiaxial diagnosis and assessment in psychiatry, including the development of several multiaxial systems for use in adult psychiatry, child and adolescent psychiatry, and old age psychiatry. Most of these systems were composed of either four or five axes and represented an elaboration of the two main aspects of mental disorders, i.e. their phenomenology, on one side, and the associated biological and psychosocial factors, on the other.

Biopsychosocial perspectives were embedded in a number of early multiaxial systems in psychiatry, including Ottosson and Perris's multidimensional classification of mental disorders [8], Strauss' pentaxial system [9], multiaxial systems and approaches to psychiatric classification proposed by Helmchen [10], Von Knorring *et al.* [11], and Bech *et al.* [12], Rutter *et al.*'s triaxial classification of mental disorders in childhood [2], and the DSM-III multiaxial system [13]. The specific axes of these multiaxial schemas covered different aspects and domains of the psychiatric patient's clinical condition, such as: general psychiatric syndromes, aetiopathogenetic formulation, personality, psychosocial stressors, physical disorders, illness course, intellectual level or mental retardation, developmental delays, illness severity and adaptive functioning. A comparative tabular presentation of early multiaxial systems in psychiatry is available elsewhere [14].

MULTIAXIAL SCHEMAS IN CURRENT DIAGNOSTIC SYSTEMS: DEVELOPMENT AND CHARACTERISTICS

ICD-10

Schema for Adults

Efforts to design an internationally based multiaxial schema for general psychiatry started during the process of developing the tenth revision of the *International Classification of Diseases (ICD-10)* [15, 16]. After a long process, including empirical studies, a schema emerged covering three different aspects of the psychiatric patient's clinical condition, intended for use in clinical work, research and training of various types of mental health professionals dealing with adult patients suffering from mental disorders. The ICD-10 multiaxial system [17, 18] uses the following three axes: Axis I—Clinical diagnoses; Axis II—Disabilities; and Axis III—Contextual factors.

   Axis I of the system is used to record diagnoses of both mental (including personality) and physical disorders [19]. Axis II covers disabilities resulting from the disorders recorded on Axis I, assessed through the World Health Organization (WHO) Short Disability Assessment Schedule (WHO DAS-S) —a brief semi-structured instrument intended for assessment and rating by clinicians of difficulties in maintaining personal care, in performance of occupational tasks, and in functioning in relation to family and broader social context due to mental and physical disorders [20].

   Axis III comprises all factors that, without being disorders themselves, contribute to the occurrence, presentation or course of the disorders recorded on Axis I or require professional attention. The factors take their origin in the ICD-10 Z categories, i.e. factors influencing health status and contact with health services [21] and are grouped in the following categories:

1. Problems related to negative events in childhood and upbringing.
2. Problems related to education and literacy.
3. Problems related to primary support group.
4. Problems related to social environment.
5. Problems related to housing or economic circumstances.
6. Problems related to (un)employment.
7. Problems related to physical environment.

8. Problems related to certain psychosocial circumstances.
9. Problems related to legal circumstances.
10. Problems related to family history of diseases.
11. Lifestyle and life-management problems.

This ICD-10 multiaxial system allows quick and simultaneous assessment of the patient's clinical condition, resulting disability and contributing contextual factors. It also minimizes the distinction between mental and "nonmental" disorders and encourages the user to employ as many ICD-10 codes as necessary to describe the patient's clinical condition. The ICD-10 multiaxial system has been suggested as potentially useful for inpatient and outpatient psychiatric settings, whenever a global and comprehensive clinical assessment of the patient is required in a limited amount of time.

Between 1993 and 1995, the cross-cultural applicability and reliability of the ICD-10 multiaxial system were explored through two WHO-coordinated international field trials involving 20 countries spanning all the regions of the world. The majority of the clinicians involved perceived the ICD-10 multiaxial system to be easy to apply and potentially useful in clinical work, research and training of mental health professionals belonging to different psychiatric schools and traditions [17].

Schema for Children

The development of an ICD-based multiaxial approach to the classification of child and adolescent psychiatric disorders was initiated by Rutter *et al.* [2]. The most recent version of this multiaxial schema for use in child and adolescent psychiatry [22] has been linked to the ICD-10 [23] and is composed of the following axes: Axis I—Clinical psychiatric syndromes; Axis II—Specific disorders of psychological development; Axis III—Intellectual level; Axis IV—Medical conditions from ICD-10 often associated with mental and behavioral disorders; Axis V—Associated abnormal psychosocial situations; and Axis VI—Global assessment of psychosocial functioning. The first four axes of this system use precisely the same diagnostic categories and codes as in ICD-10, but the categories have been placed in somewhat different order for a better fit within this multiaxial format. For example, those most applicable to children and adolescents appear first. Axis V comprises a set of selected ICD-10 Z00–Z99 categories or factors influencing health status and contact with health services. Axis VI reflects the patient's psychological, social and occupational functioning at the time of clinical evaluation and covers disabilities in functioning that have arisen as a consequence of general psychiatric disorder, specific disorders of psychological development or mental retardation.

Proposals for Old Age Patients

Since a WHO meeting on the diagnosis and classification of mental disorders held in Moscow in 1969, there have been a number of recommendations regarding development of a multiaxial classification of mental disorders in old age. The axes were to serve for the recording of clinical psychiatric syndromes, type of cognitive impairment, and severity of the patient's condition in general (i.e. dependence on others for survival). These proposals have not been formalized or field tested yet.

Schemas for Primary Health Care

In order to facilitate and stimulate the recording of psychosocial problems in primary health care, WHO developed a triaxial system that uses the following axes [24]:

1. Psychosocial problem(s).
2. Social problem(s).
3. Physical problem(s).

The design of this simple system was intended to accommodate the considerable variation in the availability and quality of primary care in various parts of the world, a wide range in the professional background, training and experience of primary care workers, and socially engendered variation in the nature and extent of psychosocial problems presented. In spite of these difficulties, the international field test of this multiaxial system, carried out as a case vignette rating exercise in seven countries, demonstrated its usefulness for compiling lists and glossaries of psychological and social problems frequently seen in primary care settings in different parts of the world.

DSM-IV

The DSM-IV multiaxial system [25] was developed to facilitate the systematic evaluation of five different domains of information that together may help the clinician plan treatment and predict outcome. The DSM-IV multiaxial schema contains the following axes: Axis I—Clinical disorders and other conditions that may be a focus of clinical attention; Axis II—Personality disorders and mental retardation; Axis III—General medical conditions; Axis IV—Psychosocial and environmental problems; and Axis V—Global assessment of functioning. The reporting of overall functioning on Axis V is based on the Global

Assessment of Functioning (GAF) Scale, which is to be rated with respect to both psychopathological status and social and occupational functioning of the patient using a single measure or score. In view of the fact that in some settings it may be useful to assess social and occupational disabilities separately and to track progress in rehabilitation independent of the severity of the psychiatric condition, three additional Axis V measures were published in the appendix of DSM-IV, i.e. the Social and Occupational Functioning Assessment Scale (SOFAS), the Global Assessment of Relational Functioning (GARF) Scale, and the Defensive Functioning Scale.

As can be seen from its structure and accompanying scales, the DSM-IV multiaxial system appears to provide a convenient format for organizing and communicating clinical information, for capturing the complexity of clinical situations, and for describing the heterogeneity of individuals presenting with the same psychiatric disorders.

Chinese Classification of Mental Disorders, third edition (CCMD-3)

A serious attempt to adapt ICD-10 to Chinese clinical reality commenced with the preparation of the *Chinese Classification of Mental Disorders*, second edition, revised (CCMD-2-R) by the Chinese Medical Association, as discussed by Lee [26]. It has been used extensively throughout China, and this experience revealed a number of problems with it [27]. On the basis of this, a new edition of the Chinese adaptation of ICD-10 has been started, under the denomination of CCMD-3 [28]. Its main objective is to improve psychiatric care, with training, research and administration as additional objectives. It includes for the first time a multiaxial schema, with seven axes. The first five axes would be similar to those in DSM-IV, although Axis IV (Psychosocial environmental problems) would be formulated as behavioral problems exacerbated by social context. Axis VI would present a global clinical impression, and Axis VII would cover interrelations among the first six axes [27].

Third Cuban Glossary of Psychiatry (GC-3)

The GC-3 is inscribed within a serial effort to adapt the latest revisions of the ICD to the Cuban reality, i.e. GC-1 was the adaptation of ICD-8, GC-2 the adaptation of ICD-9, and GC-3 that of ICD-10. It has been reported [29, 30] that the preparations of these adaptations have included the participation, through extensive consultations, of most of the psychiatrists and a large number of representatives of other mental health professionals and general practitioners in the island.

The multiaxial schema of the *Third Cuban Glossary of Psychiatry* includes six axes: Axis I—Clinical disorders; Axis II—Disabilities; Axis III—Adverse environmental and personal factors; Axis IV—Other environmental and personal factors; Axis V—Maladaptive mechanisms; Axis VI—Other significant information (tests, therapeutic response).

Attempts are under way to evaluate the usefulness of this schema for clinical care.

REVIEW OF THE USE OF MULTIAXIAL DIAGNOSIS: ITS VALUE AND LIMITATIONS

Critical Review of the Literature on Clinical Care, Training, Research and Administration

When considering the use of a multiaxial approach in daily clinical practice, the time required for routine use is crucial for its applicability on the international scene, where there is often a shortage of adequate mental health services. This concern is particularly pertinent in non-industrialized areas, where professionals frequently work in primary care settings under constraints of both limited personnel and resources. To ensure its successful application, we are faced with the problem of having to strike the right balance between the wish for richness of information, comprehensiveness of disease description, simplicity and a manageable system [16].

Despite international surveys reporting that the multiaxial approach is helpful as well as useful, the use of such systems has not been without problems. Actual use in daily clinical practice can be seen as a good test for its value as a professional instrument and here it has to be recognized that daily use by clinicians of the "non-nosological" axes has been limited, despite an expressed interest in them by the very same clinicians. The particular value in clinical settings has primarily been linked to the elucidation of complex clinical cases, and experiences have paid particular attention to the perceived use in daily clinical practice of the various multiaxial schemas [12, 31, 32].

With an increasing focus on the management of clinical care, cost reduction and efficiency of services, a multivariate approach [33] that provides a systematic scrutiny of clinical information may become increasingly demanded as a means to understand and predict service utilization and cost.

The transformation of psychiatric services, with its reduction in the number of psychiatric beds and the increasing emphasis on community care, has led to careful consideration and need for identification of those groups that either require special attention or are heavy users of mental health services. For such purposes, the utility of a measurement of adaptive functioning is evident in estimating the need for services and in providing a tool for a better allocation of the available mental health services. Yet, the level of functioning and the decision whether to hospitalize or not are found to be clearly correlated [34], and psychiatric patients who are chronically ill are reported to have the lowest premorbid level of functioning [35].

Concerning contextual factors, Salokangas et al. [36] demonstrated a clear association between unmet needs for community care and poor functional status, whereas met needs did not correlate with functional status measured by the Global Assessment Scale. Similarly, it has been demonstrated that recovery from a moderate depression is more closely related to psychosocial circumstances than to the effects of psychopharmacological treatment [37].

The routine use of a multiaxial formulation in daily practice could consequently improve outcome assessment and be a useful tool in daily clinical evaluation. Despite that, we are still seeing that limited research has focused on the interaction between the utilization of services, the severity of the condition, and ratings of adaptive functioning or psychosocial stressors/contextual factors. Also, the predictive value of a multiaxial rating for treatment outcome needs further elucidation.

Moving from the psychiatric field to that of chronic pain, certain similarities are found. It has been emphasized that only by applying a multidimensional or multiaxial (dimensional and categorical domains) approach can the complexity of the pain condition be fully captured, and a unidimensional approach is found to be inadequate in evaluating pain patients [38]. Consequently, a multidimensional perspective is necessary to ensure that adequate treatment is instituted.

Notes from the Comprehensive International Survey on the Use of ICD-10

An international survey on the use of ICD-10 was recently conducted by the WHO Committee on Evaluating and Updating the ICD-10 Mental Health Component, in collaboration with the World Psychiatric Association (WPA) Section on Classification, Diagnostic Assessment, and Nomenclature. It involved the participation of 147 respondents: for the Americas (27), Europe (83), Africa and the Middle East (9), and Asia and the South Pacific (28). A preliminary report was presented at the XI World Congress of Psychiatry [39].

Concerning the multiaxial presentation of ICD-10, 56% of the respondents found it highly or fairly valuable, 12% considered it marginally or not valuable, and 33% did not respond to the corresponding question. Problems were reported in the use of Axis I (5%), Axis II (18%), and Axis III (20%).

Also reported were general problems (12%), most of which referred to lack of access to the WHO publication [17] of the ICD-10 multiaxial schema and to lack of training resources.

Among the most highly rated recommendations for future diagnostic systems, was "to promote the use and training in multiaxial diagnostic formulations", i.e. 53% of the respondents assigned a high rating to this feature, 29% assigned it a medium rating, 5% a low rating, and 12% did not respond to this question.

RECENT DEVELOPMENTS AND PROSPECTS FOR MULTIAXIAL AND COMPREHENSIVE DIAGNOSIS

International Classification of Impairments, Disabilities and Handicaps, second edition

A multidimensional approach has recently been introduced in the second edition of the *International Classification of Impairments, Disabilities and Handicaps*, which is being developed by WHO [40] with the new title of the *International Classification of Functioning and Disability* or ICIDH-2. The new title reflects an emerging focus on social functioning and participation. It provides descriptions of various situations related to human functioning and disability as well as a framework for their recording and coding in a meaningful, interrelated and easily accessible way. ICIDH-2 organizes human functioning and disability-related information according to the following schema:

1. Body level.
2. Individual level.
3. Society level.

The specific dimensions incorporated in the ICIDH-2 are: (i) Body functions and structure; (ii) Activities; and (iii) Participation. These dimensions are reflective of various aspects of body functions and structure, performance of activities, and involvement in life situations. The ICIDH-2 dimensions are conceived as having two poles on a spectrum: at one end they can be used to indicate problems (e.g. impairment, activity limitation or participation restriction); at the other end, they can indicate non-problematic (i.e. neutral and positive) aspects of functional states.

The ICIDH-2 concept of "functioning" is used as an umbrella term for the positive or neutral aspects of dimensions at body, individual and society level. "Disability" is used as an umbrella term for the problems in these dimensions. "Functioning" and "disability" are conceived as reflecting a dynamic interaction between health conditions and contextual factors. Contextual factors include both personal and environmental factors and are seen as an essential component of the classification.

The ICIDH-2 is currently being field tested in numerous countries in different parts of the world.

Attention to the Cultural Framework of Personal Identity, Illness Experience and Clinical Care

A significant attempt to enhance a standardized multiaxial formulation by attending systematically to the cultural framework of the patient's identity, illness experience, support systems, and clinical care encounter is represented by the Cultural Formulation. This was developed by the National Institute of Mental Health (NIMH) Group on Culture, Diagnosis and Care [41] and was published as part of DSM-IV. It includes the following elements:

1. Cultural identity of the individual.
2. Cultural explanations of the individual's illness.
3. Cultural factors related to psychosocial environment and levels of functioning.
4. Cultural elements of the relationship between the individual and the clinician.
5. Overall cultural assessment for diagnosis and care.

A number of journal papers and books are now emerging on the application of the Cultural Formulation to culturally diverse cases in a variety of clinical settings [42–46]. In addition to its specific cultural value, the Cultural Formulation represents a methodological contribution towards a more comprehensive diagnostic model based on the combination of standardized and narrative components [47].

New Comprehensive Diagnostic Models: WPA and APAL Approaches

The WPA, through a multicontinental workgroup and advisors panel, is presently developing the International Guidelines for Diagnostic Assessment (IGDA). A fundamental feature of this approach is to consider the patient in his/her totality and not just as a carrier of a disease. Thus, it advises clinicians through 100 guidelines to consider all key areas of information pertinent to describing the patient's pathology, dysfunctions and problems as well as his/her assets and resources.

Its comprehensive diagnostic model is composed of a Standardized Multiaxial Diagnostic Formulation and a Personalized Idiographic Formulation. The multiaxial formulation in IGDA has four axes. The first three are those of the ICD-10 multiaxial schema [17]. The fourth axis rates quality of life, which is emerging as a major descriptor of health status as well as an outcome measure of clinical care. This Axis IV assesses the patient's self-perceived well-being concerning physical and emotional status, independent, occupational and interpersonal functioning, emotional and instrumental social supports, and a sense of personal and spiritual fulfilment.

The Personalized Idiographic Formulation involves a narrative statement reflecting the joint perspective of the clinician, the patient, and the family with regard to clinical problems and their contextualization, positive factors of the patient, and expectations on restoration and promotion of health.

The development of the IGDA was presented at the XI World Congress of Psychiatry [48] and a booklet on its essentials is scheduled to appear soon.

Reflecting the growing role of organized psychiatry in various parts of the world (consider the US, Chinese, and Cuban efforts described earlier) to respond to the challenge of adopting key international concepts and procedures for effective regional or local use, the Latin American Psychiatric Association (Asociación Psiquiátrica de America Latina, APAL) has established recently as one of its priority projects the preparation of a Latin American Guide for Psychiatric Diagnosis (GLDP) [49]. The workgroup is in the process of annotating the ICD-10 to better address the reality and needs of Latin American populations. Concerning diagnosis, the APAL workgroup plans to use the WPA IGDA diagnostic model (which is built on the ICD-10 multiaxial schema and includes both standardized and idiographic components) as basic reference, and annotate it as needed for optional Latin American use.

CONCLUSIONS

Multiaxial diagnosis represents a comprehensive approach to the fundamental task of describing the patient's condition in a manner faithful to clinical reality and useful for effective clinical care. Its roots are truly international, with growing trends for creative interaction among universal, continental and national levels. More recently, efforts to enhance the validity of diagnosis as well as the ethical responsibilities of the health professionals involved are taking the form of integrating standardized and idiographic formulations. Well-designed validation studies at both international and local levels are needed to appraise empirically the effectiveness of these proposals and guide their further development.

REFERENCES

1. Lain Entralgo P. (1982) *El Diagnóstico Médico*. Salvat, Barcelona.
2. Rutter M., Lebovici S., Eisenberg L., Sneznevskij A.V., Sadoun R., Brooke E., Lin T.Y. (1969) A triaxial classification of mental disorders in childhood. *J. Child Psychol. Psychiatry*, **10**: 41–61.
3. Mezzich J.E. (1979) Patterns and issues in multiaxial diagnosis. *Psychol. Med.*, **9**: 125–137.
4. Essen-Möller E., Wohlfahrt S. (1947) Suggestions for the amendment of the official Swedish classification of mental disorders. *Acta Psychiatr. Scand.*, **47** (Suppl.): 551–555.
5. Lecomte M., Daney A., Delage E., Marty P. (1947) Essai d'une statistique synoptique de médicine psychiatrique. *Techniques Hospitaliers*, **18**: 5–8.
6. Bilikiewicz T. (1951) Próba ukadu nozograficznego etioepigenetycznego w psychiatrii. *Neurologia i Neurochirurgia Polska*, **13**: 68–78.
7. Leme Lopes J. (1954) As dimensões do Diagnóstico Psiquiátrico. Agir, Rio de Janeiro.
8. Ottosson J.O., Perris C. (1973) Multidimensional classification of mental disorders. *Psychol. Med.*, **3**: 238–243.
9. Strauss J.S. (1975) A comprehensive approach to psychiatric diagnosis. *Am. J. Psychiatry*, **132**: 1193–1197.
10. Helmchen H. (1980) Multiaxial systems of classification. *Acta Psychiatr. Scand.*, **61**: 43–45.
11. von Knorring L., Perris C., Jacobsson L. (1978) Multiaspect classification of mental disorders: experiences from clinical routine work and preliminary studies of interrater reliability. *Acta Psychiatr. Scand.*, **58**: 401–412.
12. Bech P., Hjorts S., Lund K., Vilmar T., Kastrup M. (1987) An integration of the DSM-III and ICD-8 by global severity for measuring multidimensional outcomes in general hospital psychiatry. *Acta Psychiatr. Scand.*, **75**: 297–306.
13. American Psychiatric Association (1980) *Diagnostic and Statistical Manual of Mental Disorders*, 3rd edn (DSM-III). American Psychiatric Association, Washington.
14. Mezzich J.E. (1980) Multiaxial diagnostic systems in psychiatry. In *Comprehensive Textbook of Psychiatry*, 3rd edn (Eds H.I. Kaplan, A. Freedman, B.J. Sadock), pp. 1072–1079. Williams and Wilkins, Baltimore.
15. Sartorius N. (1988) International perspectives of psychiatric classification. *Br. J. Psychiatry*, **152** (Suppl. 1): 9–14.
16. Mezzich J.E. (1988) On developing a psychiatric multiaxial schema for ICD-10. *Br. J. Psychiatry*, **152** (Suppl. 1): 38–43.
17. World Health Organization (1997) *Multiaxial Presentation of the ICD-10 for Use in Adult Psychiatry*. Cambridge University Press, Cambridge.
18. Janca A., Kastrup M., Katschnig H., López-Ibor J.J., Jr., Mezzich J.E., Sartorius N. (1996) The ICD-10 multiaxial system for use in adult psychiatry. *J. Nerv. Ment. Dis.*, **184**: 191–192.

19. López-Ibor J.J. (1994) Axial organization of clinical diagnoses. In *Psychiatric Diagnosis: A World Perspective* (Eds J.E. Mezzich, Y. Honda, M.C. Kastrup). Springer, New York.
20. Janca A., Kastrup M., Katschnig H., López-Ibor J.J. Jr., Mezzich J.E., Sartorius N. (1996) The World Health Organization short disability assessment schedule (WHO DAS-S): a tool for the assessment of difficulties in selected areas of functioning of patients with mental disorders. *Soc. Psychiatry Psychiatr. Epidemiol.*, **31**: 349–354.
21. Janca A., Kastrup M., Katschnig H., López-Ibor J.J. Jr., Mezzich J.E., Sartorius N. (1996) Contextual aspects of mental disorders: a proposal for axis III of the ICD-10 multiaxial system. *Acta Psychiatr. Scand.*, **94**: 31–36.
22. World Health Organization (1996) *Multiaxial Classification of Child and Adolescent Psychiatric Disorders*. Cambridge University Press, Cambridge.
23. World Health Organization (1992) *International Statistical Classification of Diseases and Related Health Problems*. World Health Organisation, Geneva.
24. Clare A., Gulbinat W., Sartorius N. (1992) A triaxial classification of health problems presenting in primary health care—a World Health Organization multi-centre study. *Soc. Psychiatry Psychiatr. Epidemiol.*, **27**: 108–116.
25. American Psychiatric Association (1994) *Diagnostic and Statistical Manual of Mental Disorders*, 4th edn (DSM-IV). American Psychiatric Association, Washington.
26. Lee S. (1996) Culture in psychiatric nosology: the CCMD-2-R and the international classification of mental disorders. *Culture, Medicine & Psychiatry*, **20**: 421–472.
27. Chen Y.-F. (1999) Experience with CCMD-2-R and preparation of CCMD-3. Paper presented at the Symposium on the Third Edition of the Chinese Classification of Mental Disorders (CCMD-3), Szhen-Szhen, China, 31 May.
28. Chen Y.-F. (2000) On the development of the Third Edition of the Chinese Classification of Mental Disorders (CCMD-3). Paper presented at the Symposium "Towards Integration in the International Classification", Annual Meeting of the American Psychiatric Association, Chicago, 17 May.
29. Otero A. (1994) *Adaptación Cultural del Esquema Multiaxial de la CIE-10 a través de Ejes Complementarios*. Hospital Psiquiátrico de La Habana, Havana, Cuba.
30. Otero A. (Ed.) (2000) *Tercer Glosario Cubano de Psiquiatría (GC-3)*. Hospital Psiquiátrico de La Habana, Havana, Cuba.
31. Mezzich J.E., Fabrega H., Mezzich A.C. (1985) An international consultation on multiaxial diagnosis. In *Psychiatry—The State of the Art* (Eds P. Pichot, P. Berner, R. Wolfe, K. Thau), pp. 51–56. Plenum Press, London.
32. Williams J.B.W. (1987) Multiaxial diagnosis. In *An Annotated Bibliography of DSM-III* (Eds A.E. Skodol, R.L. Spitzer), pp. 31–36. American Psychiatric Press, Washington.
33. Mezzich J.E. (1991) Architecture of clinical information and prediction of service utilization and cost. *Schizophr. Bull.*, **17**: 469–474.
34. Mezzich J.E., Evanszuck K.J., Mathias R.J., Goffman G.A. (1984) Admission decisions and multiaxial diagnosis. *Arch. Gen. Psychiatry*, **41**: 1001–1004.
35. Gordon R.E., Gordon K.K. (1987) Relating axes IV and V of DSM-III to clinical severity of psychiatric disorders. *Can. J. Psychiatry*, **32**, 423–424.
36. Salokangas R., Palo-oja T., Ojanen M., Kalo K. (1991) Need for community care among psychotic outpatients. *Acta Psychiatr. Scand.*, **84**: 191–196.
37. Ditmann V. (1991) Modern psychiatric classification in research and clinical practice. *Arch. Suisses Neur. Psychiatry*, **142**: 341–353.

38. Turk D.C., Rudy T.E., Stieg R.L. (1988) The disability determination dilemma: toward a multiaxial solution. *Pain*, **34**: 217–229.
39. Mezzich J.E. (1999) A preliminary report on the International Survey on the Use of ICD-10. Paper presented at the WPA Classification Section Symposium on Empirical Assessment of ICD-10, XI World Congress of Psychiatry, Hamburg, 9 August.
40. World Health Organization (1999) *International Classification of Functioning and Disability (ICIDH-2), Beta-2 Draft*. World Health Organization, Geneva.
41. Mezzich J.E., Kleinman A., Fabrega H., Parron D.L. (1996) *Culture and Psychiatric Diagnosis: A DSM-IV Perspective*. American Psychiatric Press, Washington.
42. Lu F.G., Lim R.F., Mezzich J.E. (1995) Issues in the assessment and diagnosis of culturally diverse individuals. In *Annual Review of Psychiatry*, vol. 14 (Eds J. Oldham, M. Riba), pp. 477–510. American Psychiatric Press, Washington.
43. Lim R.F., Lin K.M. (1996) Psychosis following Qi-Gong in a Chinese immigrant. *Culture, Medicine & Psychiatry*, **20**: 369–378.
44. Lewis-Fernandez R. (1996) Cultural formulation of psychiatric diagnosis. *Culture, Medicine & Psychiatry*, **20**: 133–144.
45. Oquendo M.A., Graver R. (1997) Treatment of an Indian woman with major depression by a Latino therapist: Cultural Formulation. *Culture, Medicine & Psychiatry*, **21**: 115–126.
46. Caracci G. (2000) Using the DSM-IV Cultural Formulation to enhance psychodynamic understanding. *Dynamic Psychiatry*, **33**: 245–256.
47. Mezzich J.E. (1995) Cultural Formulation and comprehensive diagnosis. *Psychiatr. Clin. North Am.*, **18**: 649–657.
48. Mezzich J.E., Berganza C.E., von Cranach M., Jorge M.R., Kastrup M.C., Murthy R.S., Okasha A., Pull C., Sartorius N., Skodol A.E., Zaudig M. (1999) On the development of the International Guidelines for Diagnostic Assessment. Paper presented at the XI World Congress of Psychiatry, Hamburg, August.
49. Berganza C.E. (2000) The preparation of the Latin American Guide for Psychiatric Diagnosis (GLDP). Paper presented at the Presidential Symposium "Towards Integration in International Psychiatric Classification", Annual Meeting of the American Psychiatric Association, Chicago, 17 May.

8

Clinical Assessment Instruments in Psychiatry

Charles B. Pull[1], Jean-Marc Cloos[1] and Marie-Claire Pull-Erpelding[2]

[1]*Centre Hospitalier de Luxembourg, Luxembourg*
[2]*Centre OMS Francophone de Formation et de Référence, Luxembourg*

INTRODUCTION

Psychiatric diagnosis depends on the way mental disorders are classified, defined and assessed. In current psychiatric classifications, disorders are arranged in groups according to major common themes or descriptive likeness. Rather than diseases, most mental disorders are in fact viewed as syndromes, i.e. groupings of signs and symptoms based on their frequent co-occurrence, which may suggest a common underlying pathogenesis, course, familial pattern, or treatment selection. To help the clinician to make a diagnosis, mental disorders have been defined using explicit diagnostic criteria and algorithms. For most disorders, the definitions involve exclusion as well as inclusion criteria. To assess the signs and symptoms required for making a diagnosis, a number of clinical assessment instruments have been developed for a variety of purposes and for use by clinicians or interviewers, in different settings.

The present chapter describes the background underlying the development of clinical assessment instruments in psychiatry and reviews the major instruments that have been developed over the past 20 years for the clinical assessment of mental disorders as described in the Research Diagnostic Criteria or RDC [1], in Chapter V(F) of the *International Classification of Diseases and Related Health Problems* or ICD-10 [2, 3], and in the three latest editions of the American Psychiatric Association's *Diagnostic and Statistical Manual of Mental Disorders* [4–6]. The advantages as well as the limits of these instruments are discussed.

Psychiatric Diagnosis and Classification. Edited by Mario Maj, Wolfgang Gaebel, Juan José López-Ibor and Norman Sartorius. © 2002 John Wiley & Sons, Ltd.

PSYCHIATRIC DIAGNOSIS AND DIAGNOSES BUILT ON DIAGNOSTIC CRITERIA

Psychiatric diagnosis and the way in which psychiatric diagnoses are achieved have been considerably influenced by the way in which current diagnostic systems are constructed. Current clinical assessment instruments in psychiatry are of necessity linked to current classification systems and are, to a large degree and in some cases entirely, dependent on the way diagnoses are formulated in ICD-10 or/and DSM-IV. As a consequence, they share many of the advantages and limits that are inherent in the classification systems of today.

The classifications of mental disorders are based on two types of criteria: pathogenetic criteria and descriptive criteria. The adoption of one or the other type of criteria defines two fundamentally different psychopathological models. The first is grounded in the concept of disease and presumes the existence of natural disease entities that are defined mainly by their aetiology and their pathogenesis. The second relies on the description of syndromes, i.e. on a constellation of signs and symptoms that occur together more frequently than would be expected by a chance distribution.

The general approach taken in both ICD-10 and DSM-IV is atheoretical with regard to aetiology or pathophysiological process, except for those disorders for which this is well established and therefore included in the definition of the disorder. All of the disorders without known aetiology or pathophysiological process are grouped together on the basis of shared clinical features. The descriptive approach adopted in ICD-10 and DSM-IV to define mental disorders and to differentiate each disorder from any other disorders mainly relies on criteria such as signs and symptoms considered to be characteristic of the disorder, their duration and frequency of appearance, the order of their appearance relative to the onset of other signs and symptoms, their severity and their impact on social functioning.

Until recently, mental disorders were briefly defined in glossaries and described more extensively in textbooks. However, neither glossaries nor textbooks provided any rules for combining signs and symptoms into diagnoses. In the early 1970s, a group of clinicians associated with the Washington University in St. Louis [7] developed explicit diagnostic criteria for a limited number of disorders and proposed specific algorithms for making psychiatric diagnoses. Beginning with the third edition, the procedure has been adopted in the *Diagnostic and Statistical Manual of Mental Disorders* to define most mental disorders, and it is also used in one of the versions of ICD-10.

The procedure consists in defining mental disorders using explicit inclusion and exclusion criteria. It implies that decisions be taken concerning the nature and number of individual signs and symptoms, the frequency with which they occur, their duration as well as the importance given to each sign and symptom for making a diagnosis.

The definition of mental disorders involves monothetic as well as polythetic criteria sets. In monothetic criteria sets all of the items must be present for the diagnosis to be made, whereas with polythetic criteria sets the diagnosis may be made even if the presentation includes only a proportion of the items that are proposed to define a disorder. There are advantages as well as disadvantages in using either set of criteria. Monothetic criteria tend to enhance the homogeneity of groups of patients. They do however exclude items that may be clinically useful but which are not always present and they carry the implication that diagnostic features are more pathognomonic than is usually the case. Polythetic criteria allow for greater variation, but they also allow for more heterogeneity.

On the whole, the procedure implies a strict adherence to a "diagnostic grammar" [8], according to which any imprecision is considered a "mistake" or "error". Formulations such as "often", "persistent", "most of the time", "acute", or "several" are not exact statements, and need to be corrected.

Explicit diagnostic criteria become operational diagnostic criteria when every single operation involved in their assessment has been explicitly and comprehensively defined [9]. Individual criteria are translated into one or more questions that should allow a rigorous assessment of the various components that are included in the criterion. The questions are intended to highlight the presence or absence of a given sign or symptom, to determine whether they are clinically significant, to determine their duration and onset, to verify whether they represent a significant deviation from a previous premorbid state or whether they had always been present, and to establish that they are part of a specific mental disorder and cannot be attributed to a physical illness or the use of a psychoactive substance.

ASSESSMENT OF PSYCHIATRIC DIAGNOSES BUILT ON EXPLICIT DIAGNOSTIC CRITERIA

Psychiatric diagnoses built on explicit diagnostic criteria may be assessed using standard clinical examination, with the help of diagnostic checklists, or through semi-structured or fully structured diagnostic instruments. In some instances, it may be useful to have the patient (or proband) fill out a diagnostic questionnaire prior to a clinical examination or/and assessment with a structured or semi-structured interview.

In everyday clinical practice, clinicians examine their patients and make diagnoses following their understanding and recollection of the definitions laid down in one of the two current classification systems. From time to time, they will check the definitions of a glossary, the descriptions of a textbook or the explicit criteria provided in the manuals of current classifications prior to making a diagnosis.

Diagnostic checklists reproduce the diagnostic criteria proposed in one or the other or in both current diagnostic systems. At the end of a psychiatric examination, the clinician checks whether the criteria for one or more potential diagnoses are met.

Semi-structured interviews provide questions that are intended to help the clinician to elicit the presence or absence of any sign and symptom included in a diagnostic criterion. The interviewer, who must be a fully trained clinician, has, however, considerable leeway for asking additional questions and for proceeding with the interview as he or she deems best.

In fully structured diagnostic interviews, questions are asked as laid down in the interview. There is no need for the interviewer to ask for additional information or to interpret the answers of the respondent. As such, fully structured interviews can be administered by trained lay interviewers.

Diagnostic questionnaires are lists of items related to the diagnosis of one or more disorders. The individual items are statements that may apply to respondents and to which they are invited to respond accordingly with yes or no, true or false. The answers provide information concerning the presence or absence of psychopathology or suggest the presence or absence of a specific disorder. The clinician may use this information to guide the examination and to probe in detail for the presence of elements of psychopathology or specific disorders. Diagnostic instruments may be used as screening instruments for psychiatric diagnosis. They do not, however, provide diagnoses themselves.

In addition to the signs and symptoms required for making a psychiatric diagnosis, the clinician may wish to collect additional information that may be of interest with regard to the diagnosis of a mental disorder. In particular, the degree of disablement that is associated with specific mental disorders or with psychopathology in general can be assessed using semi-structured or fully structured interviews.

DIAGNOSTIC CHECKLISTS

Diagnostic checklists are designed to guide the clinician in the assessment of diagnosis. The clinician is, however, on his or her own for phrasing the necessary questions and for assessing the clinical significance of positive answers.

At the end of a comprehensive psychiatric interview, the clinician checks the presence or absence of the criteria required for one or more diagnoses that he or she considers to be relevant, and follows the algorithms laid down for these diagnoses in the diagnostic system(s) covered in the instrument. Diagnostic checklists do not provide any information on how to assess the individual criteria that are required for a diagnosis. In particular, they do not include any questions for assessing the signs and symptoms that have to be present for a criterion to be positive.

The Lists of Integrated Criteria for the Evaluation of Taxonomy (LICET-S and LICET-D)

The Lists of Integrated Criteria for the Evaluation of Taxonomy or LICET are polydiagnostic checklists of criteria, one for schizophrenia and other non-affective psychoses (LICET-S), the other for depressive disorders (LICET-D) [10]. LICET-S assembles all the criteria required in 12 diagnostic systems for a diagnosis of schizophrenia and other psychotic disorders. LICET-D reproduces all the criteria required in 9 diagnostic systems for a diagnosis of a number of subtypes of depressive disorder. At the end of a comprehensive examination, and using all relevant additional information that may be available, clinicians are invited to check the presence or absence of 78 (LICET-S) or 100 (LICET-D) criteria. The results are analyzed by hand, by following the flow charts corresponding to each of the systems included in the lists, or by using a simple computer program.

The lists were used in two nationwide investigations. The aim of the first survey was to elucidate the criteria used by French psychiatrists for a diagnosis of schizophrenia, as well as for other psychotic disorders that they considered to be different from schizophrenia, i.e. several types of acute and transitory psychotic disorders such as "bouffée délirante", and different types of chronic psychotic disorders, such as chronic hallucinatory psychosis [11]. The results led to definitions based on explicit criteria for a number of French diagnostic categories. The definitions proved extremely useful to explain traditional French diagnostic practices to psychiatrists outside of France. In addition, the definitions allowed French psychiatrists to understand the ways in which they differed from non-French clinicians, which in turn proved very helpful in paving the way for the acceptance of international diagnostic systems in France.

The second survey [12] was intended to elucidate French diagnostic practices in the field of depression. The results of the study led to a proposal of explicit diagnostic criteria for "depression" and for differentiating between "psychotic" and "non-psychotic" depression.

Operational Criteria Checklist (OPCRIT)

The Operational Criteria Checklist or OPCRIT is a checklist of criteria for affective and psychotic disorders [13]. It is a polydiagnostic instrument that generates diagnoses according to the explicit criteria and algorithms of 13 diagnostic systems. In addition to the criteria and algorithms of ICD-10, DSM-III, DSM-III-R and DSM-IV, the OPCRIT includes the St. Louis or Feighner criteria for schizophrenia, the RDC, Schneider's first rank symptoms [14], the Taylor and Abrams [15] criteria, the Carpenter or "flexible" criteria [16], the French empirical diagnostic criteria for non-affective psychoses, and three criteria sets for subtyping schizophrenia.

The original version of the OPCRIT has been updated several times. The current version contains 90 items. It has a glossary of descriptions for each item and instructions for coding them.

The original version as well as subsequent versions of the OPCRIT have been shown to have good inter-rater reliability within all the diagnostic systems that have been included in the instrument [17]. The concurrent validity of the OPCRIT has been investigated by Craddock et al. [18]. Good to excellent agreement was achieved between OPCRIT diagnoses and those made by consensus best-estimate procedures.

The OPCRIT checklist is included within the Diagnostic Interview for Genetic Studies (DIGS) (see below).

The ICD-10 Symptom Checklist for Mental Disorders

The ICD-10 Symptom Checklist has been developed by Janca et al. [19–21]. The checklist provides individual lists of the main psychiatric symptoms and syndromes included in the criteria that are required for making diagnoses pertaining to the F0 to F6 categories of the ICD-10. Symptoms are grouped into four modules: organic and psychoactive substance use syndromes (categories included in sections F0 and F1 of the ICD-10); psychotic and affective syndromes (F2 and F3); neurotic and behavioral syndromes (F4 and F5); and personality disorders (F6). In addition to the listing of symptoms, the modules contain items for recording onset, severity and duration of the syndrome as well as the number of episodes where applicable. The modules also list symptoms and states which should be excluded before making a positive diagnosis. Completing the checklist takes about 15 minutes. No specific training is required for an experienced clinician. The instrument is available in a dozen languages.

For checking and assessing in more detail any diagnostic categories included in the F4 section of the ICD, the authors have developed a special, expanded module, the Somatoform Disorders Symptom Checklist, which covers symptoms of somatoform disorders and neurasthenia. In addition to the listing of all relevant criteria, the module operationalizes the criteria for somatoform disorders and includes a simple algorithm that enables clinicians to score specific categories of somatoform disorders according to ICD-10.

The International Diagnostic Checklists (IDCL)

The International Diagnostic Checklists [22] are two sets of pocket-sized lists, one for checking diagnoses according to ICD-10, the other for checking diagnoses according to DSM-IV. Each list contains the criteria for a specific ICD-10 or DSM-IV category, together with coding boxes for rating their presence or absence, and instructions for making a diagnostic decision. Each list is two to four pages long. The ICD-10 set contains 30 checklists for making diagnoses according to ICD-10, the DSM-IV set contains 30 diagnostic checklists for making diagnoses according to DSM-IV.

The IDCL have been developed for use in routine clinical care. Use of the IDCL does not require that the clinician follow any standardized assessment procedure. Clinicians are free to proceed with their assessments as they would in their usual clinical practice. They are encouraged to include information obtained from informants and other sources, e.g. hospital records.

The IDCL are a revised version of the Munich Diagnostic Checklists (MDCL), which were developed for assessing diagnoses according to DSM-III-R. Reliability of MDCL diagnoses for DSM-III-R disorders was evaluated by Hiller *et al.* [23]. For most disorders, diagnostic agreement was good to excellent, with kappas ranging above 0.60.

DIAGNOSTIC SEMI-STRUCTURED INTERVIEWS FOR AXIS I DISORDERS

Several semi-structured interviews have been developed to assist the trained clinician in making diagnoses according to the RDC, DSM-IV Axis I disorders and disorders coded F1–F5 in ICD-10.

The Schedule for Affective Disorders and Schizophrenia (SADS)

The Schedule for Affective Disorders and Schizophrenia (SADS) is a semi-structured psychiatric interview developed in the mid-1970s. It merged out of the NIMH Collaborative Program on the Psychobiology of Depression, but has content derived from earlier studies such as the US–UK project [24]. It was specifically developed to provide investigators using the RDC with a clinical procedure reducing information variance in both diagnostic and descriptive evaluations of subjects [25].

The SADS is available in three major complementary versions. The *SADS regular* allows in Part I a detailed description of the features of the current episodes of illness when they were at their most severe and a similar description of the major psychopathologic features during the week prior to the evaluation, which can then be used as a measure of change. In Part II the interview allows a detailed description of past psychopathology and functioning relevant to the evaluation of diagnosis, prognosis and overall severity of disturbance, and provides a series of questions and criteria allowing the formulation of diagnoses according to the RDC (Table 8.1).

The *change version* (SADS-C) is designed for re-interviewing a previously interviewed study subject, and the *lifetime version* (SADS-L) merges the current and past symptomatology sections of the interview, allowing a more "longitudinal" completion of the interview with non-disordered or recovered respondents. Finally, *a version for children and adolescents* has recently been published [26].

The SADS has been used widely as a gold standard for clinical assessment. Its initial application was in clinical studies where accurate diagnosis is essential to treatment evaluation. The first application to a community sample was made by Weissman *et al.* in 1975 [27].

The Structured Clinical Interview for DSM-IV Axis I Disorders (SCID-I)

The Structured Clinical Interview for DSM-IV Axis I Disorders (SCID-I) is a semi-structured interview originally developed by Spitzer and Williams to assess DSM-III and DSM-III-R criteria [28, 29]. The interview was originally designed to meet the needs of both researchers and clinicians. This duality of purpose created problems for researchers because a lot of potentially useful specifiers were left out of the DSM-III-R version, and, on the other hand, clinicians still felt that the amount of detail included made the interview too long and complex. The SCID-I therefore comes in two versions: Clinician Version (SCID-CV) and Research Version.

The *Clinician Version* [30] is a streamlined version of the SCID-I available from the American Psychiatric Press (http://www.appi.org, see the category "DSM-IV library"). It is an adaptation of the SCID that is intended to introduce the benefits of structured interviewing into clinical settings. It is published in two parts: a reusable administration booklet (with color-coded tabs) and one-time-use-only scoresheets. The SCID-CV is divided into six relatively self-contained modules: (a) mood episodes; (b) psychotic symptoms; (c) psychotic disorders; (d) mood disorders; (e) substance use disorders; and (f) anxiety and other disorders. Seven diagnostic categories are not addressed (i.e. developmental disorders, sleep disorders, factitious disorders, organic mental disorders, sexual disorders, and impulse control disorders). The SCID-CV can be used partially to confirm and document a suspected DSM-IV diagnosis or be administered completely to evaluate systematically all of

TABLE 8.1 Examples of items of the Schedule for Affective Disorders and Schizophrenia (SADS)*

Example of a SADS item in Part I (current episode)

Discouragement, pessimism and hopelessness	0	No information
Have you been discouraged (pessimistic, felt hopelessness)?	1	Not at all discouraged about the future
What kind of future do you see for yourself?	2	Slight, e.g. occasional feelings of mild discouragement about the future
(How do you think things will work out?)	3	Mild, e.g. often somewhat discouraged
(Can you see yourself or your situation getting any better?)	4	Moderate, e.g. often feels quite pessimistic about future
	5	Severe, e.g. pervasive feelings of intense pessimism
	6	Extreme, e.g. delusions or hallucinations that he is doomed, or that the world is coming to an end
(What about during the past week?)	PAST WEEK 0 1 2 3 4 5 6	

Example of a SADS item in Part II (historical information)

Has had 1 or more distinct periods lasting at least 1 week during which he was bothered by depressed or irritable mood or had a pervasive loss of interest or pleasure	0	No information or not sure or part of simple grief reaction
	1	No
	2	Yes

Did you ever have a period that lasted at least 1 week when you were bothered by feeling depressed, sad, blue, hopeless, down in the dumps, that you didn't care anymore, or didn't enjoy anything?

What about feeling irritable or easily annoyed?

---

*Reproduced by permission of the American Psychiatric Press from Endicott and Spitzer (1978). A diagnostic interview: the Schedule for Affective Disorders and Schizophrenia. *Arch. Gen. Psychiatry* **35**: 837–844.

the major Axis-I diagnoses. A user's guide including role-play and homework cases provides basic training in the use of the instrument [31].

Table 8.2 presents the two columns of the SCID-CV for the assessment of the first criterion of a DSM-IV major depressive episode.

The *SCID-I Research Version* and the SCID-CV cover mostly the same disorders, although not at the same level of detail. The biggest advantage of the research version is that it is much easier to modify for a particular study and its coverage is more complete (i.e. it includes the full diagnostic criteria for the disorders and subtypes).

TABLE 8.2   Example of a question from the Structured Clinical Interview for DSM-IV Axis I Disorders, Clinician Version (SCID-CV)*

Major depressive episode—criterion 1	
In the past month . . . . . . has there been a period of time when you were feeling depressed or down most of the day, nearly every day? (What was that like?) IF YES: How long did it last? (As long as 2 weeks?)	(1) depressed mood most of the day, nearly every day, as indicated by either subjective report (e.g. feels sad or empty) or observation made by others (e.g. appears tearful). Note: In children and adolescents, can be irritable mood

*Reproduced by permission of the American Psychiatric Press from First *et al.* (1997). *User's Guide for the Structured Clinical Interview for DSM-IV Axis I Disorders—Clinician Version (SCID-CV).*

There are three editions of the SCID Research Version for DSM-IV [32]:

1. The SCID-I/P (Patient Edition) is the standard patient version with a complete coverage of psychotic symptoms.
2. The SCID-I/P (w/Psychotic Screen) (Patient Edition, with psychotic screening module) is a patient version with a highly abbreviated coverage of psychotic symptoms, which is used in some outpatient settings where psychotic disorders are expected to be rare.
3. The SCID-I/NP (Non-patient Edition) is aimed at studies of non-clinical populations (e.g. community surveys, family studies, research in primary care).

The SCID-I/P is starting with an overview section (sociodemographic data, current problems and symptoms, treatment history, and chart of significant life events), followed by a summary score sheet (lifetime and current diagnoses, and Global Assessment Functioning Scale or GAF), and nine modules for the disorders. The organization of the modules is hierarchical, with explicit decision trees to show when to discontinue administration of each module. The interviewer scores individual symptoms in the following ways: "inadequate information (?)", "absent/false (1)", "subthreshold (2)" (i.e. the criterion is nearly met), and "threshold/true (3)" (i.e. the criterion is met). Practically all symptoms are rated for the current episode. Moreover, clinicians are requested to make several additional distinctions: ratings of both current and past episodes are required for mood disorders, judgements regarding aetiology (organic/not organic) are asked for psychotic symptoms and mood syndromes. Interviewers are encouraged to use all sources of clinical data when rating the interview.

Reliability and validity of the SCID for DSM-III-R have been reported in several studies [33]. The range in reliability is enormous, depending on the nature of the sample and the research methodology (i.e. joint vs. test–retest, multi-site vs. single site with raters who have worked together, etc.). There are more than 500 reports of published studies in which the SCID was the diagnostic instrument. Major parts of the SCID have been translated into Spanish, French, German, Danish, Italian, Hebrew, Zulu, Turkish, Portuguese and Greek.

Administrating the SCID-I to a psychiatric patient usually takes between one and two hours, depending on the complexity of the psychiatric history and the subject's ability to clearly describe episodes of current and past psychopathology. A SCID-I with a non-patient takes 30 to 90 minutes.

A number of computer-based assessment tools that complement the SCID are being developed by Multi-Health Systems (http://www.mhs.com/). These include a computer-administered version of the SCID-CV and the SCID-I (Research Version), called the CAS-CV/CAS-I (Computer-Assisted SCID). Finally, a screening version of the SCID that is administered directly to patients is available (SCID-SCREEN-PQ). More details on the instrument can be obtained from the SCID website (http://cpmcnet.columbia.edu/dept/scid/).

The Schedules for Clinical Assessment in Neuropsychiatry (SCAN)

The Schedules for Clinical Assessment in Neuropsychiatry (SCAN) were developed within the framework of the World Health Organization (WHO) and the National Institute of Mental Health (NIMH) Joint Project on Diagnosis and Classification of Mental Disorders, Alcohol and Related Problems [34]. The Schedules comprise a set of instruments aimed at assessing, measuring and classifying the psychopathology and behavior associated with the major mental disorders of adult life. Administration time averages 60–90 minutes. The current version is 2.1 [35].

The structured clinical interview with semi-standardized probes is based on clinical "cross-examination". The trained clinical interviewer (a psychiatrist or clinical psychologist) decides whether a symptom has been present during the specified time and, if so, with which degree of severity. The assessed periods usually include the "present state", i.e. the month before examination, and the "lifetime before", i.e. any time previously. A "representative period", if particularly characteristic of the patient's illness, may also be chosen.

Even though for most symptoms a form of questioning is suggested, the interview offers considerable flexibility in the chronology and the phrasing of the questions. It is therefore very suitable for patients who are difficult to interview. The interviewer decides what to rate on the basis of the subject's information, always bearing the definitions and rating rules in mind. Each symptom is assessed in its own right, thus allowing comparisons of psychiatric diagnoses to be made across the world, based on the current ICD-10 and DSM-IV systems or other diagnostic systems that may develop in the future.

SCAN has four components: a semi-structured clinical interview schedule (i.e. the tenth edition of the Present State Examination (PSE-10) for SCAN version 2.1), a glossary of differential definitions, an Item Group Checklist (IGC); and a Clinical History Schedule (CHS).

The SCAN core component is the Present State Examination (PSE), which is a guide to structuring a clinical interview. There are nine earlier versions of the PSE tested globally during the past four decades. The ninth edition (PSE-9), translated into more than 35 languages, was the first of the series to be published [36]. It consisted of only 140 items, compared to the 500–600 of PSE-7 and PSE-8. Since many users regretted that the longer preceding versions were withdrawn, PSE-10 (the current SCAN 2.1 interview schedule) is now offering them a choice. PSE-10/SCAN builds on the experience of extensive tests using PSE-9. It retains the main features of PSE-9 and links together the latest two international classification systems (ICD-10 and DSM-IV).

PSE-10 itself has two main parts: Part 1 covers non-psychotic sections, such as physical health, worrying, tension, panic, anxiety and phobias, obsessional symptoms, depressed mood and ideation, impaired thinking, concentration, energy, interests, bodily functions, weight, sleep, eating disorders, alcohol and drug abuse. Part 2 covers the assessment of psychotic and cognitive disorders and abnormalities of behavior, speech and affect (Table 8.3).

TABLE 8.3 Example of a question from the Schedules for Clinical Assessment in Neuropsychiatry (SCAN)

3.00 Worrying

Have you worried a great deal during [PERIOD]?

– What is it like when you worry?
– Do unpleasant thoughts go round and round in your mind?
– Do you worry more than is necessary, given the problem?
– What happens when you try to turn your attention to something else?
– Can you stop worrying by looking at TV or reading or thinking about something you usually enjoy?

A round of painful thought which cannot be stopped and is out of proportion to the topic of worry. Worries "too much" but only in relation to real problems = mild.

The *SCAN glossary* is an essential part of SCAN. Rating is done on the basis of matching the answers of the respondent against the differential definitions of the symptoms and signs in the glossary, which is largely based on the phenomenology of Jaspers. The *Item Group Checklist (IGC)* is a list of 59 item groups rated directly, based on information derived from case notes and informants.

The *Clinical History Schedule (CHS)* consists of sections on childhood and education to age 16, intellectual level, social roles and performances, overall social handicap (disablement), as well as disorders of adult personality and behavior, and physical illnesses or disabilities not entered elsewhere.

SCAN exists in the following languages: Chinese, Danish, Dutch, English, French, German, Greek, Italian, Kannada (India), Portuguese, Spanish, Turkish, Yoruba (Nigeria).

Data from all the schedules are coded on a set of scoring sheets. A diagnostic computer program (CATEGO-5) is available to process the data and score ICD-10 and DSM-IV diagnoses. A computer-assisted PSE version, called CAPSE-2, assists the interviewer in applying SCAN and allows direct entry of ratings at the time of the interview. The program displays questions and ratings in different windows on the screen and, if needed, SCAN glossary definitions can also be referred to.

More recently, WHO developed a computerized version of SCAN 2.1 built on the top of the I-Shell system [37]. This system, which is a "computer aided personal interviewing tool" is already used for several other WHO instruments. The SCAN 2.1 for I-Shell contains all of the SCAN text and SCAN glossary as well as ICD-10 and DSM-IV diagnostic algorithms for SCAN. The SCAN program allows an easy and more accurate collection of data with the help of a user-friendly interface which also provides range checking and a context-sensitive SCAN glossary. The algorithms can be run at any time within the interview even with uncompleted data. The program can display extra information about diagnoses such as how they are calculated, which SCAN items are used for which diagnoses, etc. This kind of information is important especially for testing and improving the diagnostic algorithms. The program is available from the WHO SCAN Homepage (http://www.who.int/msa/scan) and is provided free of charge to those who have done a SCAN course in a WHO training and research center. The addresses of these centers can also be found on the SCAN Homepage.

The training courses last one week and are given by qualified trainers. The set-up is to start with an introductory talk about the "roots" of classification, followed by a walkthrough of the various sections of SCAN and the rating scales. Tapes are shown of (parts of) a SCAN interview, dealing with the various sections. The participants rate the tape and ratings are discussed. The remainder of the week is mainly spent on interviews by the participants with live patients and brief lectures on the various sections. The format of the training course may vary between centers.

Psychometric properties of SCAN 2.1 have been tested and the overall reliability was qualified as moderate to substantial [38]. More information can be found in a reference manual published at Cambridge University Press [39], which can also be used as a companion to the SCAN interview schedule and software. It describes the rationale and development of the system and provides a valuable introduction to its uses.

Other Semi-structured Diagnostic Interviews for Axis I Disorders

A number of semi-structured diagnostic interviews have been developed for specific Axis I disorders, such as the Eating Disorders Examination [40] or the Yale Brown Obsessive Compulsive Schedule [41].

The DIGS (Diagnostic Interview for Genetic Studies) [42] is a clinical interview especially designed by the NIMH Genetics Initiative for the assessment of major mood and psychotic disorders and their spectrum conditions. It has the following features: (a) polydiagnostic capacity; (b) a detailed assessment of the course of the illness, chronology of psychotic and mood syndromes, and comorbidity; (c) additional phenomenological assessments of symptoms; and (d) algorithmic scoring capability. A reliability study has been carried out with excellent sensitivity and specificity for DSM-III-R and RDC diagnoses of major depression, bipolar disorder, schizophrenia, and lower diagnostic accuracy for subtypes of schizoaffective disorder [43].

SEMI-STRUCTURED INTERVIEWS FOR PERSONALITY DISORDERS

Semi-structured interviews for the assessment of personality disorders provide questions, guidelines and instructions for the assessment of the criteria defining personality disorder in general and specific personality disorders in particular. Some of these interviews are restricted to the assessment of a single personality disorder, while others are constructed for the assessment of all the personality disorders listed in ICD-10 or/and DSM-IV.

The Diagnostic Interview for Borderline (DIB)

The Diagnostic Interview for Borderline (DIB) is a semi-structured interview for the assessment of the criteria defining borderline personality disorder.

The version published in 1981 by Gunderson [44] was constructed for the assessment of borderline personality disorder as defined in DSM-III. The interview has been revised (DIB-R) for the assessment of borderline personality disorder as defined in DSM-III-R [45].

The structure of DIB and DIB-R is, in fact, closer to the structure of a questionnaire than of a semi-structured interview. In the DIB and DIB-R, the criteria of borderline personality disorder are assessed using a comprehensive list of questions pertaining to one of four domains: affects, cognitions, impulsive behavior and interpersonal relationships. The scores computed for each domain are added and the final, global score provides information on the presence or absence of borderline personality disorder.

Investigations into the psychometric properties of the DIB have shown varying agreement with clinical and other methods of diagnosing borderline personality disorder [46, 47].

The Structured Clinical Interview for DSM-IV Axis II Personality Disorders (SCID-II)

The Structured Clinical Interview for DSM-IV Axis II personality disorders (SCID-II) is a semi-structured diagnostic interview for the assessment of the ten personality disorders described in DSM-IV [48] and for two additional personality disorders, depressive and passive aggressive, that are described in Annex B (Criteria and axes proposed for further investigation). A previous version of the instrument had been developed for the assessment of personality disorders in DSM-III-R [49, 50].

In the SCID-II for DSM-IV, the ten official and the two additional personality disorders described in DSM-IV are assessed one after the other, in the following order: avoidant, dependant, obsessive-compulsive, passive-aggressive, depressive, paranoid, schizotypal, schizoid, histrionic, narcissistic, borderline, and antisocial personality disorder.

The criteria of each disorder are assessed in the order of their appearance in DSM-IV. SCID-II is presented in three columns: the middle column lists the criteria that are to be evaluated, the left-hand column proposes questions for the assessment of each criterion, and the results of the assessment are scored in the right-hand column. SCID-II is accompanied by a user's guide which provides recommendations for the understanding of each criterion and for differentiating criteria among each other.

The assessment of personality disorders in SCID-II is based on the general criteria for personality disorders as defined in DSM-IV. The following conventions apply: for a diagnosis to be positive, characteristic signs and symptoms must persist for at least five years, at least one of the characteristics must have been present since the end of adolescence, and signs and symptoms of a personality disorder must have been present for at least the last five years.

Each criterion in the SCID-II may be scored 1 (absent, no pathology), 2 (present, but not clinically significant), or 3 (present and clinically significant). For a score of 3, the characteristics described in a criterion must be pathological, persistent, and pervasive. Decisions between a score of 2 or 3 are based on features such as the frequency or severity of a behavior, and the presence of distress or difficulties in social or occupational functioning. Criteria for which there is a discrepancy between the respondent's answers and information available from other sources are scored with a question mark.

Table 8.4 presents the three columns of the SCID-II for the assessment of the fourth criterion of DSM-IV avoidant personality disorder. The text is followed by the commentary, in the user's guide, for the same criterion.

The SCID-II interviewer may decide to use only part of the instrument, e.g. to assess only some of the DSM-IV personality disorders. He or she may also use the personality questionnaire that accompanies the SCID-II (see below) and determine which personality disorders need to be assessed in more detail, prior to administering the interview itself.

The SCID-II may be handscored. SCID-II diagnoses can also be determined using a computer scoring program, called Computer-Assisted SCID-II or CAS-II.

Inter-rater reliability of the SCID-II for DSM-III-R and the SCID-II for DSM-IV has been found quite satisfactory [51–53] when the instrument was used by trained clinicians. Results concerning concurrent validity (comparisons with clinical diagnosis and with other instruments) have been less satisfactory.

The Structured Interview for DSM-IV Personality (SIDP-IV)

The Structured Interview for DSM-IV Personality (SIDP-IV) [54] is a semi-structured diagnostic interview for the assessment of 13 personality disorders.

TABLE 8.4 Example of a question from the Structured Clinical Interview for DSM-IV Axis II Personality Disorders (SCID-II)*

4.	You've said that [Do] you often worry about being criticized or rejected in social situations	(4) is preoccupied with being criticized or rejected in social situations	? 1 2 3
	Give me some examples.	3 = a lot of time spent worrying about social situations	
	Do you spend a lot of time worrying about this?		

*Reproduced by permission of the American Psychiatric Press from First *et al.* (1997). *Structured Clinical Interview for DSM-IV Personality Disorders (SCID-II)*.

In addition to the 10 officially recognized personality disorders in DSM-IV, the SIDP-IV also allows assessment of depressive personality disorder and passive-aggressive (negativistic) personality disorder as included in Annex B of DSM-IV, as well as of self-defeating personality disorder that had been introduced and proposed for further study in DSM-III-R, but has not been retained in DSM-IV. The assessment of the three additional personality disorders is, however, relegated to the end of the interview, and as such can be easily omitted.

The SIDP was introduced as an instrument for the assessment of personality disorders in DSM-III [55]. It was subsequently adapted to take into account the changes introduced in DSM-III-R [56] and was revised again according to the criteria defined for personality disorders in DSM-IV.

In the SIDP-IV, the diagnostic criteria for the 13 personality disorders listed above are grouped together in 10 sections: (a) interest and activities; (b) work style; (c) close relationships; (d) social relationships; (e) emotions; (f) observational criteria; (g) self-perception; (h) perception of others; (i) stress and anger; (j) social conformity.

For the assessment of each criterion, the SIDP-IV follows the same basic structure: presentation of the criterion, questions to be asked to assess the presence or absence of the criterion, probes whenever the preceding questions are answered with "yes".

The use of the SIDP-IV requires that the interviewer write the answers elicited during the interview in the margins of the instrument. The answers may be a simple "yes" or "no", but consist, preferably, in a sentence and/or an example. The interviewer will proceed with the scoring itself when he or she has elicited all the available information, i.e. at the end of the interview. In the final scoring, the interviewer may take into account additional information, such as data obtained from informants, reports recorded in hospital charts, or results from other assessment instruments.

The assessment of personality disorders in the SIDP-IV is based on the general criteria for personality disorders as defined in DSM-IV. The following conventions apply: for a diagnosis to be positive, characteristic signs and symptoms must persist at least five years, and signs and symptoms of a personality disorder must have been prominent during the last five years.

Each criterion in the SIDP-IV may be scored 0 (not present or limited to rare isolated examples); 1 (sub-threshold—some evidence of the trait, but it is not sufficiently pervasive or severe to consider the criterion present); 2 (present—the criterion is clearly present for most of the last five years (i.e. present at least 50% of the time during the last five years); and 3 (strongly present—criterion is associated with subjective distress or some impairment in social or occupational functioning or intimate relationships). To be taken into account for a diagnosis of personality disorder, a criterion must be scored 2 or 3.

TABLE 8.5 Example of a question from the Structured Interview for DSM-IV Personality (SIDP-IV)*

12. Is preoccupied with being criticized or rejected in social situations	4-AVOID	0 1 2 3

In social situations, how much do you worry about being criticized or rejected by other people?
(IF A LOT): Are you able to get your mind off it?

*Reproduced by permission of the American Psychiatric Press from Pfohl et al. (1997). *Structured Interview for DSM-IV Personality (SIDP-IV)*.

Table 8.5 presents the structure, information and instructions provided in the SIDP-IV for the assessment of the fourth criterion of DSM-IV avoidant personality disorder.

The SIDP-IV is accompanied by a version which enables the interviewer to use only part of the instrument, e.g. to assess only some of the DSM-IV personality disorders. In this version, the questions are grouped according to disorders and not according to sections as in the regular SIDP-IV.

There is no screening questionnaire for the SIDP-IV. For the screening of antisocial personality disorder, the authors recommend use of the section on antisocial personality disorder included in the Diagnostic Interview Schedule. Data obtained with the SIDP-IV can be analyzed by hand or by using a computer program.

There are no results available concerning the inter-rater reliability and validity of the SIDP-IV. Inter-rater reliability of the original SIDP has been found quite satisfactory. Results concerning concurrent validity (comparisons with clinical diagnosis and comparisons with other instruments) have been less satisfactory.

The International Personality Disorders Examination (IPDE)

The International Personality Disorders Examination (IPDE) is a semi-structured diagnostic interview for the assessment of the various personality disorders described in ICD-10 and/or DSM-IV.

The IPDE has been adapted from the Personality Disorders Examination [57]. Beginning in 1985, it was first modified for international use and then further developed by an international group of experts under the auspices of the WHO. In 1995, the group decided to publish two different modules of the instrument, one for the assessment of ICD-10 personality disorders and one for the assessment of DSM-IV personality disorders. The instrument is currently available in more than 20 languages. A version for the assessment of personality disorders in both ICD-10 and DSM-IV is available in English, French and German [58].

In the IPDE, the diagnostic criteria for the ICD-10 or/and the DSM-IV personality disorders are grouped together in six domains: work, self, interpersonal relationships, affects, reality testing, and impulse control. Criteria that cannot be assessed by questions are rated on behavior observed during the interview.

Throughout the interview, each criterion and its number, together with the name of the ICD-10 and/or DSM-IV disorder, appear above the questions designed to assess it. "Yes" answers are followed by additional questions, including probes and requests for examples. A behavior or trait may be scored 0 (absent or normal), 1 (exaggerated or accentuated), and 2 (criterion level or pathological). Positive diagnoses are made on the number of criteria scored 2. A dimensional score is computed by adding scores of 1 and 2 for each disorder as well as for all ICD-10 or DSM-IV criteria assessed in the instrument.

Table 8.6 presents the structure, information and instructions provided in the combined ICD-10 and DSM-IV version of the IPDE for the assessment of two criteria that are identical in ICD-10 and DSM-IV: criterion 3 of anxious (ICD-10) and criterion 4 of avoidant (DSM-IV) personality disorder.

The assessment of personality disorders in the SIDP-IV is based on the general criteria for personality disorders as defined in ICD-10 and DSM-IV. The following conventions apply: for a diagnosis to be positive, characteristic

TABLE 8.6 Example of a question from the International Personality Disorders Examination (IPDE)

037.	0 1 2 ?	0 1 2	Is preoccupied with being criticized or rejected in social situations 30 DSM-IV Avoidant: 4
			Excessive preoccupation with being criticized or rejected in social situations 24 ICD-10 Anxious (Avoidant): 3

Do you spend a lot of time worrying about whether people like you?
If yes: Are you afraid they'll criticize or reject you when you're around them?
If yes: How much does this bother you?

There is an inclination for subjects to confuse an ordinary, understandable concern about criticism or rejection in social situations with an excessive preoccupation. It is particularly important that acknowledgement of the behavior be supported by convincing examples indicating that the concern is well beyond that experienced by most people in similar circumstances

2　Frequently is concerned about being criticized or rejected in social situations

1　Occasionally is concerned about being criticized or rejected in social situations

0　Denied, rare, or not supported by convincing examples

signs and symptoms must persist at least five years, behavior indicative of at least one criterion of a personality disorder must be present prior to age 25, and signs and symptoms of the disorder must have been prominent during the last five years.

The IPDE must be administered by a trained clinician. Information may be obtained from informants and supersedes information obtained from the proband. The data can easily be analyzed by hand, or with the help of a computer program.

From 1988 to 1989, the IPDE has been extensively investigated in a study [59] involving 14 centers from 13 countries in the United States, Europe, Africa and Asia. In this study, the instrument was tested with regard to its feasibility, acceptability, temporal stability, inter-rater reliability and validity. According to the results, the instrument proved acceptable to clinicians and demonstrated an inter-rater reliability and temporal stability roughly similar to instruments used to diagnose psychotic disorders, mood disorders, anxiety disorders, and substance use disorders.

The Personality Assessment Schedule (PAS)

The Personality Assessment Schedule (PAS) [60] inquires about 24 personality characteristics. Although the PAS was not developed to assess the personality disorders in the DSMs and the ICD-10, it provides algorithms for making diagnoses in the two systems.

FULLY STRUCTURED INTERVIEWS

Fully structured interviews can be used by trained lay interviewers and therefore are of particular importance for the assessment in psychiatric epidemiology.

The Diagnostic Interview Schedule (DIS)

The first version of the Diagnostic Interview Schedule (DIS) was developed in 1978 at the request of the Center for Epidemiological Studies at the NIMH [61, 62]. The interview was the result of an adaptation and modification of the Renard Diagnostic Instrument (RDI), an interview developed at Washington University to assess the Feighner criteria diagnoses. Questions were added to make diagnoses according to the RDC and DSM-III criteria, on both a lifetime and current basis. The interview was unique at the time of its development in allowing psychiatric diagnoses without requiring clinicians.

TABLE 8.7 Example of a question from the Diagnostic Interview Schedule (DIS)

From SECTION D—Generalized Anxiety Disorder		
D5. During the 6 months or more when you had worries like that on your mind, were you also...	*No*	*Yes*
a. *feeling restless or keyed up* or on edge a lot of the time?	1	5
b. Were you easily *tired*?	1	5
c. Did you *have* a lot of *trouble keeping your mind on what you were doing*?	1	5
d. Would your mind go blank so you *lost track of what you had been thinking* about?	1	5
e. Did you feel particularly *irritable*?	1	5
f. Were your *muscles tense*, sore, or aching?	1	5

Its questions can be asked and coded by trained lay interviewers, according to clearly stated rules [63] (see Table 8.7).

The interview has subsequently been adapted to DSM-III-R and DSM-IV. The current version DIS 4.0 focuses on DSM-IV diagnoses only and integrates many ideas that emerged in the course of field experience of the DIS and the Composite International Diagnostic Interview (CIDI), which was originally based on the DIS and uses the same strategies [64].

Both interviews have a lot in common: they have a modular diagnostic structure with fully structured questions (many with identical wording); they use reference cards to assist the interviewer and a probe flow chart to rule out symptoms without clinical significance or which are not fully explained by physical causes. A disorder is defined current if present the last two weeks, the last month, the last six months, the last year or at any time in the last year.

Each diagnosis is based on the presence of a minimum number of criteria and diagnostic labels in the left-hand margin show how each question serves the scoring algorithms. Severity may be assessed by the number of criteria met, the number of different diagnoses present, the total number of symptoms, the length of the period the subject has had these symptoms, as well as by the degree of functional impairment. The interview also asks for onset and recency for each syndrome and whether the subject sought professional help (see Table 8.8, p. 199).

A personal computer (PC) program has been developed for data entry, cleaning and scoring. It provides diagnosis, and indicates the age of onset and recency of the syndromes [65]. Support material includes mock interviews, a suggested training schedule, question-by-question specifications, a history of the interview, homework assignments and a videotape.

The DIS has been proved to work well as a screening instrument and provides acceptable classifications for epidemiological purposes [66, 67].

The instrument has been used in epidemiological studies throughout the world [68]. The present version 4.0 makes the DIS also attractive as a diagnostic instrument for clinical settings. The instrument is available through the Washington University in St. Louis, Missouri (http://epi.wustl.edu/dis/dishome.htm).

The Composite International Diagnostic Interview (CIDI)

The CIDI [69] is a comprehensive, fully structured diagnostic instrument for the assessment of mental disorders according to the definitions and criteria of ICD-10 and DSM-IV. It was developed as a joint project between the WHO and the former United States Alcohol, Drug Abuse and Mental Health Administration (ADAMHA). It has been translated into some 25 languages and thereby is the most widely used structured interview in the world, regularly revised and improved by an international advisory committee.

The CIDI has been designed for use in a variety of cultures and settings. It is primarily intended for use in epidemiological and cross-cultural studies, but can also be used for clinical and research purposes.

The interview is modular and covers presently somatoform disorders, anxiety disorders, depressive disorders, mania, schizophrenia, eating disorders, cognitive impairment, and substance use disorders.

Version 1.0 was released in December 1990, version 1.1 in May 1993, and version 2.1 in January 1997 [70]. The current version 2.1 is available in a lifetime and a 12-month form and has 15 sections: (a) Demographics; (b) Nicotine use disorder; (c) Somatoform and dissociative disorders; (d) Phobic and other anxiety disorders; (e) Depressive disorders and dysthymic disorder; (f) Manic and bipolar affective disorder; (g) Schizophrenia and other psychotic disorder; (h) Eating disorders; (j) Alcohol use disorders; (k) Obsessive-compulsive disorder and post-traumatic stress disorder; (l) Substance-related disorders; (m) Dementia, amnesic and other cognitive disorders; (o) Comments by the respondent; (p) Interviewer observations; (x) Interviewer ratings.

The highly structured CIDI questions are fully spelled out and positive responses are followed by specific probes, which aim at determining the psychiatric significance and clinical relevance of a reported symptom (see Table 8.8). Negative responses will often lead to skips within the interview. If a particular diagnosis is suspected to be present, questions about the onset and the recency of a particular cluster of symptoms will be asked. The duration and the frequency of a particular set of symptoms are also evaluated.

The CIDI is designed to be completed in a single session and lasts approximately 75 minutes. Even though the interview is quite complex in

TABLE 8.8 Examples of questions from the Composite International Diagnostic Interview (CIDI)

Example of a CIDI probe question

From SECTION C—Somatoform (F45) and dissociative (F44) disorders

SOM10D13	C4 Have you ever had *pains in your arms*	PRB: 1 2 3 4 5
PP10A	*or legs* other than in the joints?	
SOM4B1		
PAIN4A		
	MD: _____ OTHER:	

_____

Example of a CIDI "yes/no" question

from SECTION D—Phobic (F40) and other anxiety disorders (F41)

ANIM10C	D4 Was your (fear/avoidance) of	NO 1	
ANIM4C	insects, snakes, birds or other animals ever excessive, that is, much stronger than in other people?	YES 5	
ANIM10C	A. Was your (fear/avoidance) of	NO 1	
ANIM4C	insects, snakes, birds or other animals ever unreasonable, that is, much stronger than it should have been?	YES 5	
ANIM10C	B. Were you ever very upset with	NO 1	
ANIM4E	yourself for (having the fear of/ avoiding) insects, snakes, birds or other animals?	YES 5	

its decision rules, it can be administered very reliably by trained lay interviewers. Training is conducted in the regional CIDI training centers throughout the world (for addresses, see the CIDI homepage).

The interview comes with a set of manuals (both for trainers and interviewers) and a computer program. The computerized scoring algorithm gives diagnoses according to DSM-IV and ICD-10 diagnoses.

The computerized version of CIDI 2.1 is created using the I-Shell system, a "computer aided personal interviewing tool" provided by WHO. The program runs on Windows 95/98 and NT 4.0 and is available on the CIDI homepage (http://www.who.int/msa/cidi/). Alternatively, the CIDI center in Sydney has developed since 1993 a MS-DOS based program of the instrument, known as CIDI Auto [71]. The current CIDI-Auto 2.1 can be self-administered or interviewer-administered. More information is available from the CRUFAD CIDI page (http://www.unsw.edu.au/clients/crufad/cidi/cidi.htm).

The reliability and validity of the CIDI has been demonstrated in a major international field trial [72] and in other studies [73]. Inter-rater reliability has been demonstrated to be excellent, test–retest reliability good, and validity good [74].

Due to the modular architecture of the instrument, a number of alternative versions of the CIDI exist. For example, the University of Michigan version of the CIDI (CIDI-UM) is a version modified for the US National Comorbidity Survey. The CIDI-UM does not contain a section on somatoform disorders nor a section on dementia, but a section on antisocial personality disorder has been added to the instrument.

DIAGNOSTIC SCREENING QUESTIONNAIRES

A number of screening instruments are available to help identify mental disorders. These instruments are of particular importance in primary care settings.

Questionnaires for the Screening of Axis I Disorders

The General Health Questionnaire (GHQ)

The General Health Questionnaire (GHQ) is a widely used screening questionnaire for common mental disorders (depression, anxiety, social dysfunction and somatic symptoms). The GHQ is a pure state measure, evaluating how much a person feels that his or her present state is different from his or her usual one. It does not make clinical diagnoses. It can be used in community and non-psychiatric settings [75].

The GHQ has four different versions:

1. The GHQ-12 is a quick screener for survey use containing only 12 questions. As reliable, valid and sensitive as the longer versions, it takes only two minutes to complete. The results produce a single score.
2. The GHQ-28 is the most well-known and popular version of the GHQ [76]. It has 28 items divided into four subscales: (a) somatic symptoms; (b) anxiety/insomnia; (c) social dysfunction; and (d) severe depression.
3. The GHQ-30 is a quick screener with "physical" element items removed. It is the most widely validated version of the GHQ.
4. The GHQ-60 may be used to identify cases for more intensive examination.

Reliability and validity data may be found in the GHQ *User's Guide* which details six GHQ-12, twelve GHQ-28, twenty-nine GHQ-30 and sixteen GHQ-60 validity studies [77]. Each version scores high. More recently, the validity of the GHQ-12 was compared with the GHQ-28 in a WHO study of psychological disorders in general health care, showing that both instruments are remarkably robust [78, 79].

More information on the GHQ can be obtained on the GHQ homepage (http://www.nfer-nelson.co.uk/ghq/index.htm).

The Symptom Checklist-90-Revised (SCL-90-R)

The Symptom Checklist-90-Revised (SCL-90-R) is an assessment instrument initially published by Derogatis in 1975 [80, 81], now distributed by National Computer Systems, Inc. (http://assessments.ncs.com/assessments/tests/scl90r.htm). It is a brief, multidimensional self-report inventory designed to screen for a broad range of psychological problems and symptoms of psychopathology.

The instrument can be useful in the initial evaluation of patients as well as to measure patient progress during treatment. The administration time is 12 to 15 minutes.

The SCL-90-R has nine primary symptom dimensions and three global indices (Table 8.9). It is a well-researched instrument with close to 1000 studies demonstrating its reliability, validity, and utility [82].

Primary Care Evaluation of Mental Disorders (PRIME-MD)

The PRIME-MD is based on Goldberg's two-stage model: it consists of a one-page screening questionnaire with 26 questions to be completed by the patient and a 12-page structured clinical interview form to be used by

TABLE 8.9   The scales of the Symptom Checklist-90-Revised (SCL-90-R)

Primary symptom dimensions

SOM	Somatization
O-C	Obsessive-Compulsive
I-S	Interpersonal Sensitivity
DEP	Depression
ANX	Anxiety
HOS	Hostility
PHOB	Phobic Anxiety
PAR	Paranoid Ideation
PSY	Psychoticism

General indices

GSI	Global Severity Index
PSDI	Positive Symptom Distress Index
PST	Positive Symptom Total

the physician following the answers given by the patient in the question-naire.

The interview has four modules covering the four main groups of mental disorders most frequently seen in general practice (mood, anxiety, somato-form and alcohol-use disorders).

The PRIME-MD was originally developed for DSM-IV diagnostic criteria and validated in the United States [83], but there is also an international version using the ICD-10 criteria. More recently an entirely self-adminis-tered version has been tested [84].

The Symptom-Driven Diagnostic System for Primary Care (SDDS-PC)

The Symptom-Driven Diagnostic System for Primary Care (SDDS-PC) [85] is a fully computerized instrument which allows primary care physicians to screen, diagnose and track patients suffering from a mental disorder or from a substance use disorder. Like the PRIME-MD, the SDDS has two major components: (i) a five-minute patient-administered screening questionnaire; and (ii) five- to ten-minute physician-administered diagnostic interview modules based on DSM-IV criteria.

The SDDS-PC screen consists of 26 items covering six types of mental disorders commonly seen in primary care (alcohol dependence, drug dependence, generalized anxiety disorder, major depressive disorder, obses-sive-compulsive disorder and panic disorder), followed by three "impair-ment" questions (Table 8.10). Patients who screen positive for a disorder receive the corresponding interview module. The computer program of the SDDS-PC generates automatically the appropriate module interview ques-tions following the screening responses. The instrument has been validated in several major studies [86].

The Mini International Neuropsychiatric Interview (MINI)

The Mini International Neuropsychiatric Interview (MINI) [87] is a short fully structured diagnostic interview developed jointly in Europe and the United States for DSM-IV and ICD-10 psychiatric disorders. The current version 5.0 has been translated into some 35 languages and comes with a family of interviews (MINI-Screen, MINI-Plus, MINI-Kid).

The instrument can be used by lay interviewers and requires only a brief training time. For each disorder one or two screening questions rule out the diagnosis when answered negatively.

TABLE 8.10 The 26 screening questions of the Symptom-Driven Diagnostic System for Primary Care (SDDS-PC)

In the PAST MONTH have you been bothered by:

1. Unhappiness?
2. Trouble falling asleep?
3. Depression?
4. Others worried about your drinking?
5. Rapid pulse?
6. Fear of going crazy?
7. Feeling blue?
8. Wishing you were dead?
9. Trembling or shaking?
10. Palpitations?
11. Tension?
12. High or hung over from drugs?
13. Drinking too much alcohol?
14. Sudden attacks of panic or fear?
15. Cleaning things over and over?
16. Worrying?
17. Checking or counting things over and over?
18. Feeling sad?
19. Your drug use causing problems with family or at work?
20. Feeling suicidal?
21. Thoughts or images that do not make sense?
22. Drinking alcohol in the morning?
23. Your family thinking you use drugs too much?
24. Trouble staying asleep?
25. Rapid heartbeat?

In the LAST 6 months, have you been:

26. Anxious/worried?

Validation of the MINI has been done in relation to the Structured Clinical Interview for DSM-III-R, Patient Version [88], the Composite International Diagnostic Interview [89], and expert professional opinion.

Questionnaires for the Screening of Personality Disorders

Questionnaires for personality disorders consist of statements that intend to elicit the presence or absence of criteria defining a personality disorder. Probands are asked to examine each statement and to report whether it applies to their character, i.e. whether it has been typical of them throughout their lives. Negative results may usually be equated with the absence of a personality disorder. Positive results suggest the presence of a personality disorder, but they still have to be substantiated by a formal clinical examination, preferably by a semi-structured interview (see above). As a rule, personality questionnaires are used as screening instruments for personality disorders.

Classic or Traditional Personality Inventories

Traditional psychological tests continue to be routinely applied in psychiatric settings to assess patients with a potential diagnosis of personality disorder. The most widely used include questionnaires such as the Minnesota Multiphasic Personality Inventory (MMPI and MMPI-2) [90, 91] or the Sixteen Personality Factor Questionnaire (16 PF) [92], and projective tests such as the Rorschach test [93] and the Thematic Apperception Test (TAT) [94]. Traditional tests may suggest the presence of a personality disorder. The results must, however, be substantiated by a comprehensive clinical interview, preferably a semi-structured interview for personality disorders.

The Schizotypal Personality Disorder Questionnaire (SPQ)

The Schizotypal Personality Disorder Questionnaire has been developed by Raine [95] as a 74-item self-report scale modeled on DSM-III-R criteria for schizotypal personality disorder. The current version includes nine subscales to reflect the nine criteria of schizotypal personality disorder listed in DSM-IV. The SPQ includes several items for the assessment of each criterion. The results from factor analytic studies suggest that three main factors best represent schizotypal personality disorder, namely Cognitive-Perceptional Deficits (made up of ideas of reference, magical thinking, unusual perceptual experiences, and paranoid ideation), Interpersonal Deficits (social anxiety, no close friends, blunted affect), and Disorganization (odd behavior, odd speech).

SPQ-B is a brief version of the original SPQ. It includes 22 items and is proposed as a screening instrument for schizotypal personality disorder.

The Personality Disorder Questionnaire (PDQ)

The Personality Disorder Questionnaire has been developed by Hyler *et al.* [96] for the assessment of the personality disorders described in DSM-III. It has been revised and adapted for the assessment of personality disorders in DSM-III-R and DSM-IV. The latest revision of the instrument is available in two versions: PDQ-4 has been constructed for the assessment of the 10 "official" personality disorders included in DSM-IV; PDQ-4+ includes, in addition, items for the assessment of passive-aggressive (negativistic) personality disorder as well as depressive personality disorder, that are described in Annex B of DSM-IV.

The PDQ-IV includes 85 yes–no items for the assessment of the diagnostic criteria required for the 10 official DSM-IV personality disorders. The questionnaire has two validity scales to identify under-reporting, lying, or inattention. It is accompanied by a clinician-administered Clinical Significance Scale, which allows the clinician to assess the impact of any personality disorder identified by the questionnaire. The PDQ provides categorical diagnoses and an overall index of personality disturbance.

Reliability of the PDQ is good for obsessive-compulsive and antisocial personality disorder, but only fair or inadequate for the remaining personality disorders. Concurrent validity, against semi-structured interviews, is variable. The instrument has high sensitivity, but low specificity. As such it may be most useful as a screening instrument for personality disorders.

The Screening Questionnaire of the SCID-II for DSM-IV

Administration of the SCID-II interview is usually based upon the results obtained with the SCID-II Personality Questionnaire. The SCID-II Personality Questionnaire is used as a screening self-report questionnaire. It consists of a series of questions to which probands are invited to answer with "yes" or "no". The DSM-IV version of the SCID-II questionnaire has 119 questions. The formulation of the questions is such that "yes" answers always indicate the presence of a criterion for a given personality disorder.

When the SCID-II is administered, the interviewer need only to inquire about the items screened positive on the questionnaire. The assumption underlying the use of the questionnaire is that it will produce many false positives, but only few false negatives. In particular, it is assumed that a subject who responds with a "no" on a questionnaire item would also have answered "no" to the same question had it been asked aloud by an interviewer. As an example, the first criterion for DSM-IV avoidant personality disorder: "Avoids occupational activities that involve significant interpersonal contact, because of fears of criticism, disapproval, or rejection" is assessed by asking: "Have you avoided jobs or tasks that involved having to deal with a lot of people?" A "yes" answer to this question will lead to further questions included in the SCID-II interview.

The Screening Questionnaire of the IPDE

The IPDE interview is accompanied by a screening questionnaire. The ICD-10 version of the questionnaire has 59 items, the DSM-IV version 77 items and the combined version 94 items. The items of the questionnaire are statements which are to be answered by "true" or "false". The formulation of the items is such that for some items a "yes" answer indicates the presence of a personality disorder, while for others a "no" answer indicates the presence of a disorder. The IPDE screening questionnaire produces few false negative cases vis-à-vis the interview, but yields a high rate of false positives. As an example, the presence or absence of the fourth criterion of histrionic personality disorder in ICD-10 ("Continual seeking for excitement and activities in which the individual is the center of attention") and the first criterion of histrionic personality disorder in DSM-IV are assessed by the answer to the item "I would rather not be the center of attention". A "false" answer would be counted as indicating the possible presence of histrionic personality disorder.

When the scoring of three or more items suggests the presence of a personality disorder, the subject has failed the screen for that disorder and should be interviewed. Clinicians and researchers are, however, invited to adopt lower or higher screening standards, depending on the nature of the sample, and the relative importance to them of sensitivity (false negative cases) vs. specificity (false positive cases). The IPDE screening instrument should not be used to make a diagnosis.

INTERVIEWS FOR THE ASSESSMENT OF DISABLEMENT

The WHO Disability Assessment Schedule (WHODAS-II)

The WHO Psychiatric Disability Schedule (WHO/DAS) with a Guide to its Use [97] has been published to provide a semi-structured instrument for assessing disturbances in social functioning in patients with a mental disorder and for identifying factors influencing these disturbances. In order to make the instrument conceptually compatible with the revisions to the International Classification of Functioning and Disability (ICIDH-2), it has been completely revised by the WHO Assessment, Classification and Epidemiology Group.

This new measurement tool, the WHODAS-II, distinguishes itself from other measures of health status in that it is based on an international classification system and is cross-culturally applicable. It treats all disorders at parity when determining level of functioning and disability across a variety of conditions and treatment interventions. An advantage of the WHODAS II is that it assesses functioning and disability at the individual level instead of the disorder-specific level. As a result, the total impact of comorbid conditions (e.g. depression and diabetes) is straightforward to assess.

TABLE 8.11   Questions of the domain 4 of the WHO Disability
Assessment Schedule (WHODAS-II)

DOMAIN 4:   Getting along with people
In the last 30 days, how much difficulty did you have in ...
D.4.1.   Dealing with people you do not know?
D.4.2.   Maintaining a friendship?
D.4.3.   Getting along with people who are close to you?
D.4.4.   Making new friends?
D.4.5.   Sexual activities?

The WHODAS-II assesses the following domains of functioning:

1. Understanding and interacting with the world.
2. Moving and getting around.
3. Self-care.
4. Getting along with people (see Table 8.11).
5. Life activities.
6. Participation in society.

The interview also seeks information on emotional and financial burden as well as on time spent dealing with difficulties. This information can be used to identify needs, match patients to interventions, track functioning over time and measure clinical outcomes and treatment effectiveness.

Psychometric testing of the WHODAS II has been rigorous and extensive. In 1997, a Cross-cultural Applicability Research (CAR) study tested the validity of the rank ordering of disability in 14 countries [98]. In 1998, an intermediate version of the WHODAS-II (89 items) was tested in field trials in 21 sites and 19 countries. Based on psychometric analyses and further field testing in the beginning of 1999, the measure was shortened to a final version of 36 items. A 12-item screening questionnaire has also been developed. The final WHODAS-II version has undergone reliability and validity testing in 16 centers across 13 countries. Health services research studies (to test sensitivity to change and predictive validity) were carried out in centers throughout the world in 2000 and are about to be published. More information on the instrument may be obtained from the WHO WHODAS homepage (http://www.who.int/icidh/whodas).

Other Instruments for the Assessment of Disablement

During the past 30 years, many other instruments have been developed to assess disability. Table 8.12 lists some of them. The most well known and most widely used of these instruments appears to be the 36-Item Short Form

TABLE 8.12 Examples of other instruments used to assess disablement

Activities of Daily Living (ADLs)
EuroQol
Instrumental Activities of Daily Living (IADLs)
Health Utility Index (HUI)
London Handicap Scale
Quality of Well-Being Scale (QWB)
Nottingham Health Profile (NHP)
Short Form (SF-12 and SF-36)

(SF-36), a comprehensive self-administered short form with only 36 questions designed to measure health status and outcomes from the patient's point of view [99].

The SF-36 yields a profile of eight health scores:

1. Limitations in physical activities because of health problems.
2. Limitations in usual role activities because of physical health problems.
3. Bodily pain.
4. General health perceptions.
5. Vitality (energy and fatigue).
6. Limitations in social activities because of physical or emotional problems.
7. Limitations in usual role activities because of emotional problems.
8. Mental health (psychological distress and well-being).

The SF-12 [100], an even shorter survey form published in 1995, has been shown to yield summary physical and mental health outcome scores that are interchangeable with those from the SF-36 in both general and specific populations.

The instruments have been translated into more than 40 languages. The SF-36 can be used in all kinds of surveys and has been proved useful in monitoring general and specific populations, as documented in more than 2000 publications. More information can be obtained on the SF-36 homepage (http://www.sf36.com/).

RELIABILITY AND VALIDITY OF CLINICAL ASSESSMENT INSTRUMENTS IN PSYCHIATRY

A variety of semi-structured or fully structured diagnostic instruments, together with a number of screening questionnaires, are currently available for assessing probands and for making psychiatric diagnoses according to one or the other of the official classifications of mental disorders. The usefulness of such instruments is closely linked to their reliability and validity.

Inter-rater Reliability

The reliability of clinical assessment instruments is usually studied using one of the two following methods: an observer scores the interview while the interviewer also scores it and the results are compared to determine the degree to which the two raters agree (inter-rater reliability), or the interview is repeated at a later time, by the same or by a different interviewer (test–retest reliability). Good to excellent inter-rater and test–retest reliability have been reported for most interviews described in this chapter.

Validity

The best way to establish the validity of a clinical diagnostic instrument would be to measure its validity against an external "gold standard" [101]. In the absence, up to now, of any such standard for any of the disorders that are assessed in psychiatry, psychiatric diagnoses achieved using clinical assessment instruments have been compared to diagnoses derived from: i) clinician's free-form assessment; ii) other clinical assessment instruments; iii) the Longitudinal, Expert, All Data (LEAD) procedure; or iv) the consensus best-estimate diagnostic procedure.

Comparison with Clinician's Free-form Assessment

Agreement between diagnoses obtained with structured or semi-structured interviews and clinician's free-form assessment or diagnoses in medical records has generally been found to be low [102]. Such comparisons are, however, unsatisfactory for evaluating the validity of assessment instruments, since clinicians' diagnoses are unreliable themselves, as shown by lack of agreement between two clinicians assessing the same patient [103, 104].

Comparison between Assessment Instruments

Evaluating the validity of one instrument by comparing it to another instrument requires that the validity of the second instrument has been established. Up to the present, there is, however, no such instrument, although well-established instruments, such as the SCID, have been used to evaluate the validity of new instruments.

Comparisons with LEAD (Longitudinal, Expert, All Data) Diagnoses

The LEAD procedure was proposed by Spitzer in 1983 [101] for the assessment of the validity of diagnostic instruments. The LEAD procedure involves "longitudinal" evaluation, i.e. not limited to a single examination, made by "experts", i.e. by experienced clinicians, using "all data", i.e. not only data obtained during the interviews with the respondent, but also data provided from other sources, such as from family members or other significant others, hospital personnel, or case records.

The LEAD procedure has been used in a number of studies to assess the validity of diagnostic instruments, e.g. the DIS [105], or the validity of personality disorder diagnoses [106]. In recent studies, data used in the procedure have themselves been obtained using semi-structured interviews.

Comparisons with the Consensus Best-estimate Diagnostic Procedure

The best-estimate diagnostic procedure has been proposed by Leckman *et al.* [107]. Comprehensive information obtained from different methods (personal interview, family history from family informants, and medical records), including information obtained from clinical diagnostic interviews, is assessed by two or more experts to arrive independently and then by consensus at a criterion diagnosis. The procedure has been used in particular in the field of genetics [108].

CONCLUSIONS

Clinical assessment instruments in psychiatry differ in the diagnostic systems that they cover, in the training and expertise needed to administer them, in their costs—time and money—, and in the data that they yield, from screening to comprehensive diagnosis. To guide the clinician or researcher in choosing the best instrument for a given purpose or a particular study, Robins [109] has described study-specific as well as universal criteria.

Study-specific criteria include the extent to which disorders of interest are covered by the instrument (e.g. with regard to subtypes, age of onset or course), appropriateness to the study sample (e.g. clinical setting vs. general population), and appropriateness to the study resources (the financial implications varying considerably between self-administered interviews, telephone interviews, and administration by clinicians).

Universal criteria for choosing the most appropriate instrument are related to questions of efficiency (e.g. degree of difficulty or ease to ask and to understand the interview questions), format (e.g. interviewer instructions, coding procedures), transparency of computer programs (allowing the user to understand the diagnostic algorithms followed in a given program), acceptability (to both respondents and interviewers), support available (e.g. instruction manuals, data entry programs, videotapes) and reliability and validity of the instrument.

ACKNOWLEDGEMENT

The authors wish to thank Isabelle Heuertz and Myriam Kolber for their help with the manuscript.

REFERENCES

1. Spitzer R.L., Endicott J., Robins E. (1978) *Research Diagnostic Criteria (RDC) for a Selected Group of Functional Disorders*, 3rd edn. New York State Psychiatric Institute, New York.
2. World Health Organization (1992) *The ICD-10 Classification of Mental and Behavioural Disorders: Clinical Descriptions and Diagnostic Guidelines*. World Health Organization, Geneva.
3. World Health Organization (1993) *The ICD-10 Classification of Mental and Behavioural Disorders: Diagnostic Criteria for Research*. World Health Organization, Geneva.
4. American Psychiatric Association (1980) *Diagnostic and Statistical Manual of Mental Disorders*, 3rd edn (DSM-III). American Psychiatric Association, Washington.
5. American Psychiatric Association (1987) *Diagnostic and Statistical Manual of Mental Disorders*, 3rd edn, revised (DSM-III-R). American Psychiatric Association, Washington.
6. American Psychiatric Association (1994) *Diagnostic and Statistical Manual of Mental Disorders*, 4th edn (DSM-IV). American Psychiatric Association, Washington.
7. Feighner J.P., Robins E., Guze S., Woodruff R.A., Winokur G., Munoz R. (1972) Diagnostic criteria for use in psychiatric research. *Arch. Gen. Psychiatry*, **26**: 57–63.
8. Robins L.N. (1989) Diagnostic grammar and assessment: translating criteria into questions. *Psychol. Med.*, **19**: 57–68.
9. Pull C.B., Guelfi J.D. (1995) L'opérationnalisation du diagnostic psychiatrique. In *Psychopathologie Quantitative* (Eds J.D. Guelfi, V. Gaillac, R. Dardennes), pp. 1–8. Masson, Paris.
10. Pull C.B., Pull M.C., Pichot P. (1984) Les Listes Intégrées de Critères d'Evaluation Taxonomiques: L.I.C.E.T.-S et L.I.C.E.T.-D. *Acta Psychiatr. Belg.*, **84**: 297–309.

11. Pull C.B., Pull M.C., Pichot P. (1987) Des critères empiriques français pour les psychoses: III. Algorithmes et arbres de décision. *Encéphale*, **13**: 59–66.
12. Pull C.B., Pull M.C., Pichot P. (1988) French diagnostic criteria for depression. *Psychiatrie et Psychobiologie*, **3**: 321–328.
13. McGuffin P., Farmer A., Harvey I. (1991) A poly-diagnostic application of operational criteria in studies of psychotic illness: Development and reliability of the OPCRIT system. *Arch. Gen. Psychiatry*, **48**: 764–770.
14. Schneider K. (1950) *Klinische Psychopathologie*. Thieme, Stuttgart.
15. Taylor M.A., Abrams R. (1978) The prevalence of schizophrenia: a reassessment using modern diagnostic criteria. *Am. J. Psychiatry*, **16**: 467–478.
16. Carpenter W.T., Strauss J.S., Bartko J.J. (1973) Flexible system for the diagnosis of schizophrenia: Report from the WHO International Pilot Study of Schizophrenia. *Science*, **182**: 1275–1278.
17. Williams J., Farmer A.E., Ackenheil M., Kaufmann C.A., McGuffin P. (1996) A multi-centre inter-rater reliability study using the OPCRIT computerized diagnostic system. *Psychol. Med.*, **26**: 775–783.
18. Craddock M., Asherson P., Owen M.J., Williams J., McGuffin P., Farmer A.E. (1996) Concurrent validity of the OPCRIT diagnostic system: comparison of OPCRIT diagnoses with consensus best-estimate lifetime diagnoses. *Br. J. Psychiatry*, **169**: 58–63.
19. Janca A., Üstün T.B., van Drimmelen H., Dittmann V., Isaac M. (1995) *The ICD-10 Symptom Checklist for Mental Disorders*. Huber, Bern.
20. Janca A., Hiller W. (1996) ICD-10 checklists: a tool for clinicians' use of the ICD-10 classification of mental and behavioural disorders. *Compr. Psychiatry*, **37**: 180–187.
21. Janca A., Üstün T.B., Early T.S., Sartorius N. (1993) The ICD-10 Symptom Checklist: a companion to the ICD-10 Classification of Mental and Behavioural Disorders. *Soc. Psychiatry Psychiatr. Epidemiol.*, **28**: 239–242.
22. Hiller W., Zaudig M., Mombour W. (1990) Development of diagnostic checklists for use in routine clinical care. A guide designed to assess DSM-III-R diagnoses. *Arch. Gen. Psychiatry*, **47**: 782–784.
23. Hiller W., Zaudig M., Mombour W. (1995) *International Diagnostic Checklists for ICD-10 and DSM-IV*. Huber, Bern.
24. Endicott J., Spitzer R.L. (1978) A diagnostic interview: the Schedule for Affective Disorders and Schizophrenia. *Arch. Gen. Psychiatry*, **35**: 837–844.
25. Endicott J., Spitzer R.L. (1979) Use of the research diagnostic criteria and the Schedule for Affective Disorders and Schizophrenia to study affective disorders. *Am. J. Psychiatry*, **136**: 52–56.
26. Kaufman J., Birmaher B., Brent D., Rao U., Flynn C., Moreci P., Williamson D., Ryan N. (1997) Schedule for Affective Disorders and Schizophrenia for School-Age Children—Present and Lifetime Version (K-SADS-PL): initial reliability and validity data. *J. Am. Acad. Child Adolesc. Psychiatry*, **36**: 980–988.
27. Weissman M.M., Myers J.K. (1980) Psychiatric disorders in a US community: the application of research diagnostic criteria to a resurveyed community sample. *Acta Psychiatr. Scand.*, **62**: 99–111.
28. Spitzer R.L., Williams J.B.W., Gibbon M., First M.B. (1992) The Structured Clinical Interview for DSM-III-R (SCID): I. History, rationale, and description. *Arch. Gen. Psychiatry*, **49**: 624–629.
29. Spitzer R.L., Williams J.B.W., Gibbon M., First M.B. (1990) *Structured Clinical Interview for DSM-III-R: Patient Edition/Non-patient Edition (SCID-P/SCID-NP)*. American Psychiatric Press, Washington.

30. First M.B., Spitzer R.L., Gibbon M., Williams J.B.W. (1996) *Structured Clinical Interview for DSM-IV Axis I Disorders, Clinician Version (SCID-CV)*. American Psychiatric Press, Washington.
31. First M.B., Spitzer R.L., Gibbon M., Williams J.B.W. (1997) *User's Guide for the Structured Clinical Interview for DSM-IV Axis I Disorders—Clinician Version (SCID-CV)*. American Psychiatric Press, Washington.
32. First M.B., Spitzer R.L., Gibbon M., Williams J.B.W. (1997) *Structured Clinical Interview for DSM-IV Axis I Disorders, Research Version: (1) Patient Edition (SCID-I/P); (2) Non-patient Edition (SCID-I/NP); (3) Patient Edition with Psychotic Screen (SCID-I/P W/ PSY SCREEN)*. Biometrics Research, New York State Psychiatric Institute, New York.
33. Williams J.B.W., Gibbon M., First M.B., Spitzer R.L., Davis M., Borus J., Howes M.J., Kane J., Pope H.G., Rounsaville B., Wittchen H. (1992) The Structured Clinical Interview for DSM-III-R (SCID): II. Multi-site test–retest reliability. *Arch. Gen. Psychiatry*, **49**: 630–636.
34. Wing J.K., Babor T., Brugha T., Burke J., Cooper J.E., Giel R., Jablensky A., Regier D., Sartorius N. (1990) SCAN: Schedules for Clinical Assessment in Neuropsychiatry. *Arch. Gen. Psychiatry*, **47**: 589–593.
35. World Health Organization (1997) *Schedules for Clinical Assessment in Neuropsychiatry (SCAN)*. World Health Organization, Geneva.
36. Wing J.K., Cooper J.E., Sartorius N. (1974) *Measurement and Classification of Psychiatric Symptoms: An Instruction Manual for the PSE and CATEGO Program*. Cambridge University Press, Cambridge.
37. Celik C. (1999) *SCAN I-Shell: Computer Assisted Personal Interviewing Application for the Schedules for Clinical Assessment in Neuropsychiatry Version 2.1 and Diagnostic Algorithms for WHO ICD-10 Chapter V DCR and for American Psychiatric Association Diagnostic and Statistical Manual Version IV*. World Health Organization, Geneva.
38. Rijnders C.A., van den Berg J.F., Hodiamont P.P., Nienhuis F.J., Furer J.W., Mulder J., Giel R. (2000) Psychometric properties of the Schedules for Clinical Assessment in Neuropsychiatry (SCAN-2.1). *Soc. Psychiatry Psychiatr. Epidemiol.*, **35**: 348–352.
39. Wing J.K., Sartorius N., Üstün T.B. (1998) *Diagnosis and Clinical Measurement in Psychiatry: A Reference Manual for SCAN*. Cambridge University Press, Cambridge.
40. Cooper Z., Fairburn C. (1987) The Eating Disorder Examination: a semi-structured interview for the assessment of the specific psychopathology of eating disorders. *Int. J. Eating Disord.*, **6**: 1–8.
41. Goodman W.K., Price H., Rasmussen S., Mazure C., Fleischman R., Hill C., Heninger G., Charney D. (1989) The Yale Brown Obsessive Compulsive Scale: Part I—Development, use and reliability. *Arch. Gen. Psychiatry*, **46**: 1006–1011.
42. Nurnberger J.I., Blehar M.C., Kaufmann C.A., York-Cooler C., Simpson S.G., Harkavy-Friedman J., Severe J.B., Malaspina D., Reich T. (1994) Diagnostic interview for genetic studies: rationale, unique features, and training. *Arch. Gen. Psychiatry*, **51**: 849–859.
43. Faraone S.V., Blehar M., Pepple J., Moldin S.O., Norton J., Nurnberger J.I., Malaspina D., Kaufmann C.A., Reich T., Cloninger C.R. *et al.* (1996) Diagnostic accuracy and confusability analyses: an application to the Diagnostic Interview for Genetic Studies. *Psychol. Med.*, **26**: 401–410.
44. Gunderson J.G., Kolb J.E., Austin V. (1981) The Diagnostic Interview for Borderline Patients. *Am. J. Psychiatry*, **138**: 896–903.

45. Zanarini M.C., Gunderson J.G., Frankenburg F.R., Chauncey D.L. (1989) The revised Diagnostic Interview for Borderlines: discriminating BPD from other Axis II disorders. *J. Personal. Disord.*, **3**: 10–18.
46. Frances A., Clarkin J.F., Gilmore M., Hurt S.W., Brown R. (1984) Reliability of criteria for borderline personality disorder: a comparison of DSM-III and the Diagnostic Interview for Borderline Patients. *Am. J. Psychiatry*, **141**: 1080–1084.
47. Hurt S.W., Clarkin J.F., Koenigsberg H.W., Frances A., Nurnberg H.G. (1986) Diagnostic Interview for Borderlines: psychometric properties and validity. *J. Consult. Clin. Psychol.*, **54**: 256–260.
48. First M.B., Spitzer R.L., Gibbon M., Williams J.B.W. (1997) *Structured Clinical Interview for DSM-IV Personality Disorders (SCID-II)*. American Psychiatric Press, Washington.
49. First M.B., Spitzer R.L., Gibbon M., Williams J.B.W. (1995) The Structured Clinical Interview for DSM-III-R Personality Disorders (SCID-II): I. Description. *J. Personal. Disord.*, **9**: 83–91.
50. First M.B., Spitzer R.L., Gibbon M., Williams J.B.W., Davies M., Borus J., Howes M.J., Kane J., Pope H.G., Rounsaville B. (1995) The Structured Clinical Interview for DSM-III-R Personality Disorders (SCID-II): II. Multi-site test–retest reliability study. *J. Personal. Disord.*, **9**: 92–104.
51. Dreessen L., Hildebrand M., Arntz A. (1998) Patient-informant concordance on the Structured Clinical Interview for DSM-III-R Personality Disorders (SCID-II). *J. Personal. Disord.*, **12**: 149–161.
52. Dreessen L., Arntz A. (1998) Short-interval test–retest interrater reliability of the Structured Clinical Interview for DSM-III-R Personality Disorders (SCID-II) in outpatients. *J. Personal. Disord.*, **12**: 138–148.
53. Maffei C., Fossati A., Agostoni I., Barraco A., Bagnato M., Deborah D., Namia C., Novella L., Petrachi M. (1997) Interrater reliability and internal consistency of the Structured Clinical Interview for DSM-IV Axis II Personality Disorders (SCID-II), version 2.0. *J. Personal. Disord.*, **11**: 279–284.
54. Pfohl B., Blum N., Zimmerman M. (1997) *Structured Interview for DSM-IV Personality: SIDP-IV*. American Psychiatric Press, Washington.
55. Stangl D., Pfohl B., Zimmerman M., Bowers W., Corenthal C. (1985) A structured interview for the DSM-III personality disorders: a preliminary report. *Arch. Gen. Psychiatry*, **42**: 591–596.
56. Pfohl B., Blum N., Zimmerman M., Stangl D. (1989) *Structured Interview for DSM-III-R Personality: SIDP-R*. Department of Psychiatry, University of Iowa, Iowa City.
57. Loranger A.W., Susman V.L., Oldham J.M., Russakoff L.M. (1987) The Personality Disorder Examination: a preliminary report. *J. Personal. Disord.*, **1**: 1–13.
58. Loranger A.W., Janca A., Sartorius N. (1997) *Assessment and Diagnosis of Personality Disorders: The ICD-10 International Personality Disorder Examination (IPDE)*. Cambridge University Press, Cambridge.
59. Loranger A.W., Sartorius N., Andreoli A., Berger P., Buchheim P., Channabasavanna S.M., Coid B., Dahl A., Diekstra R., Ferguson B. *et al.* (1994) The International Personality Disorder Examination: IPDE. The WHO/ADAMHA International Pilot Study of Personality Disorders. *Arch. Gen. Psychiatry*, **51**: 215–224.
60. Tyrer P. (1988) *Personality Disorders: Diagnosis, Management and Course*. Wright, Boston.

61. Robins L.N., Helzer J.E., Croughan J.L., Ratcliff K.S. (1981) National Institute of Mental Health diagnostic interview schedule: its history, characteristics, and validity. *Arch. Gen. Psychiatry*, **38**: 381–389.
62. Helzer J.E., Robins LN. (1988) The diagnostic interview schedule: its development, evolution, and use. *Soc. Psychiatry Psychiatr. Epidemiol.*, **23**: 6–16.
63. Helzer J.E. (1985) A comparison of clinical and Diagnostic Interview Schedule diagnoses: physician reexamination of lay-interviewed cases in the general population. *Arch. Gen. Psychiatry*, **42**: 657–666.
64. Robins L.N. (1988) An overview of the Diagnostic Interview Schedule and the Composite International Diagnostic Interview. In *International Classification in Psychiatry: Unity and Diversity* (Eds J.E. Mezzich, M. von Cranach), pp. 205–220. Cambridge University Press, New York.
65. Erdman H.P., Klein M.H., Greist J.H., Skare S.S., Husted J.J., Robins L.N., Helzer J.E., Goldring E., Hamburger M., Miller J.P. (1992) A comparison of two computer-administered versions of the NIMH Diagnostic Interview Schedule. *J. Psychiatr. Res.*, **26**: 85–95.
66. Helzer J.E., Spitznagel E.L., McEvoy L. (1987) The predictive validity of lay Diagnostic Interview Schedule diagnoses in the general population: a comparison with physician examiners. *Arch. Gen. Psychiatry*, **44**: 1069–1077.
67. Robins L., Helzer J.E. (1994) The half-life of a structured interview: the NIMH Diagnostic Interview Schedule (DIS). *Int. J. Methods Psychiatr. Res.*, **4**: 95–102.
68. Hwu H.G., Compton W.M. (1994) Comparison of major epidemiological surveys using the Diagnostic Interview Schedule. *Int. Rev. Psychiatry*, **6**: 309–327.
69. Robins L.N., Wing J., Wittchen H.U., Helzer J.E., Babor T.F., Burke J., Farmer A., Jablensky A., Pickens R., Regier D.A. *et al.* (1988) The Composite International Diagnostic Interview: an epidemiologic instrument suitable for use in conjunction with different diagnostic systems and in different cultures. *Arch. Gen. Psychiatry*, **45**: 1069–1077.
70. WHO (1997) *Composite International Diagnostic Interview, version 2.1.* World Health Organization, Geneva.
71. Peters L., Andrews G. (1995) Procedural validity of the computerized version of the Composite International Diagnostic Interview (CIDI-Auto) in the anxiety disorders. *Psychol. Med.*, **25**: 1269–1280.
72. Wittchen H.U., Robins L.N., Cottler L.B., Sartorius N., Burke J.D., Regier D. (1991) Cross-cultural feasibility, reliability and sources of variance of the Composite International Diagnostic Interview (CIDI). *Br. J. Psychiatry*, **159**: 645–653.
73. Wittchen H.U. (1994) Reliability and validity studies of the WHO-Composite International Diagnostic Interview (CIDI): a critical review. *J. Psychiatr. Res.*, **28**: 57–84.
74. Andrews G., Peters L. (1998) The psychometric properties of the Composite International Diagnostic Interview. *Soc. Psychiatry Psychiatr. Epidemiol.*, **33**: 80–88.
75. Johnstone A, Goldberg D. (1976) Psychiatric screening in general practice: a controlled trial. *Lancet*, **i**: 605–608.
76. Goldberg D.P., Rickels K., Downing R., Hesbacher P. (1976) A comparison of two psychiatric screening tests. *Br. J. Psychiatry*, **129**: 61–67.
77. Goldberg D.P., Williams P. (1988) *The User's Guide to the General Health Questionnaire.* NFER–Nelson, Windsor.
78. Goldberg D.P., Gater R., Sartorius N., Üstün T.B., Piccinelli M., Gureje O., Rutter C. (1997) The validity of two versions of the GHQ in the WHO study of mental illness in general health care. *Psychol. Med.*, **27**: 191–197.

79. Werneke U., Goldberg D.P., Yalcin I., Üstün B.T. (2000) The stability of the factor structure of the General Health Questionnaire. *Psychol. Med.*, **30**: 823–829.
80. Derogatis L.R., Lipman R.S., Covi L. (1973) SCL-90: an outpatient psychiatric rating scale—preliminary report. *Psychopharmacol. Bull.*, **9**: 13–28.
81. Derogatis L.R., Rickels K., Rock A.F. (1976) The SCL-90 and the MMPI: a step in the validation of a new self-report scale. *Br. J. Psychiatry*, **128**: 280–289.
82. Derogatis L.R. (1994) *Symptom Checklist-90–Revised (SCL-90–R): administration, scoring and procedures manual*, 3rd edn. National Computer Systems, Minneapolis.
83. Spitzer R.L., Williams J.B., Kroenke K., Linzer M., deGruy F.V., Hahn S.R., Brody D., Johnson J.G. (1994) Utility of a new procedure for diagnosing mental disorders in primary care: the PRIME-MD 1000 study. *JAMA*, **272**: 1749–1756.
84. Spitzer R.L., Kroenke K., Williams J.B. (1999) Validation and utility of a self-report version of PRIME-MD: the PHQ primary care study. *JAMA*, **282**: 1737–1744.
85. Weissman M.M., Olfson M., Leon A.C., Broadhead W.E., Gilbert T.T., Higgins E.S., Barrett J.E., Blacklow R.S., Keller M.B., Hoven C. (1995) Brief diagnostic interviews (SDDS-PC) for multiple mental disorders in primary care. A pilot study. *Arch. Fam. Med.*, **4**: 220–227.
86. Broadhead W.E., Leon A.C., Weissman M.M., Barrett J.E., Blacklow R.S., Gilbert T.T., Keller M.B., Olfson M., Higgins E.S. (1995) Development and validation of the SDDS-PC screen for multiple mental disorders in primary care. *Arch. Fam. Med.*, **4**: 211–219.
87. Sheehan D.V., Lecrubier Y., Sheehan K.H., Amorim P., Janavs J., Weiller E., Hergueta T., Baker R., Dunbar G.C. (1998) The Mini-International Neuropsychiatric Interview (MINI): the development and validation of a structured diagnostic psychiatric interview for DSM-IV and ICD-10. *J. Clin. Psychiatry*, **59** (Suppl. 20): 22–33.
88. Dunbar G.C., Sheehan M.F., Sheehan D.V., Lecrubier Y., Sheehan K.H., Janavs J., Weiller E., Keskiner A., Schinka J., Knapp E. (1997) The validity of the Mini International Neuropsychiatric Interview (MINI) according to the SCID-P and its reliability. *Eur. Psychiatry*, **12**: 232–241.
89. Lecrubier Y., Sheehan D., Weiller E., Amorim P., Bonora I., Sheehan K.H., Janavs J., Dunbar G.C. (1997) The Mini-International Neuropsychiatric Interview (MINI). A short diagnostic interview: reliability and validity according to the CIDI. *Eur. Psychiatry*, **12**: 224–231.
90. Hathaway S.R., McKinley J.C. (1943) *The Minnesota Multiphasic Personality Inventory (MMPI)*. University of Minnesota, Minneapolis.
91. Butcher J.N., Dahlstrom W.G., Graham J.R., Tellegen A., Kaemmer (1990) *The Minnesota Multiphasic Personality Inventory-2 (MMPI-2)*. University of Minnesota Press, Minneapolis.
92. Cattell H.E.P., Cattell A.K., Cattell H.E. (1993) *Sixteen Personality Factor Questionnaire*, 5th edn. Institute for Personality and Ability Testing, Champaign.
93. Rorschach H. (1921) *Psychodiagnostik*. Huber, Bern.
94. Morgan C.D., Murray H.A. (1938) Thematic Apperception Test (TAT) In *Explorations in Personality: A Clinical and Experimental Study of Fifty Men of College Age* (Eds H.A. Murray, W.G. Barrett, E. Homburger), pp. 530–545. Oxford University Press, New York.
95. Raine A. (1991) The SPQ: a scale for the assessment of schizotypal personality based on DSM-II-R criteria. *Schizophr. Bull.*, **17**: 555–564.

96. Hyler S.E., Skodol A.E., Kellman H.D., Oldham J.M., Rosnick L. (1990) Validity of the Personality Diagnostic Questionnaire—revised: comparison with two structured interviews. *Am. J. Psychiatry*, **147**: 1043–1048.

97. World Health Organization (1988) *WHO Psychiatric Disability Assessment Schedule*. World Health Organization, Geneva.

98. Üstün T.B., Chatterji S., Bickenbach J.E., Trotter R.T., Room R., Rehm J., Saxena S. (2001) *Disability and Culture: Universalism and Diversity*. Hogrefe & Huber, Göttingen.

99. Ware J.E., Snow K.K., Kosinski M., Gandek B. (1993) *SF-36 Health Survey: Manual and Interpretation Guide*. Health Institute, New England Medical Center, Boston.

100. Ware J.E., Kosinski M., Keller S.D. (1996) A 12–Item Short-Form Health Survey: construction of scales and preliminary tests of reliability and validity. *Med. Care*, **34**: 220–233.

101. Spitzer R.L. (1983) Psychiatric diagnosis: are clinicians still necessary? *Compr. Psychiatry*, **24**: 399–411.

102. Steiner L.S., Kraemer T.J., Sledge W.H., Walker M.L. (1995) A comparison of the Structured Clinical Interview for DSM-III-R and Clinical Diagnoses. *J. Nerv. Ment. Dis.*, **183**: 365–369.

103. Kosten T.A., Rounsaville B.J. (1992) Sensitivity of psychiatric diagnosis based on the best estimate procedure. *Am. J. Psychiatry*, **149**: 1225–1227.

104. Robins L. (1985) Epidemiology: reflections on testing the validity of psychiatric interviews. *Arch. Gen. Psychiatry*, **42**: 918–924.

105. Griffin M.L., Weiss R.D., Mirin S.M., Wilson H., Bouchard-Voelk B. (1987) The use of the Diagnostic Interview Schedule in drug-dependent patients. *Am. J. Drug Alcohol Abuse*, **13**: 281–291.

106. Pilkonis P.A., Heape C.L., Ruddy J., Serrao P. (1991) Validity in the diagnosis of personality disorders: the use of the LEAD standard. *Psychol. Assessment*, **3**: 46–54.

107. Leckman J.L., Sholomskas M.A., Thompson W.D., Belanger A., Weissman M.M. (1982) Best estimate of lifetime psychiatric diagnosis. *Arch. Gen. Psychiatry*, **39**: 879–883.

108. Roy M.A., Lanctôt G., Mérette C., Cliche D., Fournier J.P., Boutin P., Rodrigue C., Charron L., Turgeon M., Hamel M. *et al.* (1977) Clinical and methodological factors related to reliability of the best-estimate diagnostic procedure. *Am. J. Psychiatry*, **154**: 1726–1733.

109. Robins L. (1995) How to choose among the riches: selecting a diagnostic instrument. In *Textbook in Psychiatric Epidemiology* (Eds M.T. Tsuang, M. Tohen, G.E.P. Zahner), pp. 243–271. Wiley, New York.

9

Psychiatric Diagnosis and Classification in Primary Care

David Goldberg[1], Greg Simon[2] and Gavin Andrews[3]

[1]*Institute of Psychiatry, King's College, London, UK*
[2]*Center for Health Studies, Group Health Cooperative, Seattle, WA, USA*
[3]*School of Psychiatry, University of New South Wales at St. Vincent's Hospital, Darlinghurst, Australia*

INTRODUCTION

Karl Jaspers stressed that:

> when we design a diagnostic schema, we can only do so if we forego something at the outset...and in the face of facts we have to draw the line where none exists...A classification therefore has only a provisional value. It is a fiction which will discharge its function if it proves to be the most apt for the time [1].

Different professional groups quite legitimately need classifications for different purposes, and it is most unlikely that the purposes of psychiatrists working mainly in private practice will be remotely the same as those of primary care physicians working in community settings.

Where family doctors are concerned, they can avoid diagnosis altogether, or take one of three major official choices when they are confronted by a mentally ill patient:

1. They can use adaptations of those classifications produced by their colleagues such as the ICHPPC-2 (International Classification of Health Problems in Primary Care) of the WONCA (World Organization of National Colleges, Academies and Academic Associations of General Practitioners) or, in the United Kingdom, the Read codes.
2. They can use tri-axial classifications, with separate assessments of physical health, psychological adjustment and social adjustment.
3. They can use what are essentially classifications designed by psychiatrists (such as the ICD-10 or the DSM-IV).

Psychiatric Diagnosis and Classification. Edited by Mario Maj, Wolfgang Gaebel, Juan José López-Ibor and Norman Sartorius. © 2002 John Wiley & Sons, Ltd.

APPROACHES TO CLASSIFICATION OF MENTAL DISORDERS IN PRIMARY CARE

Classifications Produced by General Practitioners

The WONCA System (ICHPPC-2)

General practitioners (GPs) have produced a simplified version of the WONCA system, but this has troubles of its own, since the 21 conditions recognized are sometimes over-inclusive, and at other times do not allow recognition of important syndromes [2]. For example, dementia and delirium are included together as "organic psychoses", and all childhood disorders are grouped together; while chronic neurosis, fatigue syndromes, and even chronic psychosis are nowhere to be found.

The designers of ICHPPC-2 were clearly correct to focus their classification on a couple of dozen disorders that are commonly encountered in primary care, but it seems likely that the borders between the various disorders could be drawn in a more useful way, and it would be of great importance to ensure that primary care workers were given assistance in recognizing disorders for which there are treatments.

The Read Codes

An alternative approach in the United Kingdom is to use the Read codes. This is a system derived from computerized records in the doctor's office, and is used for central data collection within the National Health Service concerned with all morbidity, including psychological. Since many consultations in primary care do not result in a firm diagnosis, it is a classification of: (a) complaints (e.g. "tearful", "loss of confidence", "worried", "tired all the time"); (b) abnormalities noticed by the doctor (e.g. "disoriented", "flight of ideas", "poor insight into neurotic condition"); (c) circumstances surrounding the consultation (e.g. "life crisis", "marital problems"); (d) investigations (e.g. "depression screen", "psychological testing"); (e) treatment given or stopped (e.g. "lithium stopped", "grieving counseling"); (f) referral decisions (e.g. "refer to counselor", "refer to psychologist") and, finally, (g) diagnosis where one is known (e.g. "alcoholic psychosis", "schizophrenic psychosis") [3]. The system allows [11] diagnoses corresponding to the ICD-10, all relating to organic psychoses and psychotic illnesses, as well as codes for non-psychotic conditions (e.g. anorexia nervosa, drug dependency) and quasi-diagnostic terms (e.g. attempted suicide, emotional problem).

With such logical heterogeneity, and so little help in deciding which code to use, it is hardly surprising that there is great variation between practices in the way in which the system is used. Nonetheless, about 97% of practices have clinical systems that use Read codes, and of these, probably 30% use clinical terms (and their associated codes) to record every consultation, and many more than that use the terms at some consultations or at least in recording prescribing.

Avoiding Psychological Diagnoses

Many GPs try to avoid classification wherever possible, and do this because they wish to remain "patient-centered". Doctors who do this will only diagnose depression by *agreeing with the patient* after the patient has himself suggested the possibility. They tend to use vague umbrella terms like "emotional distress" to cover the multiplicity of psychological disorders which confront them in primary care settings. There is, of course, no necessary antithesis between being patient-centered and finding out what is actually wrong with the patient, but there is a real risk that such taxophobic doctors may miss, and therefore under-treat, many cases of emotional distress.

Tri-axial Classifications

Another approach is to use tri-axial classifications—using psychological illness, physical illness, and social circumstances as the axes. This was shown to produce better agreement between observers than the use of official classifications [4]. The three axes were mental disorders; physical disorders; and social circumstances. Despite the obvious attractions of this procedure, the obstinate fact is that GPs will not use tri-axial systems in their routine work, so such methods seem destined for use by researchers.

Classifications Produced by Psychiatrists

Classifications designed by psychiatrists, such as ICD-10 or DSM-IV, are generally found to be over-complicated for use in general medical settings. GPs do not really need to recognize 26 varieties of major depressive episode, or 31 different kinds of mood, anxiety and somatoform disorder. It is clear that such classifications need to be adapted to the clinical environment of primary care—with the need to make: (a) accurate physical assessments; (b) a rough psychological assessment; and above all (c) a management plan. This must be achieved in much less time than is generally available to psychiatrists. This necessitates adapting the schemes created by psychiatrists to suit the conditions of primary care.

IS PRIMARY CARE DIFFERENT?

Comparisons between Illnesses Seen in Primary Care and those Seen by the Specialist Services

The typical presentation of anxiety and depressive symptoms in primary care does differ from that seen in specialist clinics. Primary care patients are more likely to present with somatic complaints or concerns regarding undiagnosed medical illness [5, 6]. A useful primary care classification should give greater emphasis to these somatic presentations. While primary care patients may present with somatic symptoms, many will readily acknowledge psychological distress when asked—a process referred to as "facultative somatization" [5–7]. Somatic symptoms may serve as a "ticket of admission" to the primary care consultation, because the patient believes that such symptoms are a more legitimate reason for seeking health care. Overt presentation of psychological distress can be facilitated (or discouraged) by specific physician behaviors during the consultation [6, 8]. The much-described "somatization" of primary care patients might be more accurately described as a collaboration between patients and doctors [7].

While the presentation of anxiety or depressive disorders may differ significantly between primary care and specialist services, the form or structure of common mental disorders does not appear to. Epidemiological surveys in primary care find that the DSM and ICD criteria used to define common mental disorders in specialty care appear equally valid and reliable in primary care [9, 10]. The latent structure of anxiety and depressive symptoms does not seem to vary significantly across different levels of care (community, primary care, or specialty practice). This consistency of syndromes or symptom patterns has important implications for the development of primary care classifications. Adaptation of existing specialist classifications for use in primary care should not require definition of new syndromes or significant revision of existing ones. Instead, adaptation should focus on condensation or simplification to make specialist classifications more useful in primary care practice.

Patients' tendencies to present with psychological or somatic symptoms may also be influenced by education or by linguistic and cultural differences. We should recognize that physicians as well as patients bring their educational and cultural backgrounds to the doctor–patient encounter.

Comparisons between Primary Care Physicians' Diagnoses and Research Diagnoses

Studies where independent assessments have been made by research psychiatrists typically show two sorts of discrepancy—patients who are deemed by their GPs to have mental disorders but who do not meet standard diagnostic criteria for mental disorders; and those thought mentally ill by the researchers but treated symptomatically for physical symptoms by their GPs [11]. Little harm comes from the first sort of discrepancy other than unnecessary prescriptions of psychotropic drugs: the fact that the disorder has been recognized, together with the active therapeutic stance of the GP, probably speeds resolution of symptoms. It must also be admitted that not all of those who are found to be mentally unwell by the researchers actually want their GP to see them as mentally ill. Many know that they have transient disorders; some do not wish to have treatment for symptoms such as panic attacks even when it is offered; while others are mainly concerned to have their doctor exclude serious physical causes for the somatic symptoms which are troubling them. Failure to detect disorder can therefore be a collusive phenomenon between a reluctant patient and a GP who is unsure what to do about any disorder that is detected. Despite the exceptions mentioned, it is nevertheless important that staff in primary care settings are able to detect psychological disorders, since several different surveys have shown that detected disorders have a better outlook than those that remain undetected.

The Clinical Realities of Primary Care

Clinical utility should be the most important measure of a diagnostic system. A clinically useful classification should both reflect the current state of practice and facilitate necessary improvement. The development of the DSM and ICD classifications for specialists illustrates this conversation between clinical practice and official diagnostic classifications. The development of specific treatments for affective and anxiety disorders motivated the division of amorphous neurotic disorders into specific syndromes. The dissemination of these more specific classifications (DSM-III and ICD-9) was a major factor in the dissemination of more specific, evidence-based treatments.

For example, the World Health Organization (WHO) study of psychological disorders in general medical settings [10] produced the diagnoses shown in Table 9.1. We can see from this table that, if the taxonomically vague concept of "neurasthenia" is disregarded, the commonest disorders seen in primary care are depression, various anxiety disorders, and alcohol problems. However, these data express the mental disorders of primary care in the language of psychiatrists: in practice, combinations of anxiety and depressive symptoms are much more common than either disorder on its own, and "unexplained somatic symptoms" are a frequent presentation of mental disorder, more common than the psychiatrist's concept of "somatization disorder". In this chapter, we consider the specific needs of a

TABLE 9.1. Predicted prevalence of ICD-10 mental disorders among consecutive attenders in 15 centers, showing proportion recognized by physicians in 4 centers (after Üstün and Sartorius [10])

ICD-10 diagnosis	Predicted prevalence (%) (15 centers)	Proportion detected by physicians (%) (4 centers)[a]
Current depression	10.4	60.5
Generalized anxiety disorder	7.9	50.1
Neurasthenia (chronic fatigue)	5.4	61.1
Harmful use of alcohol	3.3	9.6
Alcohol dependence	2.7	66.6
Somatization disorder	2.7	64.4
Dysthymia	2.1	73.5
Agoraphobia	1.5	65.7
Panic disorder	1.1	59.2
Hypochondriasis	0.8	73.1
Proportion with at least one diagnosis	24.0	58.8

The 15 centers were Ankara, Athens, Bangalore, Berlin, Groningen, Ibadan, Mainz, Manchester, Nagasaki, Paris, Rio de Janeiro, Santiago de Chile, Seattle, Shanghai and Verona.
[a]These 4 centers (Manchester, Seattle, Verona and Bangalore) had somewhat better detection rates than all 15.

classification of psychological disorders presenting in primary care. We focus on symptoms and disorders most commonly encountered in primary care: anxiety, depression, and unexplained somatic symptoms.

Across different health care systems, primary health providers may range from physicians with specialist qualifications (internists or pediatricians) to paraprofessionals with quite limited training. Even in developed countries, physicians may delegate recognition and assessment of psychological disorders to nurses or other clinical staff. A practical primary care classification system should be appropriate for use by a wide range of health care providers. As discussed below, the ICD-10 primary care taxonomy is actually a family of classifications for use by a range of health care providers (a more complex system for physicians and a simplified system for non-professional or paraprofessional providers). Two primary care modifications of the DSM system (also discussed below) have been adapted for use by primary care nursing staff.

A classification of mental disorders should both consider the realities of current primary care practice and direct attention toward important short-comings. In other words, an appropriate classification system must remain relevant and accessible to primary care providers while emphasizing areas of need for more specific diagnosis and management. Like any good educational program, a classification system will target clinical areas where both the need for improvement and the potential for change are great. Given the competing demands and limited resources of primary care, the number of such targets should be relatively small. Psychiatric specialists must recall that cardiologists, endocrinologists, and rheumatologists all have their own agendas for improving diagnosis and management in primary care.

As discussed above, common and treatable mental disorders often go unrecognized in primary care. In addition, recognition may be non-specific (e.g. "stress reaction" rather than "depressive episode"). Specific recognition and diagnosis are associated with improved outcome, while non-specific recognition is not [7, 12]. Consequently, any useful classification for primary care should be designed to increase recognition and specific diagnosis of common anxiety and depressive disorders. In addition to providing diagnostic criteria, a classification tool should emphasize the presenting symptoms or complaints most often seen in primary care.

A classification scheme for primary care should emphasize diagnostic distinctions with clear implications for primary care management. This is especially important in the discussion of syndromes or conditions which often co-occur. No primary care classification would be complete without a discussion of unexplained somatic symptoms. Such a discussion, however, must mention the need to evaluate depressive symptoms in all patients with unexplained somatic complaints [13, 14]. The additional diagnosis of a depressive episode has clear and important implications for management. Similarly, any discussion of the diagnostic evaluation of depression should mention assessment of drug and alcohol use.

The clinical utility of a primary care classification is best illustrated by examining a typical presentation of psychological distress in primary care. Consider a patient presenting with fatigue, abdominal pain, insomnia, and persistent worry or "nerves" following a marital separation. In this situation, we would hope the physician would consider a series of specific diagnostic questions:

- Is a depressive syndrome present?
- (If yes) Is the depressive syndrome severe enough to warrant specific treatment (antidepressant pharmacotherapy or referral for depression-specific psychotherapy)?
- Is there a significant risk of suicide or self-harm?
- Is there a history suggesting manic or hypomanic episodes?
- Are psychotic symptoms present?
- Is there evidence of alcohol or other drug abuse or dependence?

Each of these questions has clear implications for immediate management options in primary care (antidepressant prescription, hospitalization, referral to specialist services). We would give much lower priority to other diagnostic distinctions not linked to immediate primary care management. The list of second-order diagnostic questions might include:

- Is depression superimposed on dysthymic disorder?
- Are diagnostic criteria met for recurrent major depression?
- Do psychotic symptoms indicate a diagnosis of unipolar depression with psychosis, schizoaffective disorder, bipolar disorder, or some other condition?
- Are criteria met for diagnosis of bipolar disorder?

While all of these questions may be relevant to specialist management, they have little influence on the primary care physician's immediate management decisions. To specialists, it may seem heretical (or negligent) to sacrifice these diagnostic distinctions. For better or worse, improving the management of mental disorders in primary care will require that classification systems and educational efforts focus on a brief list of clinical priorities.

Comorbidity and Overlap with General Medical Illness

The diagnostic responsibilities of the primary care physician are inherently more complicated than those of specialists. Many presentations involve a mix of somatic and psychological symptoms. This co-occurrence of somatic and psychological symptoms may reflect several different underlying relationships.

Common mental disorders may present with somatic symptoms suggesting general medical illness. Somatic distress is a universal component of anxiety and depressive disorders. The structure and expectations of primary care practice often encourage the expression of somatic distress and discourage open expression of psychological symptoms [5–7].

In some cases, general medical disorders—or side effects of medications used to treat those disorders—may mimic psychiatric disorders. Textbooks of psychiatry and general medicine invariably contain extensive lists of these medical mimics of psychiatric illness. Conditions commonly included range from relatively common (e.g. hypothyroidism) to extremely rare (e.g. pheochromocytoma). The intended message to students and practitioners is that a covert medical condition may be the primary cause of psychological symptoms such as depressed mood or anxiety. Detection and treatment of that covert medical condition (or discontinuation of the offending medication) is expected to definitively treat the accompanying psychopathology. Providers are cautioned that a premature focus on psychiatric symptoms may lead to overlooking a hidden medical diagnosis. It is striking that such lists of the medical mimics of psychiatric illness are rarely balanced by the converse—lists of the psychiatric mimics of common medical disorders. This asymmetry suggests an implicit judgement that a missed diagnosis of depressive illness is less significant than a missed diagnosis of an analogous general medical disorder. Such a judgement seems questionable given ample evidence for the prevalence, burden, and frequent non-recognition of depression. Overemphasis of psychiatric diagnosis in primary care at the expense of medical diagnosis does not seem to be a major priority for education or quality improvement.

In addition, chronic medical disorders are associated with increased prevalence of psychiatric illness. Non-specific mechanisms may account for much of this association. Persistent symptoms such as pain or sleep disturbance may precipitate or maintain depression. Activity limitations resulting from chronic medical illness may also contribute to depression, especially among the elderly. In addition, some specific disorders are associated with increased risk of psychiatric illness. Central nervous system disorders associated with increased risk of depression or other psychiatric illness include cerebrovascular disease, multiple sclerosis, and lupus. A diagnostic classification for primary care should direct special attention to those medical conditions associated with a higher risk of psychiatric disorder. It is also essential to distinguish this co-occurrence of psychiatric and general medical illness from the "medical mimics" of psychiatric illness mentioned above. True co-occurrence of psychiatric and general medical illness implies that each requires assessment and treatment. In this situation, psychiatric symptoms should not be viewed as diagnostic clues or "red herrings".

Anxiety and depression can have a major influence on the burden and outcomes of general medical illness. Even when there is no causal link between psychiatric and general medical illness, anxiety and depression are associated with greater disability, greater use of medical services, and increased mortality [15–18]. For example, depression co-occurring with ischemic heart disease has a significant negative impact on both disability and mortality [19, 20]. In this case, depression may exert a direct physiologic effect on platelet aggregation. In other cases, depressive or anxiety disorders may exert a more general effect on health behaviors such as smoking, diet, alcohol use, or adherence to medical treatment [21]. It is reasonable to assume (but remains to be proved) that recognition and appropriate management of anxiety could have significant impact on the course of chronic medical illness. For this reason, any classification of mental disorders designed for primary care must not view mental and general medical disorders as mutually exclusive possibilities. Depressive symptoms in the setting of chronic illness should not automatically be viewed as secondary to medical illness or prescribed medication. Such an "either–or" view can lead primary care physicians to overlook important opportunities for treatment. In some primary care surveys, presence of a chronic medical illness has been associated with decreased likelihood that anxiety or depressive disorders will be recognized.

ADAPTING PSYCHIATRISTS' CLASSIFICATIONS TO THE NEEDS OF PRIMARY CARE

The Special Version of the Mental Disorders Section of ICD-10 for Use in Primary Care (ICD-10-PHC)

The tenth revision of the ICD has some important differences from its predecessor where mental disorders are concerned. The traditional dichotomy between "psychosis" and "neurosis" is no longer recognized; the user is provided with clear diagnostic criteria for use in research projects; and special versions of the classification are available for use in specialized settings.

The ICD-10-PHC classification [22] is unusual in a number of important respects. It is user-friendly, consisting of about 26 rather than 440 different disorders; it gives clear advice about probable presenting complaints and the differential diagnosis of such complaints; and, most important of all, it gives clear advice about the management of each disorder. The set of disorders found useful in one country may well be different from that found useful in another, and each country is allowed to make its own selection of disorders to be adopted. It may not be necessary to include eating disorders in India, or conversion hysteria in Scandinavia. However, most of the disorders will be common to all countries, and the categories will correspond broadly to those recognized by the more detailed ICD-10 used by psychiatrists [23]. The ICD-10-PHC classification is not simply a condensed version of the larger classification system for specialists. It is a separate system created for primary care, but designed to be compatible with the classification system used by specialists.

The classification is accompanied by a choice of other supporting materials: a glossary giving definitions of all technical terms used; advice on the way in which psychological inquiries should be fitted into the course of the usual medical consultation, and the circumstances which should act as "triggers" for the GP to focus upon psychological adjustment; and a diagnostic flow chart showing how the various diagnoses logically relate to one another. The conditions which have been suggested for inclusion in ICD-10-PHC are shown in Table 9.2.

TABLE 9.2 List of 26 conditions included in the primary care version of ICD-10 (ICD-10-PHC)

	Nearest ICD-10 equivalent
Disorders in childhood	
Enuresis	F 98.0
Conduct disorder	F 91
Hyperkinetic (attention deficit) disorder	F 90
Mental retardation	F 70
Adult disorders	
Alcohol misuse	F 10
Drug use disorders	F 11
Acute psychosis	F 23
Chronic psychosis	F 20
Bipolar disorder	F 31
Depression	F 32
Mixed anxiety and depression	F 41.2
Generalized anxiety	F 41.1
Unexplained somatic symptoms	F 45
Phobic disorders	F 40
Panic disorder	F 41.0
Dissociative (conversion) disorder	F 44
Sexual disorders—male	F 52
Sexual disorders—female	F 52
Eating disorders	F 50
Neurasthenia	F 48.0
Post-traumatic stress disorder	F 43.1
Adjustment disorders	F 43.2
Sleep problems	F 51
Bereavement	Z 63
Organic disorders	
Dementia	F 00
Delirium	F 05

Field Trials of the New Classification

Field trials were conducted in 40 different countries, and the experiences of doctors using the classification in these trials led to extensive modifications to the classification. Several new disorders were included (for example, bereavement and chronic anxious depression), some were discarded (tobacco use disorder) and others were split into separate disorders (male and female sexual disorders). Many comments by GPs allowed WHO to modify the advice given about each disorder. Reliability studies showed that the classification had acceptable inter-rater reliability.

The field trial in the United Kingdom reported by Goldberg *et al.* [24] showed that doctors had reduced their prescriptions of antidepressants while using the new classification, and now required their patients to report more symptoms of depression before advising an antidepressant. The categories most often thought excellent were depression (60%), adjustment disorder (43%), unexplained somatic symptoms (38%), anxiety state (38%), acute psychotic disorder (33%) and panic disorder (30%).

The guidance on depression given by ICD-10-PHC has been evaluated in Bristol with a superior group of experienced GPs [25]. Independent assessments were made of patients treated by the doctors before and after the guidance was provided. There was no improvement in the detection of depression, or change in prescriptions of antidepressants. However, there was an increase in numbers diagnosed with depression, and with unexplained somatic symptoms, and the GPs made increased use of psychological interventions, and more of these cases were treated without antidepressant drugs.

Recent Refinements in the United Kingdom

A meeting of psychiatrists and GPs in Bristol suggested the inclusion of local sources of help, of information leaflets for patients, of self-help groups and other voluntary organizations, as well as making many suggestions for local amendments [26]. A national group with representatives of both groups of doctors then discussed these proposals further, adding information about the evidence base for each assertion in the guidelines, using Cochrane criteria as far as possible.

These materials have been published by the Royal Society of Medicine (RSM) [27] (www.roysocmed.ac.uk), and can also be found on the website www.whoguidemhpcuk.org. The RSM publication includes two floppy disks, one for downloading into the GP's computer, the other for the patient information leaflets.

The Adaptation of DSM-IV for Use in Primary Care

The DSM series produced by the American Psychiatric Association is now in its fourth edition with a "text revision" (DSM-IV-TR) released in 2000. This most recent version of the DSM classification includes 896 pages (without appendices). Clinical descriptions and diagnostic criteria are provided for several hundred disorders, grouped in 16 major diagnostic categories. For each disorder, DSM-IV provides a clinical description and specific diagnostic criteria—but no specific information regarding management. As stated in its introduction, the DSM classification was designed primarily for mental health specialist clinicians and researchers. Several recent modifications of the DSM-IV were intended to facilitate and promote its use in primary care.

DSM-IV-PC

A primary care version of DSM-IV (DSM-IV-PC) was published by the American Psychiatric Association in 1995 [28]. This abbreviated (208 pages) version of the DSM classification was developed through a collaborative effort of psychiatrists, other mental health specialists, and primary care physicians. The DSM-IV-PC focuses on a limited number of conditions found to be prevalent in primary care practice. The overall format is generally the same as that of the parent DSM classification—clinical descriptions followed by diagnostic criteria. Clinical descriptions emphasize the presenting symptoms and differential diagnostic questions most commonly encountered in primary care. No specific information is provided regarding management. The primary care version of DSM does, however, include some diagnostic aids not found in the DSM classification for specialists. A series of nine diagnostic algorithms give specific guidance for diagnostic assessment of common symptomatic presentations (e.g. depressed mood, anxiety, unexplained physical symptoms, cognitive disturbance, sleep disturbance). A symptom index (arranged in both alphabetical and topical order) links common presenting symptoms to the appropriate diagnostic criteria and diagnostic algorithms.

No empirical research has examined the reliability, validity or utility of the DSM-IV-PC system in primary care practice. Considerable research, however, supports the validity and reliability of the major diagnostic categories in the parent DSM-IV. For many disorders, the DSM-IV field trials included primary care as well as specialist settings. Given that the diagnostic criteria in DSM-IV-PC are completely consistent with those in the parent classification, it seems reasonable to apply data from DSM-IV field trials to the primary care version. The utility of DSM-IV-PC in primary care practice, however, has not been addressed by research. Outstanding questions include: Does introduction of the DSM-IV-PC system improve the overall rate of recognition of mental disorders or the accuracy of diagnosis for specific disorders (depressive episode, alcohol use disorders)? How does introduction of DSM-IV-PC affect indicators of mental health treatment (use of antidepressants, use of benzodiazepines, referral to specialist care)?

PRIME-MD

The Primary Care Evaluation of Mental Disorders (PRIME-MD) system was developed by Spitzer *et al.* [29] to facilitate recognition and specific diagnosis of mental disorders in primary care. It is less a revision of the DSM-IV classification than an assessment tool to facilitate use of DSM-IV in primary care. It is most directly descended from the Structured Clinical Interview for

DSM III/IV (SCID) [30] developed to facilitate standardized diagnosis in specialist practice and research. The original version of PRIME-MD included a brief self-report screening questionnaire (the Patient Questionnaire) and a clinician-administered semi-structured interview (the Clinician Evaluation Guide) for follow-up of positive screening results. Both the screening questionnaire and the semi-structured interview adhere closely to DSM-IV criteria and resemble simplified versions of the SCID. The system allows diagnosis of several common mental disorders (major depressive episode, panic disorder, generalized anxiety disorder, alcohol abuse/dependence, bulimia, somatoform disorders). No specific advice is provided regarding management. An evaluation of the original system among 1000 US primary care patients [9] found that trained primary care physicians using the PRIME-MD system showed excellent diagnostic agreement with a subsequent telephone SCID assessment by a mental health specialist. Average physician time required was 8.4 minutes. Nearly half of patients identified by the PRIME-MD were not previously recognized, and a new treatment or referral was initiated for over 60% of those not already in treatment. Subsequent studies have supported utility and validity of the PRIME-MD among German, Spanish, and Native American primary care patients [31–33]. Kobak et al. [34] described an adaptation of the PRIME-MD for computer-assisted telephone administration (using interactive voice response technology). The automated system showed good to excellent agreement with both the standard clinician-administered PRIME-MD and a SCID assessment by a mental health specialist. The computer-administered system may have somewhat better sensitivity for detection of substance abuse. The most recent adaptation of the PRIME-MD is a self-administered version (the Patient Health Questionnaire) suitable for either paper-and-pencil or computer-assisted administration. The self-administered version showed excellent agreement with the clinician-administered version. Physician time required to review the self-report assessment was typically less than three minutes—considerably less time than required to administer the original PRIME-MD semi-structured interview.

Symptom-Driven Diagnostic System for Primary Care (SDDS-PC)

The Symptom-Driven Diagnostic System for Primary Care (SDDS-PC) is an assessment tool developed by Weissman et al. [35] to facilitate recognition and diagnosis of common mental disorders in primary care. Like the PRIME-MD, the SDDS-PC is a tool to facilitate use of the DSM-IV diagnostic system rather than a separate set of diagnostic criteria (see Table 9.3). The assessment covers symptoms of depressive episodes, generalized anxiety, panic disorder, alcohol or drug dependence, and obsessive-compulsive

TABLE 9.3 Diagnoses covered by the Symptom-Driven Diagnostic System for Primary Care (SDDS-PC) and the Primary Care Evaluation of Mental Disorders (PRIME-MD)

	SDDS-PC	PRIME-MD
Depressive episode	Yes	Yes
Generalized anxiety disorder	Yes	Yes
Panic disorder	Yes	Yes
Alcohol abuse/dependence	Yes	Yes
Drug abuse/dependence	Yes	
Obsessive-compulsive disorder	Yes	
Dysthymia		Yes
Bulimia		Yes
Multisomatoform disorder		Yes

disorder as well as evaluation of suicidal behavior. An initial 16-question screening instrument is suitable for paper-and-pencil or computer-assisted administration (via telephone or computer screen). Six clinician-administered diagnostic interview modules may be used to evaluate positive screening results. Time required to administer each interview module is typically two to three minutes. In two validation studies among US primary care patients, the SDDS-PC system (with diagnostic modules administered by a trained nurse) showed excellent agreement with a SCID assessment by a mental health specialist.

Other Systems

In addition to the classification systems described above, a large number of questionnaires and screening scales have been evaluated for use in primary care. For example, Mulrow *et al.* [36] have reviewed the use of several depression screening measures, finding that all perform reasonably well. Most of these measures, however, are intended for screening rather than diagnosis. All are focused on one or few disorders, and none could be considered diagnostic or classification systems.

Diagnosis and Disability

Most people who meet criteria for a diagnosis of a mental disorder are disabled to some degree. Some, especially some people with severe psychosis, depression or dementia, are severely disabled and are unable to maintain themselves in employment, unable to do required daily tasks, and unable to sustain a relationship with others. Doctors have little difficulty identifying this level of disability and responding appropriately. Some people with a mental disorder are not disabled by their disorder, either because it is so mild that it does not interfere with their lives, or because they are able to live in such a way that the disorder does not impinge on work or personal relationships. The example usually quoted is of a person with an incapacitating fear of heights who is not disabled provided he or she lives and works in low rise buildings. Most doctors are also familiar with people with potentially severe mental illnesses, like schizophrenia or mania, who are able to compartmentalize the psychosis and continue their work and personal relationships in an appropriate manner. But most people with a mental disorder have some disability as a consequence. In epidemiological surveys for instance, the average person who meets criteria for a substance use or personality disorder will report mild disability, while the average person with an anxiety, depressive, or somatoform disorder will report moderate disability. People with psychosis and dementia describe themselves as being only moderately impaired, as if their remembrance of being well is hazy and their judgement of disability relates to day-to-day changes in their well-being. Self-reported disability in these disorders is of dubious value.

How is disability assessed? Ideally one should observe the person and note the degree to which he or she is unable to work or get on with others, and then establish that this inability is directly related to the person's mental disorder. Obviously such direct observation is impracticable and one has to rely on what the patients say, supplemented by some knowledge of the usual level of disability associated with that disorder. The WHO burden of disease project used groups of experts to establish the average disability weights associated with various disorders. They used a scale where a score of zero means a health status consistent with perfect health (e.g. epilepsy was weighted 0.1) and a score of 1 means a health status akin to death (e.g. the terminal phase of malignant neoplasms was weighted 0.9). Paraplegia was given a disability weight of 0.6. The disability weights for mental disorders [37] are distributed over the range of the scale (for example severe depression 0.8, moderate depression 0.3, mild depression 0.1), making it clear that mental disorders are as disabling as chronic physical disorders, and that the degree of disability expected in the average patient would vary according to diagnosis.

When clinicians assess a patient, such average measures are of little use and one usually has to rely on patient self-report measures. The most widely used measures are the short forms derived from the Rand Corporation Medical Outcomes Study in the 1970s. The Short Form 12 (SF-12) [38] is appropriate for routine use in general practice and gives separate mental and physical competency scores. The population mean on both scales is 50, and scores above this indicate no disability. Scores of 40–50 indicate mild disability, 30–40 moderate disability, and below 30 severe disability. The WHO is also developing a brief disability measure (WHODAS II) that should be applicable for use in primary care (www.who.int/icidh/whodas). Many primary care physicians will not find it easy to use either of these scales and there are two questions that can be asked of patients that correlate with the scores on these two measures. They are:

> Beginning yesterday and going back four weeks, how many days out of the past four weeks were you totally unable to work or carry out your normal activities because of your health?

Record this number as total disability days. The next question is:

> Apart from those days, how many days in the past four weeks were you able to work and carry out your normal activities, but had to cut down on what you did, or did not get as much done as usual because of your health?

Record this as "cut down days". The sum of cut down days and total disability days is the disability days attributed to illness. The disability day measure correlates highly with the formal SF-12 and DAS-II questionnaires. Normative data on disability days for the common mental disorders are displayed in Table 9.4.

Why bother about assessing disability? The usual reply is that such measures provide a basis for sickness certificates and the like. But doctors have been writing sickness certificates for years without feeling the need for external measures. The proper answer is that a reduction in disability, especially in the number of cut down days, is a very good indication that the patient is responding to treatment, and is a much better indicator of

TABLE 9.4 Self-reported disability by one-month ICD-10 diagnosis. Data from the Australian National Survey of Mental Health and Wellbeing (Andrews et al. [39])

	Disability by diagnosis	
	Short Form 12 (SF-12) Mental health summary score Mean (SE)	Disability days Mean (SE)
One-month ICD-10 diagnosis		
Affective disorder	33.4 (0.7)	11.7 (0.7)
Anxiety disorder	39.2 (0.5)	8.9 (0.7)
Substance use disorder	44.4 (0.7)	5.2 (0.5)
Personality disorder	42.0 (0.6)	7.4 (0.5)
Neurasthenia	34.6 (1.3)	14.1 (1.3)
Psychosis	39.7 (1.1)	6.3 (1.9)

Worse disability is indicated by lower SF-12 mental health summary scores and higher disability days.

improvement than a question about symptom severity. Disability assessment has another advantage: it acts as a qualifier on complaints of symptoms. That is, a person who complains of many and varied symptoms, but who is not disabled, is probably in need of less treatment than their symptoms would indicate. Conversely, a person who says stoically "I'm just a bit down and find it hard to get started", has no other symptoms but has missed days at work and has had to cut down on most other days in the past month, is certainly in need of treatment.

SPECIAL GROUPS

Children and Adolescents

Children and adolescents do have emotional and behavioral disorders that should be recognized and treated. The recognition of the externalizing or acting out youth requires little skill, the parents or school will complain about the behavior, but the recognition of the internalized anxious or depressed child is difficult. Epidemiological surveys in many countries have shown that one in five children and adolescents will have experienced significant emotional problems in the previous six months. At any point in time, one in ten children will meet criteria for a mental disorder and warrant treatment if education and vocational choice is not to be impaired by what may well be a chronic mental disorder. Thus, the task for the clinician is to decide whether the symptoms being reported by the parent or complained of by the older child are evidence of normal variation, are problems related to intercurrent stressors, or are evidence of an ICD-10 or DSM-IV-PC defined mental disorder.

There are well established risk factors that should raise the index of suspicion in clinicians that the child is at risk of developing a mental disorder. Mental disorders are more frequent in children of low intelligence, and in children with chronic physical disease, especially if that disease involves the central nervous system, e.g. epilepsy. Temperament, evident from infancy, is another good predictor. Easy children tend to be happy, regular in feeding and sleeping patterns, and they adapt easily to new situations. Difficult children are irritable, unhappy, intense, and have difficulty adjusting to change. Children with difficult temperaments are at higher risk of developing emotional and behavioral problems. Children are very sensitive to their direct family environment and, while the preceding factors are intrinsic to the child, poor family environments are not. Clinicians must be alert to families that are characterized by lack of affection, parental conflict, overprotection, inconsistent rules and discipline, families in which there is parental mental illness such as depression or substance use disorders, and above all to families in which physical or sexual abuse of the child is a possibility.

When the index of suspicion is high, clinicians should attempt to obtain information from several informants: the child, the parents and sometimes the teachers or other family members. The following is a checklist of areas that should be covered, differentiating between symptoms and behaviors that are within normal variation, or consistent with problems that are likely to remit, or indicative of mental disorder [40]:

- Achievement of developmental milestones
- Fears, phobias and obsessions
- Depressive symptoms, including suicidal thoughts
- Inattention, impulsivity, excessive activity
- Aggressive, delinquent and rule breaking conduct
- Problems with learning, hearing, seeing
- Bizarre or strange ideas or behavior
- Use of alcohol or drugs
- Difficult relationships with parents, siblings or peers.

Studies indicate that less than 30% of children with substantial dysfunction are recognized by primary care physicians. Recognition of conduct or attention problems is reasonably good because of the clarity of the parental complaint or school report, but recognition of the anxiety and depressive syndromes or of physical or sexual abuse is poor. There is a 35 item Pediatric Symptom Checklist (PSC) that has demonstrated reliability and validity as a screening instrument for use with cooperative parents. According to the author [41], it can be given to parents in the waiting room and completed in a few minutes before seeing the doctor. The scale is reproduced in Table 9.5. The PSC is scored by assigning two points for every "often" response, one point for every "sometimes" response and no points to the "never" answers. Adding the points yields the total score. If the PSC score is 28 or above, there is a 70% likelihood that the child has a significant problem. If the score is below this, then there is a 95% likelihood that the child does not have serious difficulties. Interested clinicians should consult the original articles or access the website (www.healthcare.partners. org/psc).

Diagnosis in the Elderly

Across all ages, common mental disorders are much more likely to present in primary care than in specialist clinics. Among the elderly, primary care accounts for an even greater proportion of mental health care [42]. Even in

TABLE 9.5 Pediatric Symptom Checklist (PSC; Jellinek [41], reproduced by permission)

Please mark under the heading that best describes your child:

	Never	Sometimes	Often
Complains of aches and pains			
Spends more time alone			
Tires easily, has little energy			
Fidgety, unable to sit still			
Has trouble with a teacher			
Less interested in school			
Acts as if driven by a motor			
Daydreams too much			
Distracted easily			
Is afraid of new situations			
Feels sad, unhappy			
Is irritable, angry			
Feels hopeless			
Has trouble concentrating			
Less interested in friends			
Fights with other children			
Absent from school			
School grades dropping			
Is down on him or herself			
Visits doctor with doctor finding nothing wrong			
Has trouble sleeping			
Worries a lot			
Wants to be with you more than before			
Feels he or she is bad			
Takes unnecessary risks			
Gets hurt frequently			
Seems to be having less fun			
Acts younger than children of his or her age			
Does not listen to rules			
Does not show feelings			
Does not understand other people's feelings			
Teases others			
Blames others for his or her troubles			
Takes things that do not belong to him or her			
Refuses to share			

those countries relatively well supplied with mental health specialists, initial presentation to specialist care is relatively rare. Consequently, the need to improve recognition and diagnosis of mental disorders in primary care applies even more to older adults. A few diagnostic issues specific to the elderly deserve mention.

Community and primary care surveys typically show that prevalence rates for anxiety and depressive disorders are lower among the elderly than in middle age [43, 44]. While this pattern is seen for a wide range of disorders, most attention has been directed at age differences in rates of depressive disorders. Application of standard DSM or ICD criteria for depressive episode leads to the conclusion that depressive disorders are only half as frequent above age 60 as below. This has led to questions regarding the validity of DSM and ICD criteria in the elderly [45, 46]. Some have proposed that older adults are less likely to endorse emotional symptoms such as depressed mood or sadness, leading to an under-estimation of the true prevalence of depression [46]. Others have found that elders are less likely to report symptoms of all types, and that this may reflect a general tendency to under-report distressing experience [47]. Either of these views would suggest use of a somewhat lower threshold for diagnosis of depression in the elderly. Primary care physicians in the United States and Western Europe may, in fact, already use such an adjustment. Though epidemiological data suggest a decreasing prevalence of depressive disorder with age, rates of antidepressant prescription are generally as high or higher in the elderly [48].

The overlap between depressive symptoms and symptoms of chronic medical illness has also led to questions regarding appropriateness of depression diagnostic criteria in the elderly. Symptoms such as fatigue, loss of weight or appetite, and poor concentration may reflect medical illness rather than depression, especially among older primary care patients. This concern has led to development of alternative depression measures that rely more on "psychic" and less on "somatic" symptoms [49]. Such a change in emphasis, though, would probably be inappropriate for a primary care classification. Depressed primary care patients are especially likely to present with somatic symptoms or complaints. Given concerns about under-diagnosis of depression in primary care, changes to decrease diagnostic sensitivity would probably be ill-advised.

CROSS-NATIONAL ADAPTATION OF DIAGNOSTIC SYSTEMS

Adaptation of a diagnostic system for use in different countries and cultures must consider several of the same issues important to adaptation from specialist to primary care practice. First, the form or structure of mental disorders may differ significantly across countries or cultures. Second, the prevalence of specific disorders may vary. Finally, the importance of specific clinical questions—and specific diagnostic distinctions—may differ widely according to the resources available.

Available evidence does not suggest that the form or structure of common mental disorders in primary care varies widely across countries or cultures. The common anxiety and depressive syndromes originally defined in Western Europe and the United States are also seen among primary care patients in economically developing countries [10]. Consequently, adaptation of a classification system should not usually require redefinition of core syndromes or development of new diagnostic criteria.

Cross-national epidemiological data, however, find some areas of significant variation. Overall morbidity rates show significant variability across countries and cultures. Both community and primary care surveys find that overall rates of psychiatric morbidity are typically highest in Latin America and lowest in Asia, with intermediate rates in North America and Western Europe [10, 50]. When a primary care classification is adapted for local use, some disorders may require less emphasis (or be omitted altogether). In addition, the typical presentation of anxiety and depressive disorders varies across countries and cultures [7]. While somatic presentations of psychological distress are the norm worldwide, overtly psychological presentations may be relatively common in some settings and quite rare in others. Local adaptation of a generic classification must consider culture-specific somatic presentations.

Variation across countries and health systems in availability of treatments has important implications for the utility of a primary care classification. In some cases, resource limitations may argue for simplification of a diagnostic classification. If antidepressant drugs are unavailable, the distinction between major depressive episodes and less severe depression becomes less important. In other cases, resource limitations may require an expanded scope of primary care practice. When no specialist services are available, management of psychotic disorders becomes a primary care responsibility. In this situation, distinguishing among various agitated or psychotic states (delirium, mania, and schizophrenia) becomes more relevant to primary care practice.

TRAINING AND IMPLEMENTATION

Accurate diagnosis of mental disorders in primary care is a multi-step process involving initial recognition, diagnostic assessment, and (in some cases) diagnostic confirmation. Each of these steps has unique requirements and potential difficulties. Quality improvement efforts will need to address each of these stages differently.

The initial stage in diagnosis is recognition of the presence of psychological distress or mental disorder. Abundant evidence suggests that a large number of anxiety and depressive disorders go unrecognized in the typical primary care visit. Recognition is strongly related to presenting complaint, so the most straightforward approach to improving recognition is to encourage the presentation of psychological complaints [5, 6]. Presentation of psychological complaints is associated with specific physician behaviors, and those behaviors are modifiable through training [8]. In some cases, a focus on physician awareness and interviewing style may be sufficient. Even the most skillful physician, however, will fail to recognize some cases of significant psychological disorder.

Any systematic program to increase recognition should be inexpensive, convenient, and acceptable to patients. Ideally, this initial stage of diagnosis should require little or no time from physicians and minimal time from other clinical staff. The least expensive and intensive approach is a passive screening program allowing patients to self-screen and self-identify. Examples include pamphlets or posters in the waiting room or consulting room. These approaches are probably the least expensive and least intrusive, but evidence of effectiveness is lacking. A range of options is available for active screening. While visit-based screening is the most common approach, mail screening allows a clinic or practice to target specific high-risk groups or screen those who make infrequent visits. Various modes of administration are available: paper and pencil, computer screen, telephone, or face-to-face live interview. The choice of methods should depend on local availability and acceptability to patients. Finally, a large number of measures have been proved sufficiently sensitive and specific for primary care screening. The PRIME-MD [9] and SDDS-PC [51] described above are examples of multipurpose measures intended to screen for a number of specific mental and substance use disorders. The General Health Questionnaire (GHQ) [52] and the Mental Health Inventory (MHI-5) [53] are examples of a "broad spectrum" screener for common anxiety and depressive disorders. The Center for Epidemiologic Studies Depression Scale (CES-D) [54] and the Alcohol Use Disorders Identification Test (AUDIT) [55] are examples of disorder-specific screeners.

A substantial literature suggests that screening alone (or simple recognition of psychological distress) is probably not sufficient to improve outcomes [56–59]. Screening must be followed by specific diagnosis and effective treatment [12, 60, 61]. Several studies have examined the diagnostic performance of trained primary care providers [8, 9]. Specific diagnostic tools (algorithms, criteria, semi-structured interviews) are acceptable to primary care providers and feasible for use in busy primary care practices. Diagnoses made by trained primary care staff agree well with those made by mental health specialists [9, 35]. Research supports the accuracy of diagnoses by trained physicians and nurses, with no data necessarily favoring one type of provider over the other. Two recent studies with the PRIME-MD system [29, 34] suggest that completely automated administration may agree well with a face-to-face assessment by a trained physician. Despite this evidence, it seems unlikely that most primary care physicians (or mental health specialists) would choose to initiate treatment on the basis of an automated assessment. Computerized assessment tools may be most useful for "ruling out" a specific diagnosis among those with positive screening results.

In the case of less common or more severe disorders, the primary care physician or practice should focus on screening with referral to specialist services for diagnostic confirmation. In the case of rare disorders (such as Tourette's syndrome), training primary care physicians or nurses in specific diagnosis (or treatment) does not seem a worthwhile investment. In the case of more severe disorders (such as bipolar disorder or schizophrenia), definitive diagnosis and management will usually be the responsibility of specialist services. When specialist consultation is available, training of the primary care team should focus on screening for severe disorders rather than definitive diagnostic evaluation (i.e. sensitivity rather than diagnostic specificity).

Training Other Primary Care Staff

Receptionists and Practice Nurses

It is difficult to attend a primary care physician for a regular check-up and not have blood and urine tests, and one's blood pressure estimated. So it should be. It should be equally difficult to attend and not have one's emotional well-being estimated. Unfortunately it is not. The GHQ is probably the world standard measure used for this purpose [62]. All patients, apart from those on regular repeat visits, should be given a GHQ (and for that matter an SF-12) by the receptionist or practice nurse on arrival. If parents are bringing children to see the doctor, they should be asked to fill in the parent screening for children (PSC) before the consultation begins. All receptionists and practice nurses should be trained to score these questionnaires and to flag, with a discrete code, whether the score is above the established threshold, exactly as abnormal laboratory tests are flagged to aid easy recognition by the doctor who is responsible for diagnostic decisions.

Psychologists

Psychologists are, or should be, mental health specialists. They should be capable of administering and interpreting the standard diagnostic tests, including the Composite International Diagnostic Interview (CIDI)

[63], a structured diagnostic interview for DSM-IV and ICD-10 that includes the Mini Mental State Examination [64], the Equivalent Diagnostic Interview Schedule for Children [65] and the Child Behavior Checklist [66]. They should be able to administer the Wechsler Intelligence Scale for Children [67] to any child who has a problem at school. In addition, the psychologist should be familiar with a range of questionnaires used to identify symptoms specific to the various mental disorders. Once such self-report measures are established in a clinic, the practice nurse can administer and score most of them. In fact, in many practices, clinical information systems can be used to administer most of the tests used to assess mental well-being.

Volunteers, NGO Staff and other Multipurpose Care Workers

These people, who often function with people at considerable risk of mental abnormality, need ways of identifying people who should be referred to a primary care physician for further assessment. Again, they should be trained to administer and score the GHQ and the SF-12, and to recognize when a person's score is above the accepted threshold. Furthermore, because their clientele are underserviced, they may need some understanding of the ways that people with the common mental disorders behave. *The Management of Mental Disorders* is a very accessible workbook (see www.crufad. org/books) that is published in the UK, Australia, New Zealand and Canada, with Italian and Chinese language versions in preparation. All primary care staff, from doctors to care workers, should have access to this resource.

CONCLUSIONS

We have shown that primary care needs to use a simplified system of classification, aimed at choosing appropriate management for the individual patient. The main problems in the development of the mental health aspect of primary care are finding the time to deal with the sheer mass of psychological problems in care, and training suitable staff in the specific skills they need to deal with the various problems that are of high prevalence in this setting. Across the world, many patients can now be offered treatment where previously no help would have been forthcoming, and there is a growing appreciation of the contribution that can be made by other staff, with the doctor responsible for initial triage.

REFERENCES

1. Jaspers K. (1963) *General Psychopathology*. Manchester University Press, Manchester.
2. World Organization of National Colleges, Academies and Academic Associations of General Practitioners (WONCA) (1988) *ICHPCC-2-Defined International Classification of Health Problems in Primary Care*, 3rd edn. Oxford Medical Publications, Oxford.
3. NHS Information Authority (2000) *The Clinical Terms (The Read Codes). Version 3 Reference Manual*. NHS Information Authority, Loughborough.
4. Jenkins R., Smeeton N., Shepherd M. (1988) Classification of mental disorders in primary care. *Psychol. Med.*, Suppl. 12.
5. Bridges K.W., Goldberg D.P. (1985) Somatic presentations of DSM-III psychiatric disorders in primary care. *J. Psychosom. Res.*, **29**: 563–569.
6. Goldberg D.P., Bridges K. (1988) Somatic presentations of psychiatric illness in primary care. *J. Psychosom. Res.*, **32**: 137–144.
7. Simon G.E., VonKorff M., Piccinelli M., Fullerton C., Ormel J. (1999) An international study of the relation between somatic symptoms and depression. *N. Engl. J. Med.*, **341**: 1329–1335.
8. Scott J., Jennings T., Standart S., Ward R., Goldberg D. (1999) The impact of training in problem-based interviewing on the detection and management of psychological problems presenting in primary care. *Br. J. Gen. Pract.*, **443**: 441–445.
9. Spitzer R.L., Williams J.B.W., Kroenke K., Linzer M., deGruy F.V., Hahn S.R., Brody D., Johnson J.G. (1994) Utility of a new procedure for diagnosing mental disorders in primary care: the PRIME-MD 1000 study. *JAMA*, **272**: 1749–1756.
10. Üstün T., Sartorius N. (1995) *Mental Illness in General Health Care*. Wiley, New York.
11. Goldberg D.P., Huxley P.J. (1991) *Common Mental Disorders—A Biosocial Model*. Routledge, London.
12. Goldberg D.P., Privett M., Üstün T.B., Gater R., Simon G. (1998) The effects of detection and treatment on the outcome of major depression in primary care: a naturalistic study in 15 cities. *Br. J. Gen. Pract.*, **48**: 1840–1844.
13. Kroenke K., Spitzer R.L., Williams J.B.W., Linzer M., Hahn S.R., deGruy F.V., Brody D. (1994) Physical symptoms in primary care: predictors of psychiatric disorders and functional impairment. *Arch. Fam. Med.*, **3**: 774–779.
14. Simon G.E., VonKorff M. (1991) Somatization and psychiatric disorder in the NIMH Epidemiologic Catchment Area Study. *Am. J. Psychiatry*, **148**: 1494–1500.
15. Wells K.B., Stewart A., Hays R.D., Burnam M.A., Rogers W., Daniels M., Berry S., Greenfield S., Ware J. (1989) The functioning and well-being of depressed patients: results from the Medical Outcome Study. *JAMA*, **262**: 914–919.
16. Simon G.E., VonKorff M., Barlow W. (1995) Health care costs of primary care patients with recognized depression. *Arch. Gen. Psychiatry*, **52**: 850–856.
17. Penninx B.W., Geerlings S.W., Deeg D.J., van Eijk F.T., van Tilburg W., Beekman A.T. (1999) Minor and major depression and the risk of death in older persons. *Arch. Gen. Psychiatry*, **56**: 889–895.
18. Penninx B.W., Leveille S., Ferrucci L., van Eijk J.T., Guralnik J.M. (1999) Exploring the effect of depression on physical disability: longitudinal evidence from the established populations for epidemiologic studies of the elderly. *Am. J. Public Health*, **89**: 1346–1352.

19. Sullivan M.D., LaCroix A.Z., Spertus J.A., Hecht J. (2000) Five-year prospective study of the effects of anxiety and depression in patients with coronary artery disease. *Am. J. Cardiol.*, **86**: 1135–1138.
20. Pratt L.A., Ford D.E., Crum R.M., Armenian H.K., Gallo J.J., Eaton W.W. (1996) Depression, psychotropic medication, and risk of myocardial infarction. Prospective data from the Baltimore ECA follow-up. *Circulation*, **94**: 3123–3129.
21. DiMatteo M.R., Lepper H.S., Croghan T.W. (2000) Depression is a risk factor for noncompliance with medical treatment: meta-analysis of the effects of anxiety and depression on patient adherence. *Arch. Intern. Med.*, **160**: 2101–2107.
22. World Health Organization (1996) *Diagnostic and Management Guidelines for Mental Disorders in Primary Care*. Hogrefe & Huber, Gottingen.
23. Üstün B., Goldberg D.P., Cooper J., Simon G., Sartorius N. (1995) A new classification of mental disorders based upon management for use in primary care. *Br. J. Gen. Pract.*, **45**: 211–215.
24. Goldberg D.P., Sharp D., Nanayakkara K. (1995) The field trial of the mental disorders section of ICD-10 designed for primary care (ICD10–PCH) in England. *Family Practice*, **12**: 466–473.
25. Upton M., Evans M., Goldberg D.P., Sharp D. (1999) Evaluation of ICD10-PHC mental health guidelines in detecting and managing depression in primary care. *Br. J. Psychiatry*, **175**: 476–482.
26. Wilkinson E., Sharp D., Crilly C., Croudace T., Evans J., McCann G., Harrison G. (2001) A method for developing local guidelines from an international template: the UK experience with ICD10-PHC. *Family Practice*, in press.
27. World Health Organisation (2000) *The WHO Guide to Mental Health in Primary Care*. Royal Society of Medicine, London.
28. American Psychiatric Association (1995) *Diagnostic and Statistical Manual of Mental Disorders, 4th edn (DSM-IV), Primary Care Version*. American Psychiatric Association, Washington.
29. Spitzer R.L., Kroenke K., Williams J.B. (1999) Validation and utility of a self-report version of PRIME-MD: the PHQ primary care study. *JAMA*, **282**: 1737–1744.
30. First M., Spitzer R., Gibbon M., Williams J. (1997) *Structured Clinical Interview for DSM-IV Axis I Disorders (SCID-I), Clinician Version*. American Psychiatric Press, Washington.
31. Baca E., Saiz J., Aguera L. (1999) Validation of the Spanish version of the PRIME-MD: a procedure for diagnosing mental disorders in primary care. *Actas Esp. Psiquiatr.*, **27**: 375–383.
32. Loerch B., Szegedi A., Kohnen R., Benkert O. (2000) The primary care evaluation of mental disorders (PRIME-MD), German version: a comparison with the CIDI. *J. Psychiatr. Res.*, **34**: 211–220.
33. Parker T., May P.A., Maviglia M.A., Petrakis S., Sunde G., Gloyd S.V. (1997) PRIME-MD: its utility in detecting mental disorders in American Indians. *Int. J. Psychiatry Med.*, **27**: 107–128.
34. Kobak K.A., Taylor L.H., Dottl S.L., Greist J.H., Jefferson J.W., Burroughs D., Mantle J.M., Katzelnick D.J., Norton R., Henk H.J. *et al.* (1997) A computer-administered telephone interview to identify mental disorders. *JAMA*, **278**: 905–910.
35. Weissman M.M., Olfson M., Leon A.C., Sheehan D.V., Hoven C., Conolly P., Fireman B.H., Farber L., Blacklow R.S., Higgins E.S. *et al.* (1995) Brief diagnostic interviews (SDDS-PC) for multiple mental disorders in primary care. *Arch. Fam. Med.*, **4**: 208–211.

36. Mulrow C.D., Williams J.W., Gerety M.B., Ramirez G., Montiel O.M., Kerber C. (1995) Case-finding instruments for depression in primary care settings. *Ann. Intern. Med.*, **122**: 913–921.
37. Mathers C., Vos T., Stevenson C. (1999) *The Burden of Disease and Injury in Australia.* AIHW, Canberra.
38. Ware J.E., Kosinski M., Keller S.D. (1996) A 12-item short form health survey. *Med. Care*, **34**: 220–233.
39. Andrews G., Henderson S., Hall W. (2001) Prevalence, comorbidity, disability and service utilisation: overview of the Australian National Mental Health Survey. *Br. J. Psychiatry*, **178**: 145–153.
40. Andrews G., Jenkins R. (Eds) (1999) *Management of Mental Disorders*, United Kingdom edn. World Health Organization Collaborating Centre in Mental Health, London.
41. Jellinek M. (1998) Approach to the behavior problems of children and adolescents. In *The MGH Guide to Psychiatry in Primary Care* (Eds T.A. Stern, J.B. Herman, P.L. Slavin), pp. 437–443. McGraw-Hill, New York.
42. Unutzer J., Simon G., Belin T.R., Datt M., Katon W., Patrick D. (2000) Care for depression in HMO patients aged 65 and older. *J. Am. Geriatr. Soc.*, **48**: 871–878.
43. Regier D.A., Boyd J.H., Burke J.D., Rae D.S., Myers J.K., Kramer M., Robins L.N., George L.K., Karno M., Locke B.Z. (1988) One-month prevalence of mental disorders in the United States. *Arch. Gen. Psychiatry*, **45**: 977–986.
44. Simon G.E., VonKorff M., Üstün T.B., Gater R., Gureje O., Sartorius N. (1995) Is the lifetime risk of depression actually increasing? *J. Clin. Epidemiol.*, **48**: 1109–1118.
45. Blazer D. (1989) The epidemiology of depression in late life. *J. Geriatr. Psychiatry*, **22**: 35–52.
46. Gallo J., Anthony J.C., Muthen B.O. (1994) Age differences in the symptoms of depression: a latent trait analysis. *J. Gerontol.*, **49**: 251–264.
47. Simon G.E., VonKorff M. (1992) Reevaluation of secular trends in depression rates. *Am. J. Epidemiol.*, **135**: 1411–1422.
48. Mamdani M., Hermann N., Austin P. (1999) Prevalence of antidepressant use among older people: population-based observations. *J. Am. Geriatr. Soc.*, **47**: 1350–1353.
49. Yesavage J.A., Brink T.L., Rose T.L. (1983) Development and validation of a geriatric depression screening scale. *J. Psychiatr. Res.*, **17**: 37–49.
50. Weissman M.M., Bland R.C., Canino G.J. (1996) Cross-national epidemiology of major depression and bipolar disorder. *JAMA*, **276**: 293–299.
51. Weissman M.M., Broadhead W.E., Olfson M., Faravelli C., Greenwald S., Hwu H.G., Joyce P.R., Karam E.G., Lee C.K., Lellouch J., *et al.* (1998) A diagnostic aid for detecting DSM-IV mental disorders in primary care. *Gen. Hosp. Psychiatry*, **20**: 1–11.
52. Goldberg D., Williams P. (1988) *A User's Guide to the General Health Questionnaire: GHQ.* National Foundation for Educational Research, Windsor.
53. Berwick B.H., Murphy J.M., Goldman P.A., Ware J.E., Barsky A.J., Weinstein M.C. (1991) Performance of a five-item mental health screening test. *Med. Care*, **29**: 169–176.
54. Radloff L.S. (1977) The CES-D Scale: a self-report depression scale for research in the general population. *Appl. Psychol. Measurement*, **1**: 385–401.
55. Babor T., de la Fuente J., Saunders J., Grant M. (1989) *AUDIT: The Alcohol Use Disorders Identification Test, Guidelines for Use in Primary Care.* World Health Organization, Geneva.

56. Dowrick C., Buchan I. (1995) Twelve month outcome of depression in general practice: does detection or disclosure make a difference? *Br. Med. J.*, **311**: 1274–1277.
57. Mathias S.D., Fifer S.K., Mazonson P.D., Lubeck T.D., Buesching D.P., Patrick D.L. (1994) Necessary but not sufficient: the effect of screening and feedback on outcomes of primary care patients with untreated anxiety. *J. Gen. Int. Med.*, **9**: 606–615.
58. Callahan C.M., Hendrie H.C., Dittus R.S., Brater D.C., Hui S.L., Tierney W.M. (1994) Improving treatment of late life depression in primary care: a randomized clinical trial. *J. Am. Geriatr. Soc.*, **42**: 839–846.
59. Katon W., VonKorff M., Lin E., Bush T., Lipscomb P., Russo J. (1992) A randomized trial of psychiatric consultation with distressed high utilizers. *Gen. Hosp. Psychiatry*, **14**: 86–98.
60. Schulberg H.C., Block M.R., Madonia M.J., Scott C.P., Rodriguez E., Imber S.D., Perel J., Lave J., Houck P.R., Coulehan J.L. (1996) Treating major depression in primary care practice: eight-month clinical outcomes. *Arch. Gen. Psychiatry*, **53**: 913–919.
61. Katzelnick D.J., Simon G.E., Pearson S.D., Manning W.G., Helstad C.P., Henk H.J., Cole S.M., Lin E.H.B., Taylor L.V.H., Kobak K.A. (2000) Randomized trial of a depression management program in high utilizers of medical care. *Arch. Fam. Med.*, **9**: 345–351.
62. Goldberg D.P. (1972) *The Detection of Psychiatric Diagnosis by Questionnaire*. Oxford University Press, London.
63. World Health Organization (1997) *Complete International Diagnostic Interview— Version 2.1*. World Health Organization, Geneva.
64. Folstein M.F., Folstein S.E. McHugh P.R. (1975) Mini-Mental State: a practical method for grading the cognitive ability of patients for the clinician. *J. Psychiatr. Res.*, **12**: 189–198.
65. Shaffer D., Fisher P., Lucas C.P., Dulcan M.K., Schwab-Stone M.L. (2000) NIMH Diagnostic Interview Schedule for Children (Version IV). *J. Am. Acad. Child Adolesc. Psychiatry*, **39**: 28–38.
66. Achenbach T.M., Edelbrock C. (1983) *Manual for the Child Behaviour Checklist and Revised Behaviour Profile*, 2nd edn. University of Vermont, Burlington.
67. Wechsler D. (1991) *Wechsler Intelligence Scale for Children*, 3rd edn. Psychological Corporation, New York.

10

Psychiatric Diagnosis and Classification in Developing Countries

R. Srinivasa Murthy[1] and Narendra N. Wig[2]

[1]National Institute of Mental Health, Bangalore, India
[2]Postgraduate Institute of Medical Education and Research, Chandigarh, India

INTRODUCTION

Psychiatric services and psychiatry as a medical discipline in developing countries are of recent origin. Less than 50 years ago, most of the developing countries had very few mental health professionals. The only available sources of help were the traditional systems of care and an extremely limited number of mental hospitals. Most of these hospitals were large in size, often located far away from the general population, and played a custodial role rather than the therapeutic function. The majority of developing countries depended on European and North American countries for training of mental health professionals. Modern psychiatry was usually started by expatriate mental health professionals. The limitations of language and the cross-cultural differences in the expression of mental distress often led to interpretation of the psychiatric phenomenon on the basis of Western orientations. A common expression of this was the concept of "culture bound syndromes", with colorful names [1–3]. Currently most of these syndromes have retreated to the background of psychiatric classification. This is one of the expressions of the growth of modern psychiatry in developing countries. Though some of the recent developments are positive, there is still a great amount of deprivation in services and professionals in most developing countries. In a large number of countries the available resources for care are less than 1% of those available in Europe and North America.

In addition to the practitioners of traditional medical systems, in developing countries there are numerous religious healers or faith healers providing help to people for psychological and psychosocial problems. They are a

Psychiatric Diagnosis and Classification. Edited by Mario Maj, Wolfgang Gaebel, Juan José López-Ibor and Norman Sartorius. © 2002 John Wiley & Sons, Ltd.

large and heterogeneous group. Some of them use magical and occult practices. They may make astrological predictions, use trance-like experience in which spirits are supposed to "possess" the healers or the sufferer, and use various means to remove the evil spirits or the effects of black magic done to a person. Others in this group are members of the priestly class or leaders of the established religious order, to whom people go for advice and counseling, and who on the basis of prevailing religious teachings provide psychological counseling [4]. There is considerable overlap between practices used by the various groups. Common to all the religious and faith healers, however, is a culturally approved belief system shared by the healer and the patient and a powerful personality of the healer. Although most countries of the world accept modern scientific medicine as the basis for their public health action as well as for their preventive and curative medical services, in many developing countries the governments also provide patronage and financial support to other well-established traditional systems. These include the Chinese traditional medicine (including acupuncture) in China; Ayurveda in India, Sri Lanka and countries of South Asia; and Unani or Arabic medicine in India, Pakistan and other countries in the Middle East and Africa.

Classification is an essential part of scientific thinking. It brings order in the otherwise confusing mass of information which is gathered through observation. It identifies the similarities and differences between various categories. It helps to communicate meaningfully with other observers of a similar phenomenon. It also helps to generate hypotheses for further experiment and observation. Thus, classification is not a closed static system but an open-ended dynamic system, which goes on changing with addition of new knowledge.

In present-day psychiatry, classification has become even more important than it is in many other medical specialities. The knowledge about the aetiology of most psychiatric conditions is still unsatisfactory. Multiple factors acting together at a given time seem to be a more likely explanation than a single causative factor. It is still not known how to measure these complex interactions between different factors. Reliable laboratory tests and radiological diagnostic procedures are relatively few. Most of the time, for the diagnosis, a clinician has to depend on a good history and mental state examination. Under these circumstances, a reliable system of classification becomes a priority without which it is not possible to communicate with others, or to plan research or even to efficiently organize the treatment of the patient and compare it with others. In this sense, classification has become the common language of communication in psychiatry today.

The present review of psychiatric diagnosis and classification in developing countries is presented under the following broad headings: (a) historical development of psychiatric classification in developing countries as re-flected in the medical and historical texts; (b) conceptual differences in psychiatric diagnosis and classification in developing vs. Western countries; (c) clinical research in developing countries relating to modern psychiatric classification; (d) some classification systems from developing countries; (e) the *International Classification of Diseases*, tenth edition (ICD-10) field trials in developing countries; (f) the shortcomings of existing classifications and future needs of developing countries in psychiatric classification; and (g) conclusions.

HISTORICAL ASPECTS OF PSYCHIATRIC CLASSIFICATION IN DEVELOPING COUNTRIES

In developing countries, apart from modern European medicine, there exist at least three major medical traditions, those of: (a) China and the Far East, (b) India and South Asia, (c) Middle East and North Africa. Sub-Saharan Africa has its own medical traditions, but they are not so well documented. The Chinese and Indian civilizations have a continuous history of more than 3000 years. Islamic civilization is also over 1400 years old. Each one of these major civilizations has a rich heritage and traditions in various branches of sciences and arts, like mathematics, astronomy, architecture, music and literature. They have also a very long and continuous historical tradition in medicine, with numerous medical texts preserved from the past.

Traditional Medical Systems in India and South East Asia

In India and the neighboring countries, like Nepal, Bangladesh and Sri Lanka, a highly developed and elaborate system of medicine has flourished for nearly 3000 years. It is generally known by the name of Ayurveda (the science of life) [5].

There are many medical texts dating back to the first and second century AD which describe in detail the principles of Ayurveda. The two best known medical works are by the Ayurvedic physicians Caraka and Susruta. These books were originally compiled sometime between the third century BC and the third century AD. The principles of Ayurvedic medicine, as in other Indian philosophical systems, were probably well developed by the third century BC. In Ayurveda, the fundamental principle of health is the proper balance between five elements (Bhutas) and three humors (Dosas). The balance occurs at different levels: physical, physiological, psychological and finally spiritual—the state of bliss in which the ultimate goal is tran-quility [5, 6]. The human being is considered an integral part of the nature and is made up of the same five elements (Bhutas) that constitute the universe: water, air, fire, earth, and sky. The three humors or Dosas recognized in Ayurvedic medicine are kapha (phlegm), pitta (bile) and vata (wind). People in India, to describe the states of health and disease, still popularly use these terms for the three Dosas. Another concept that is very central to Ayurvedic medicine and Indian philosophy is the Tri-guna or the theory of three inherent qualities or modes of nature. These three gunas are Sattva (variously translated as light, goodness or purity), Rajas (action, energy, passion) and Tamas (darkness, inertia). In the medical and religious texts, the theory of the three gunas is used repeatedly to describe different types of personalities, food, action, etc. [7].

All the major Ayurvedic texts, like Caraka Samhita and Susruta Samhita, have a separate section dealing with insanity (unmada). In addition, there are chapters on spirit possession (bhutonmada) and epilepsy (apasmara). Different types of convulsions, paralysis, fainting, intoxications are also well described. There is detailed description of different types of spirit possessions. Twenty-one subtypes based on three groups of sattva, rajas, and tamas are described. Though at times the descriptions appear artificial, some of them have clear resemblance to some modern descriptions of personality disorders, psychosis, and mental retardation [8]. The chapters on unmada (insanity) are very well written, both in Caraka Samhita and Susruta Samhita. Six types of mental disorders are well recognized: vatonmad, caused by vata dosa; kaphonmad, caused by kapha dosa; pittonmad, caused by pitta dosa; sampattonmad, caused by combined dosas; vishaja onamad, caused by intoxications and poisons; and shokaja unmad, caused by excessive grief.

Many psychiatrists in India have made serious attempts to equate some of these Ayurvedic descriptions to modern psychiatric diagnostic terms [8–10]. The results are neither uniform nor comparable. In Ayurveda there are no separate chapters on neurosis or stress-related somatic illness. However, there are numerous references suggesting that the influence of psychological and environmental factors on health and disease was well recognized [11, 12].

Traditional Chinese Medicine

Like other ancient systems of medicine, Chinese medicine is intimately linked with the prevailing religious and philosophical thought, which is difficult to grasp by one unfamiliar with Chinese culture. It is generally accepted that the main core of Chinese medicine separated itself from magico-religious concepts of diseases earlier than in other cultures. The three major religious philosophies in Chinese culture have been Taoism,

Buddhism, and Confucianism. One central concept in Chinese medicine is that of the Yin and Yang as two parts, in a perennial state of opposition and attraction. The *Canon of Internal Medicine*, one of the sourcebooks of Chinese medicine, dating back to the fourth century, refers to mental disorders like insanity, dementia, violent behavior, convulsions and possession by spirits. In the field of treatment, one of the important contributions of Chinese medicine is acupuncture, which still retains its popularity.

Arabic or Islamic Medicine

Health sciences greatly flourished during the rise of Islamic civilization between the seventh and twelfth centuries in the Middle East, Central Asia, North Africa and Spain. The Arab or Islamic medical system is still widely practiced in Pakistan, India, Bangladesh, and many Arab countries of the Middle East and Africa, particularly in the rural areas. In the Indian subcontinent, this system of medicine is called Tib-E-Unani or "Greek Medicine", which points to its early roots.

The original source for Islamic medicine was the existing Greek and Latin medical texts based on the theories of Hippocrates and Galen and other well-known scholars. Islamic medicine has also been influenced by Indian medical texts. During the early Islamic centuries, numerous medical texts from Greece and India were translated into Arabic. Soon the famous physicians belonging to the Arabic tradition, like Al Razi (Rhazes, 865–925 AD) and Ibn Sena (Avicena, 980–1037 AD), not only refined the old medical knowledge, but also gave it the present shape. The Arabic medical books, particularly Avicena's *Canon of Medicine*, had a deep impact on European medical traditions. It was an essential medical text in many universities in Europe until the seventeenth century.

A number of Islamic medical authorities have described in detail the existing psychiatric classification in their books. Some of the best known examples are Haly Abbas in his book *Kamil-Us-Sinaa* (second half of tenth century) and Samarqandi (died 1227) [5]. Most of these classifications follow the pattern of the earlier Greek and Latin texts. Conditions like epilepsy, dementia, melancholia and hysteria are well described. In the medical works of Ibn-Jazlah, written in the eleventh century, we find a beautiful example of medical description and the Arabic art of calligraphy. Recently this has been published as a new book in English [13]. The section on mental disorders consists of a one-page table that concisely lists the names of the eight common neuropsychiatric diseases on one side, while on the other side age, sex, season of occurrence, cause, main symptoms, routine treatment and treatment for royalty and nobles are described. In the limited space of one table, all the important known facts have been summarized [5].

The eight diseases, in their original Arabic names together with English translations are: Al Sadr (confusion and dizziness; ? delirium); Al Dawar (vertigo); Al Saraa (epilepsy, fits); Al Sakta (stroke); Al Qaboos (nightmare, anxiety state); Al Malikhoulia, Al Maraqiyah (melancholia and hypochondriac obsession); Al Qatrat or Al Qutrub (insanity; ? psychosis); and Al Ishq (sickness due to love, wasting away in love).

The last illness, Al Ishq or wasting away in love, is described as being common among youth. It is interesting to note that this remained a well-recognized medical entity in Islamic medicine for many centuries.

Medical Traditions in Africa

While the northern part of Africa came greatly under the influence of Muslim empires, Sub-Saharan Africa remained largely free of the influence of other civilizations till the arrival of European colonial powers in the eighteenth century or so. Though there were at times large powerful African empires, like the Masai of East Africa, African society largely remained divided into various tribes, each one having its separate traditions and culture. It is generally accepted that the dominant feature of traditional medicine in Africa has been the beliefs in gods, spirits of ancestors and supernatural powers. In many parts of Africa, nearly all forms of illness, personal catastrophes, accidents, and unusual happenings were generally attributed to machinations of the enemy and malicious influence of spirits that inhabit the world around, though according to Lambo this is not the whole story [14, 15]. Many of the tribes were also aware of the concept of the natural causation. This was particularly true of the Masai tribe of East Africa and the Shona tribe of present-day Zimbabwe. The Shona people identify four general causes of mental illness, which is diagnosed when a person does not talk sense or behaves in a strange or foolish manner. Such a person may be restless, violent or very quiet. These four causes are the influence of spirits, old age, worry or guilt for a wrong or immoral act and the improper development of the brain.

CONCEPTUAL DIFFERENCES IN PSYCHIATRIC DIAGNOSIS

There are a number of differences between the classifications in traditional and modern systems of medicine. Magico-religious traditions still persist in many developing countries, particularly in the rural societies. As a result many of the psychotic, neurotic and personality disorders are often understood by the general population as being the result of spirit possession or witchcraft. However, if the patient consults a practitioner of well-organized traditional medical systems like Ayurveda, Chinese or Islamic medicine, the explanation provided is usually on the lines of "scientific" theory of that system, e.g. imbalance of body humors, etc.

The concept of insanity as a grossly disturbed behavior with loss of insight seems to be well recognized in most of the ancient medical texts. However, such a diagnosis was based predominantly on observation of external behavior. The intrapsychic processes as such were neither given prominence nor used as a basis of diagnosis or classification. For example, in Indian Ayurvedic texts there is no clear recognition of separate affective or mood disorders, nor is there any clear description of insanity resembling paranoid psychosis, while states of excitement, severe withdrawal and socially inappropriate behavior are well described. Many people in the developing countries, including health personnel, easily recognize conditions like acute or chronic psychosis as clear examples of mental illness, but conditions like depression, hypomania and paranoid states are less easily accepted as psychiatric problems.

In the European philosophical tradition there is a strong tendency to think in terms of duality or "polarity of contrasting opposites" [6]. In modern psychiatry this has often led to an undue preoccupation with controversies like nature/nurture, body/mind, conscious/unconscious, organic/functional and so on. This has also influenced modern psychiatric classifications. Other cultures have looked at the nature differently, often "by juxtaposition and identification of polarities" [6]. The Chinese theory of Yin–Yang principles is a beautiful example of this. In Indian philosophy, instead of bipolar models, there are often three dimensions of a phenomenon, e.g. the Tri-Guna theory of inherent qualities of nature as sattva, rajas and tamas, or the triumvirate of Gods, Brahma, Vishnu and Shiva, controlling the three aspects of creation, preservation and destruction of the universe.

The current division of functional psychoses into affective disorders and schizophrenia seems to be based on the nineteenth century European understanding of human mind into arbitrary divisions of "feeling" and "thinking". Such concepts do not find recognition in traditional medical systems.

Unlike modern medicine, the traditional systems of medicine do not maintain a strict division between body and mind. For example, the imbalance between body humors can affect both physical and mental functions. As a result, the practitioners of traditional medical systems tend to have a more holistic approach towards their patients. A neurotic patient feels more comfortable with a traditional healer because there is no tendency to be labeled as having "no physical" illness as is common with the practitioners of modern medicine.

The concept of "subconscious" processes is relatively new in modern psychiatry. It has no roots in traditional medicine. Subconscious processes are often mentioned as the underlying cause for illnesses such as hysteria and somatoform disorders. In developing countries, lay persons as well as health workers find such concepts often difficult to comprehend.

In the traditional medical systems there is no unified concept of neurosis as has emerged in psychiatry during the last 100 years. Though feelings of fear and grief are recognized by all cultures, in modern medicine the excess of these two emotions has been given the status of medical disorders like anxiety and depression. It is difficult to explain, if the excess of anxiety or depression is a medical disorder, why an excess of anger or greed or lust should not be considered as pathological.

The classification of personality types and personality disorders has received considerable attention in the traditional medical system. In general, the classification of personality was closely modeled on the prevailing religious and moral codes of human behavior. A major difference in the classification of personality disorders of traditional medical systems vs. modern psychiatry is that while the latter uses the concept of average norm (i.e. whatever is markedly deviant is abnormal), the former prefers the ideal norm (i.e. whatever is less than ideal is inadequate and thus, in a sense, abnormal). In modern psychiatry personality disorders, especially antisocial personality, are seen as deeply ingrained patterns of behavior, which do not easily change. Other cultures do not seem to share this pessimistic view. As depicted in the old Indian epic stories as well as in the present-day Indian films, in popular imagination a bad person can often turn good under a strong emotional impact.

CLINICAL RESEARCH IN DEVELOPING COUNTRIES

Information on the use of psychiatric classification in developing countries is available from a number of sources. Though these studies are not systematic and do not use standardized assessment tools, and their samples are most often purposive, they provide the ground experience of psychiatrists in developing countries. Reports are available on the clinical diagnosis of patients seen in general hospital psychiatric wards in Singapore [16, 17]; and patients referred to psychiatric services in Nigeria [18–22], Malaysia [23], Tanzania [24], Libya [25], Ghana [26], Papua New Guinea [27], India [28–33], Ethiopia [34, 35], Israel [36], Turkey [37], Pakistan [4], Bahrain [38], Egypt [39] and Japan [40].

Information from routine psychiatric services demonstrates that the groups of patients seeking care are mostly suffering from different forms of psychoses and depressive disorders. Strikingly, there are limited numbers of persons suffering from personality disorders and adjustment disorders seeking help. Most probably, the public perception that severe disorders are those relevant to psychiatric care and the limited availability of services leads to a greater attention to severe forms of mental disorders.

Acute Psychosis

During the last 50 years, many reports from countries in Asia, Africa, and Latin America have confirmed the occurrence of acute and transient psychotic disorders which do not fit into the traditional subdivision of psychoses into schizophrenia and manic-depressive illness. Many more reports of acute psychoses from India have appeared in recent years [41–46].

Kapur and Pandurangi [42] studied reactive psychosis and acute psychosis without precipitating stress to compare the antecedent factors, phenomenology, treatment and prognosis in 30 cases of each category matched on age and sex, and followed up for seven months. The two groups differed markedly on several dimensions. The reactive psychotic group had more hysterical and affective symptoms, a more vulnerable personality, higher stressful experiences prior to illness and a relatively better prognosis compared to the other group. The difference still persisted when cases receiving a diagnosis of schizophrenia or affective psychoses during follow-up were excluded from the analysis.

In a major multicenter study conducted by the Indian Council of Medical Research (ICMR) [45], more than 300 individuals with acute onset psychotic illnesses from four centers in India were investigated in detail and followed up for one year. The most striking feature of this study was that more than 75% of the patients had fully recovered with no relapse of psychotic illness at one-year follow-up. In a similar study sponsored by the World Health Organization (WHO) and conducted in New Delhi with cases of acute first episode psychosis, Wig and Parhee [46] reported that nearly 70% of the cases suffered from only a single episode of illness during the course of one-year follow-up.

The ICD-9 diagnosis at the time of initial assessment did not differentiate cases with good recovery from those with poor outcome in either the ICMR or the WHO study. Irrespective of the initial diagnosis (schizophrenia, manic-depressive psychosis, or non-organic psychosis), more than 70% of the cases had completely recovered after one year. Another striking feature of these studies was the difficulty in classifying acute psychotic cases into either schizophrenia or manic-depressive psychosis. Only 49% of the sample in the WHO study and 60% in the ICMR study were given a diagnosis of schizophrenia or manic-depressive psychosis at the initial assessment.

The ICMR study made an attempt to develop purely descriptive diagnostic categories on the basis of the presenting clinical picture. Ten categories were chosen and operationally defined to cover the entire range of observed behavior. These were: (a) predominantly excited, (b) predominantly withdrawn, (c) predominantly depressed, (d) predominantly elated, (e) predominantly paranoid, (f) predominantly confused, (g) predominantly hysterical, (h) predominantly spirit possession, (i) mixed, and (j) others. More than 50% of the cases belonged to predominantly excited and paranoid types. The next two common categories were withdrawn and depressed types (25%).

The WHO launched a "cross-cultural study of acute psychosis" as part of the larger study called "Determinants of outcome of severe mental disorders" (DOSMED). Varma *et al.* [47] reported on 109 cases of acute psychosis seen in the Chandigarh center. These were assessed by the Schedule for Clinical Assessment of Acute Psychotic States (SCAAPS) and the Present State Examination. A conventional diagnosis like manic-depressive psychosis or schizophrenia was seen in 60% of cases, and was less often associated with stress. About 40% of all cases presented with CATEGO subtypes which were not indicative of a specific diagnosis.

The salient features of acute transient psychosis collated from the above studies are: (a) acute onset (full blown psychotic illness within two weeks); (b) short-lasting course; (c) good outcome: more than two-thirds of cases recover fully with no relapse in one year; (d) no uniform clinical picture; (e) no major physiological or psychological stress at the beginning of psychosis; and (f) the initial diagnosis according to standard classifications does not seem to be significantly correlated with the outcome.

Susser and Wanderling [48] re-examined the data from the WHO DOSMED study [49], which had included 13 sites in two contrasting socio-cultural settings, the developing country and the industrialized country [47]. For this study, Susser *et al.* [50] introduced the term *non-affective acute remitting psychoses* (NARP) to describe non-affective psychoses that were characterized by a very acute onset within one week and a full remission during a two-year follow-up period, received an ICD-9 diagnosis of schizophrenia and did not show or had only minimum affective symptoms. There were 794 patients who met all criteria for inclusion in their study: 140 (18%) had NARP and 654 (82%) had other ICD-9 schizophrenia. For NARP, the incidence in men was about one-half the incidence in women, and the incidence in the developing country setting was about 10-fold higher than in the industrialized setting.

These associations with sex and setting were sharply different from those of schizophrenia. The authors concluded that NARP represented a distinct disorder, and that the epidemiological pattern could yield clues to its causes. To verify the above findings, Susser *et al.* [50] examined 46 cases of acute and transient psychotic disorders or NARP from the Chandigarh center [47], and confirmed that acute transient psychoses conform neither with schizophrenia of brief duration nor with atypical affective syndromes. To explore the long-term course of these psychotic disorders, subjects who continued to receive treatment were studied at 12-year follow-up [51]. Though the original diagnoses of this cohort were made using ICD-9 criteria, for the latter study the patients were rediagnosed using the ICD-10 diagnostic criteria for research. Acute transient psychosis had an excellent long-term outcome, which was distinctly better than that of other remitting psychoses.

The above studies have important implications for ICD-10 diagnosis of acute and transient psychotic disorders, code F23. They suggest that the creation of a separate diagnostic grouping for such disorders in the ICD-10 represents a significant step forward in diagnostic classification. However, these data indicate that the ICD-10 duration criteria for these disorders are too restrictive. The ICD-10 allows a duration up to one month when schizophrenic symptoms are present, and up to three months when these symptoms are absent. In the above studies, these disorders typically lasted more than one month and sometimes more than three months. Thus, the ICD-10 criteria are likely to exclude a large proportion of the very conditions for which the grouping of acute and transient psychotic disorders was intended.

For reasons which are not properly understood, these illnesses represent a very small fraction of psychiatric morbidity in industrialized countries today, but are relatively common in developing countries. Their correct and timely recognition is important because of their benign prognosis. The ICD-10 now contains a major rubric (F23) with five subdivisions and diagnostic guidelines which should help to differentiate the typical polymorphic acute states from schizophrenia. Since very little is known about this group of disorders, it is likely to be a rewarding field for clinical and epidemiological research [52].

The symptomatology and outcome of acute psychosis were studied in 50 Egyptian patients [53]. In 74% of cases an identifiable stressor was present before the onset of acute psychosis. After three months, 54% of cases showed a full remission, 28% had residual symptoms, 4% were in a relapse and 14% were still in the index episode. After one year, the corresponding figures were 64% remission, 12% residual symptoms, 14% relapse and 10% in index episode. In terms of social outcome, 54% reported improvements, 30% worsening and 16% severe social impairment. The symptoms that were most common in the Indian sample and not so prevalent in the Egyptian sample included agitation and excitement, hostile irritability, lack of initiative, overactivity, loss of appetite, delusions of reference, and tangential speech.

Depressive Disorders

The phenomenology and classification of depressive disorders have been studied in individual centers as well as in international cross-cultural studies. Depression was reported to be manifesting as masked depression with somatic complaints in Nigeria [19]. The core depressive symptoms were somatic complaints in patients in Ethiopia [34, 54].

A large amount of information on the diagnosis and classification is available from cross-cultural studies of groups of patients with the same diagnosis. Though there were some studies in this area prior to 1990 [55–60], the number of studies during the last decade is remarkable. This could be a reflection of the availability of the ICD-10 and DSM-IV for comparative studies.

The pre-1990 studies have focused on: depressive symptoms in students of Japanese, Chinese and Caucasian ancestry [55]; the reliability of diagnosis across countries in a WHO international collaborative study from Colombia, Brazil, Sudan, Egypt, India and Philippines [56]; the characteristics of depressed patients contacting services in Basel, Montreal, Nagasaki, Teheran and Tokyo [57]; the diagnosis of mental disorders among Turkish and American clinicians [58]; the symptomatology of depression in the black and white groups and overseas Chinese [59]; affective disorders in Nagasaki, Shanghai and Seoul [60]; and hysterical manifestations in patients of Africa and Europe. A number of studies showed a more frequent somatic presentation in patients with depression from developing countries.

Jablensky *et al.* [57] reported the existence of a common core of depressive symptomatology across centers. However, feelings of guilt and self-reproach were present in 68% of cases in Basel, 58% in Montreal, 48% in Tokyo, 41% in Nagasaki and only 32% in Teheran. Suicidal ideas were less frequent in Teheran (46%) and Tokyo (41%) as compared to Montreal and Nagasaki (70%). Various somatic symptoms (including vital signs like lack of appetite, loss of weight, loss of libido, constipation) were present in 40% of all patients. They were less frequent in Montreal (27%) and Basel (32%) and more frequent in Teheran (57%). Chang [59] reported a mixture of affective and somatic complaints in the black group, existential and cognitive concerns in the white group, and somatic complaints in the overseas Chinese group.

Turkish patients scored higher in the vegetative-somatic syndrome scale as compared to German patients [61]. True somatization was significantly more common in Chinese American patients. The Chinese Americans complained predominantly with cardiopulmonary and vestibular symptoms, whereas Caucasians had more symptoms of abnormal motor functions [62].

Hysterical Dissociative Disorders

Saxena and Prasad [31] studied the utility of DSM-III sub-classification of dissociative disorders in 62 cases. They found that 90% of cases fell into the atypical subcategory. They suggested to include the categories of simple dissociative disorder and possession disorder in future revisions. Alexander *et al.* [63] studied the prevalence of ICD-10 and DSM-IV categories of dissociative (conversion) disorders in their clinical population and found the need for a category they called "brief depressive stupor". They also called for the inclusion of the category of dissociative convulsions.

Anorexia Nervosa

Lee [64] focused on the question of Western psychiatry's ethnocentricity using the example of anorexia nervosa. A mixed retrospective–prospective study of 70 Chinese anorexic patients in Hong Kong showed that, although they were similar to Western anorexics, 58.6% did not exhibit any fear of fatness throughout the course of their illness. Instead, these non-fat phobic patients used epigastric bloating, no appetite, or simply eating less as legitimizing rationales for food refusal and emaciation. Authors argue that anorexia nervosa may display phenomenological plurality in a Westernizing society, and its identity may be conceptualized without invoking the explanatory construct of fat phobia exclusively.

Culture Bound Syndromes

As early as in 1960, Wig [65] described cases of young adult males complaining of involuntary passage of white discharge (which patients described as dhat) per urethra during micturation or defecation, leading to multiple somatic symptoms along with anxiety and depressive features. Many subsequent workers have confirmed the presence of this phenomenon, which is perhaps unique to the culture of South Asia [66–68]. Varma [69], while proposing a classification of neurosis for use in India, included Dhat syndrome in his scheme. ICD-10 has finally accepted the presence of this disorder and classified it under the category of neurotic disorders, other, code F48.

Miscellaneous Studies

A number of other studies have reported on the presentation of mental disorders and their classification in developing countries. Somatization complaints formed the basis of distress of the mentally ill in Nigeria [19, 20]; 75% of patients seen were suffering from psychoses, with antisocial personality as the most common personality disorder in Libya [25]; 49% of the patients seen in Papua New Guinea were diagnosed as suffering from schizophrenia [27]; flight of ideas was rarely seen in patients suffering from mania in Eastern India [32]; 97% of patients with common mental disorders presented with somatic complaints in Harare [33]; the core depressive symptoms were somatic complaints in Ethiopia [34, 54]; the majority of the refugees presented with anxiety, depressive or somatic symptoms in Delhi [29, 30]; 61% of the 139 attendees at a faith healing center in Pakistan had a psychiatric diagnosis (major depressive episode 24%, generalized anxiety disorder 15%, and epilepsy 9%) and there was little agreement between the faith healers' classification and DSM-III-R diagnosis [4]. A limited number of case reports of Amok [70], brain-fag syndrome [71], and culture bound syndromes from South Africa have been published. Saxena and Prasad [31] applied DSM-III criteria to 123 Indian psychiatric outpatients with predominantly somatic symptoms. They found that the most common Axis I diagnoses were dysthymic disorder and generalized anxiety disorder. More than one-third of the patients fitted only into atypical diagnostic categories.

The area of personality disorders has been the focus of study only recently. Loranger *at al.* [72] reported on 716 patients from 14 centers in 11 countries of North America, Europe, Africa and Asia. They found that the assessment instrument (International Personality Disorder Examination, IPDE) proved acceptable to clinicians across cultures. Moriya *et al.* [73] reported on the differences in the borderline personality disorder in the East and West.

Kortmann [35] studied the applicability of DSM-III in 40 Ethiopian patients and found that the categories of psychotic and affective disorders were congruent with DSM-III categories but the classes of somatoform and fictitious disorders did not fit the DSM-III system.

In a study of the relationship between neurotic and personality disorders involving 200 neurotic patients, personality disorders and personality abnormalities were significantly more frequent in neurotic patients than in controls [74].

A striking lacuna in clinical research carried out in developing countries is the almost total absence of diagnostic work in children and adolescents. There are just few clinical studies focusing on psychoses or mania [75, 76]. There are also few studies reporting on the experience of other mental health professionals, like clinical psychologists, psychiatric social workers, psychiatric nurses and occupational therapists [77]. Though mental health care in primary health care is a widely accepted approach in developing countries, systematic studies of psychiatric diagnosis and classification at that level are scarce [78, 79].

EXPERIENCES OF APPLYING AND USING MODERN PSYCHIATRIC CLASSIFICATION IN DEVELOPING COUNTRIES

China

China has a national system of psychiatric classification called the Chinese Classification of Mental Disorders (CCMD) [80–84]. The first published classificatory scheme appeared in 1979. This was revised and named the CCMD-1 in 1981, and was further modified in 1984. The CCMD-1 was subsequently revised and tested on 22 285 outpatients and 8061 inpatients in 77 mental health facilities all over China. These efforts culminated in the publication of the CCMD-2, which represented a marked change from the previous classificatory schemes. For the first time in China, operationalized criteria for a broad range of diagnostic categories became available [82].

The CCMD-2-R and the ICD-10 share a broadly comparable architecture. Many Chinese psychiatrists believe that the CCMD-2-R has special advantages such as simplicity, stability, the inclusion of culture-distinctive and serviceable forensic categories, and the exclusion of otiose Western diagnostic categories. Linguistically, it is easier to use than the Chinese version of the ICD-10, which contains excessively long sentences, awkward terms, and syntactical problems. Unlike the ICD-10, which is divided into clinical, research and primary care versions, the CCMD-2-R is an all-purpose document.

CCMD-2-R is published in the form of a handbook of 238 pages. It contains operationalized criteria for all diagnostic categories and the equivalent or closest ICD-9 and ICD-10 codes alongside the diagnostic headings. The CCMD-2-R strategy of classification is both aetiological and symptomatological. Zheng *et al.* [85] have demonstrated that the reliability and validity of the CCMD-2 and the DSM-III-R were closely compatible in most diagnostic categories, such as schizophrenia, bipolar disorder and most depressive disorders. Discrepancies, however, remain in the diagnosis of neurasthenia and hysteria.

The CCMD-2-R duration criterion for the diagnosis of schizophrenia remains three months. The Chinese Task Force felt that the ICD-10 criterion of one month will not adequately exclude transient psychoses that turn out to be non-schizophrenic in nature. The CCMD-2-R preserves "paranoid psychosis" and "simple schizophrenia", but excludes "schizotypal disorders". As "reactive psychosis" has long been a popular diagnostic concept in China, the category "acute and transient psychotic disorders" of the ICD-10 (F23) has been welcomed by Chinese psychiatrists.

In affective (mood) disorders, the CCMD-2-R maintains a simple notion of depression, and uses the term yi yu zheng (depressive syndrome) without any sub-classification. Although the CCMD-2-R duration criterion (two weeks or more) for the diagnosis of depression is the same as that of the ICD-10 and DSM-IV, depressed mood is required as the "main characteristic" of the condition.

Neurosis and psychogenic mental disorders are preserved in the CCMD-2-R, which emphasizes as their main characteristics the presence of predisposing personality and social factors and the preservation of "insight". Both "hysteria" and "hysterical psychosis" are retained.

Chinese psychiatrists are far from being impressed by the category of somatoform disorders. With the exception of hypochondriacal neurosis, the whole category of somatization disorders of the ICD-10 is excluded in the CCMD-2-R. The ICD-10 definition of neurasthenia, which requires fatigue (or weakness) as the mandatory core symptom, misrepresents the reality of Chinese neurasthenic patients. In Hong Kong, insomnia and headache are usually the core symptoms of neurasthenic patients, while fatigue is commonly an accessory symptom. In the CCMD-2-R, the diagnosis of neurasthenia requires the presence of three out of five symptoms (weakness, dysphasia, excitement, nervous pain and sleep symptoms). Consonant with an aetiologically based classification, depressive neurosis (or dysthymia) is grouped under neurosis rather than mood disorders.

The CCMD-2-R includes three "culture-related mental disorders" under "neurosis and psychogenic mental disorders". They include koro, qigong-induced mental disorders, and superstition- and witchcraft-induced mental disorder.

Since the DSM-IV and ICD-10 diagnostic criteria for anorexia nervosa may be inadequate when applied in a Chinese setting, more culture-flexible diagnostic criteria that take into account the local meanings of food refusal will be adopted in the next version of the CCMD. Another point of cross-cultural interest pertains to the amount of weight loss. The CCMD-2-R requires a weight loss of 25% or more of standard body weight for a diagnosis of anorexia nervosa to be made. Given the generally slim body shape of Chinese females, this is a stringent requirement compared to that of the ICD-10 and DSM-IV, where a weight loss of 15% is required. It implies that mild forms of anorexia nervosa will be excluded.

Two of the eight types of personality disorders listed in ICD-10 are excluded in the CCMD-2-R. These are anxious and dependent personality disorders. This may be because many of their defining features are normative or tolerated in the Chinese culture. The category of pathological gambling is also absent in Chinese classification.

The somewhat pejorative heading of sexual perversion is used to include disorders of sexual orientation, sexual preference, and gender identity. The whole ICD-10 block of psychological and behavioral disorders associated with sexual development and orientation is excluded. Pedophilia is excluded. In mental retardation, a borderline intelligence category is added.

The part relating to mental disorders in childhood and adolescence of the CCMD-2-R classification is a condensed version of the ICD-10 and DSM-IV. Because complex classifications are believed to be perplexing to Chinese psychiatrists, subtypes and novel categories are deleted. Examples are hyperkinetic disorder, conduct disorder, oppositional defiant disorder, reactive/disinhibited attachment disorder of childhood. The category of sibling rivalry disorder is not included, apparently because of the one-child-per-couple family plan enforced in China since 1980.

Cuba

The development of the various editions of the Cuban glossary of psychiatry started in 1975. They have attempted to reflect the realities and needs of Cuba in particular within the general framework of Latin America culture [86].

The third edition includes a number of contributions on the diagnosis of mental disorders as experienced in Cuba, covering adult and child psychiatry. A basic principle in the development was to be similar to ICD-10, with minimal differences. In line with this, the coding system was faithfully followed. Contributions and changes were incorporated through the employment of the fifth digit in the diagnostic code or through the utilization of codes not used in ICD-10. The diagnostic guidelines were also respected to the largest possible extent. In some cases, supplemental text was added.

There is a chapter on "syndromes of difficult placement", often referred to as culture bound syndromes. This includes widely known folk syndromes, such as amok, brain fag rust, as well as syndromes and idioms of distress reported by Cuban psychiatrists. Illustrative of the latter is obriu, which refers to certain children believed to have the power to exercise a malign supernatural influence on their relatives, particularly siblings, who as a consequence can experience various illnesses and even die.

The multiaxial scheme uses six axes. Axis I refers to clinical diagnosis including both mental and non-mental disorders. Axis II refers to disabilities. Disablements in personal care, occupational functioning, functioning in the family and broader social functioning are included. Axis III refers to psycho-environmental (adverse) factors. Axis IV includes other psycho-environmental factors such as living alone. Axis V refers to maladaptive behavior and psychological needs, which includes conditions such as hypertrophic affective needs, indecisiveness and difficulties managing hostility. Axis VI includes other significant factors such as those resulting from laboratory tests and responses to therapeutic interventions.

A significant outcome of the Cuban classification is the stimulation of the first Latin American glossary of psychiatry as a Latin American annotation of ICD-10.

Africa

In 1986 three African psychiatrists from Algeria, Morocco and Tunisia edited the first *Manual for North African Practitioners*, which reflects the influence of the French psychiatric diagnostic system. A prominent feature of the manual is its emphasis on organic problems that are not part of the Anglo-Saxon definition of mental disorders. In general, somatization seems to dominate the psychiatric picture reflected in the manual. The listing of chronic delusional psychoses, confusional psychoses and "bouffées délir-antes" as major types of mental illness reflect the influence of French nosology [87].

India

Wig and Singh [88] first reported their experience with the existing classifi-cations (ICD-7 and DSM-I) and suggested some modifications derived from their clinical observations. They mostly found both systems useful in India. However, they suggested the landmark inclusion of a category which they named "acute psychosis of uncertain etiology", with subdivisions (with predominantly confusional picture and with predominantly paranoid-hallucinatory picture). It is noteworthy that they differentiated it from hysterical psychosis, which they included in the category of reactive psych-osis, which had further subdivisions. Later, Wig and Narang [89] described cases of acute short-lived hysterical psychosis following some major life event. This kind of psychosis was seen more often in people with hysterical personality, or who had suffered from hysterical illness in the past. The psychosis began suddenly and dramatically with onset related to an event which was profoundly upsetting for the individual. It terminated abruptly leaving no residual defect, and recurrences were possible if the stress was not alleviated.

ICD-10 FIELD TRIALS IN DEVELOPING COUNTRIES

The international field trial of ICD-10 included 97 centers involving 568 clinicians. They examined 2460 patients and made a total of 9276 evalu-ations. [90]. Of these, 26 centers (27%), 98 clinicians (17%), 706 evaluated patients (29%), and 2144 assessments (23%) were from 14 developing countries (Bahrain, Brazil, China, Colombia, Egypt, India, Republic of Korea, Mexico, Nigeria, Pakistan, Peru, Sudan, Turkey and Uruguay). Most clinicians reported that the draft document was easy to understand and use and that the classification provided a good fit for the vast majority of the clinical conditions encountered in clinical settings. The trial also provided valuable indications about changes needed for subsequent versions.

Some of the developing countries have analyzed the country experiences of the field trial. The WHO Study Group from India [91] had nine centers participating in the trial. The field trial's investigators made a total of 671 assessments. Of these, nearly 58% were joint assessments, while 42% were case summary assessments. The most common diagnoses covered were mood disorders, schizophrenia, neurotic disorders, and drug dependence. Organic disorders and mental retardation were very few in numbers. The results showed that the ICD-10 was quite adequate in its face validity, reliability, applicability, and ease of use. In Kuwait, the draft guidelines were applied in 63 patients diagnosed as suffering from schizophrenia [92]. They found that first rank symptoms (FRS) were present in 62% of patients. Delusional perception was the most common FRS. They cautioned about the need for clinicians in eliciting FRS, in view of the socially shared beliefs about the influence of God's will, the devil and/or sorcery. Okubo et al. [93] found the interdiagnostician reliability in the ICD-10 field trial in Japan to be high for schizophrenia and mood disorders. The reliability in ratings on neurotic, stress related and somatoform disorders was less good. They also found that the subtyping of schizophrenia in ICD-10 was more reliable than that made using DSM-III.

The experience of psychiatrists from the Arab countries is available from clinical studies and ICD-10 field trials. As part of the field trials of ICD-10, eight centers evaluated 233 patients with 614 assessments. The inter-rater reliability was found to range between an almost perfect (0.81–1) to substantial agreement (0.61–0.80) in diagnosing organic disorders, substance use disorders, schizophrenic, schizotypal and delusional disorders, affective disorders and neurotic and stress related disorders. The categories of psychological development and child and adolescent disorders were diagnosed less frequently and the agreement between raters was lower. Difficulties in using the research criteria were identified in the domain of simple schizophrenia and dissociative vs. conversion disorders [94].

One category that did not find a place in the ICD-10 was that of patients presenting with bizarre, inappropriate behavior, with marked acting out and emotional outbursts. The condition is frequently precipitated by an intrapsychic or external stress and associated with perceptual disorders that do not satisfy the criteria for true hallucinations. These are usually wish fulfilling, seem to be under the control of the patient and are usually vivid, reflecting the cultural experiences of the patient for his or her emotional state. The condition may also be complicated by temporary motor or sensory disability and occasionally a sense of being possessed. These clusters of symptoms are referred to as hysterical. The classical division into conversion and dissociation is arbitrary and unsatisfactory. It might be more useful to identify acute and chronic hysterical conditions rather than conversion and dissociation, as the latter division does not help either in management or in predicting outcome. Another domain in which Arab psychiatrists found a difficulty in using the ICD-10 was that of negative symptoms in schizophrenia.

A number of authors have reviewed the adaptability of current classifications to the needs of the developing countries [85, 95–110].

There are three broad streams of ideas that emerge from the review of experience of use of the ICD-10 in developing countries. Firstly, there is a recognition of the importance of psychiatric classification among the psychiatrists of developing countries. This is reflected in a large number of efforts to use and evaluate the classification in the different clinical settings. Secondly, the majority of the efforts to modify the classification system are sporadic and cross-sectional. A number of important leads have been identified but not adequately followed up with systematic studies to influence the classification. Thirdly, there is evidence that the classification can be moulded to meet the needs of the developing countries when sufficient new experiences and information are generated and shared with the international community. A good example is the category of acute psychoses. Future efforts should be systematic and longitudinal.

SHORTCOMINGS OF CURRENT CLASSIFICATORY SYSTEMS

The shortcomings of current classificatory systems arise from three areas: (a) cultural differences, (b) health services and (c) clinical needs.

Shortcomings Related to Cultural Differences

The contemporary psychiatric diagnosis and classification has evolved in Europe and America in the last 100 years and reflects the thinking and cultural bias of that society. Many observers have stressed that patients in developing countries express themselves more easily in somatic than in psychological terms [111–117]. As a result, many categories based on psychological symptoms are difficult to apply in the countries of the Third World. Many conditions commonly seen in developed countries, like anorexia nervosa, phobic and panic disorders, sexual deviations, personality disorders, etc., are uncommon in developing countries. On the other hand, acute transient psychotic disorders, hysterical symptoms and multiple somatic symptoms are very common here.

The need for a culturally sensitive international classification is expressed differently by the different researchers. Some emphasize the need for cultural sensitivity of the professionals [61, 72]. Two views reflect this position: "In the African group a tendency to externally oriented direct expression prevails in contrast with more direct and self-oriented expression patterns in the occidental group" [118]; "Psychiatrists who examine patients should be aware of the details and boundaries of socioculturally shared beliefs in order to be able to filter out pathological, i.e. culture-alien beliefs from the repertoire of beliefs expressed by patients" [92].

Some view the cultural differences in a positive manner. Howard *et al.* [117], studying disaster related mental health problems, conclude as follows: "By comparing and contrasting diverse populations with culturally valid instruments, investigators can hope to discover which types of psychopathology and mental illness are 'common', that is prevalent, reliable, and valid in all populations; which are 'shared' by some but not all populations; and which, if any, may be 'unique' to only one population."

On the other hand, others consider cultural factors as so significant that the current classifications are inadequate and totally inappropriate. An example of the view is: "These endeavours strengthen the biomedical ideology that psychiatric disorders are uniform cross-culturally. In so doing, projects undermine the possibility that workers will conceptualise descriptions of patient life circumstances in culturally meaningful terms, and give credence to locally controlled modes of solving problems of human distress" [119].

However, recognizing the need for an international classification, the way ahead would be to systematically document the differences and integrate the experiences of developing countries into the international systems. The responsibility for this mainly lies on the psychiatrists of developing countries [115].

Shortcomings on Health Service Grounds

A large number of mental health problems, including severe mental disorders, in developing countries do not reach psychiatrists and are cared for by non-psychiatrists. With recent emphasis on incorporation of psychiatric services into primary health care, primary care workers and physicians will use psychiatric diagnoses increasingly. The existing classifications are obviously too complex for such use. It is also to be kept in mind that, for the majority of the routine psychiatric cases in developing countries, there are only a limited number of diagnostic categories that are regularly and frequently used. A survey done in India is illustrative of this point [96]. A questionnaire was sent to psychiatric specialists of general hospitals and mental hospitals regarding the use of ICD-9 during the year 1983. A total of 48 respondents, who had seen 11 430 cases in general and mental hospital settings, considered the ICD-9 as "mostly suitable" for their needs. None of them felt that it was useless or unsuitable for the majority of their cases. Four diagnostic categories of ICD-9, 296 (affective psychoses), 295 (schizophrenia), 300 (neurotic disorders), and 298 (other non-organic psychosis), covered 85% of all cases seen. Organic psychoses and mental retardation added another 5% to the cases. Some of the least used categories were 305 (non-dependent use of drugs), 302 (sexual deviations), 301 (personality disorders) and 297 (paranoid states). Of the respondents, 37% felt there was a need for an additional category of "acute psychoses" not well covered at present under categories of 295, 296, or 298.

Shortcomings on Clinical Grounds

The contemporary psychiatric classifications are far from perfect, as the aetiology of most psychiatric disorders remains unknown. Many severe disorders have diffuse boundaries, and their clinical pictures merge into each other, for example, schizophrenia and affective disorders.

There are still many areas in ICD-10 which are inadequate for developing countries, e.g. classification of acute and transient psychotic disorders, somatoform disorders, culture bound symptoms, child and personality disorders, etc. Only good research work done in developing countries can provide a framework for better classification than available at present.

FUTURE NEEDS OF DEVELOPING COUNTRIES IN PSYCHIATRIC CLASSIFICATION

The observation of Stengel [120] 40 years ago, that the lack of a common classification of mental disorders has defeated attempts at comparing psychiatric observations and the results of treatments undertaken in various countries or even in various centers in the same country, is relevant even today.

It is true that the field has come quite far from the complex and confusing scenario of the 1950s. There are now classifications which have evolved taking into consideration multicentered collaborative efforts, field trials, validity exercises, follow-up studies, and data from all recent advances in the field of genetics, biochemistry, neuroimaging, etc. The most recent revisions of classificatory systems, ICD-10 and DSM-IV, have come out with far greater clarity and applicability, making their use almost universal. However, as previous sections of this chapter have demonstrated, there is still a vast scope for improvement to meet the expectations and aspirations of the international community, especially practitioners, carers, and sufferers from mental disorders in the Third World countries. With the ever increasing emphasis in recent times on globalization, and easier and faster accessibility of information and communication, the benefit of advances in modern health care systems should be available in equal measures all over the world. A reliable and valid expression or language in psychiatry will be a major step forward in that direction, if it can be understood across all regions and cultures of the world. A classification system which serves this purpose in the field of mental health is expected to meet a variety of needs of its potential users, including clinicians, researchers and administrators.

ICD-10 is an "international" classification developed by WHO with the help of experts from both the developing and developed countries. DSM-III and IV are essentially "national" classifications for use in the United States. All countries of the world (including the United States) are required to submit health data for international purposes to WHO using the existing international classification of diseases—at present ICD-10. It is all right for any department of psychiatry in an Asian or African country to use DSM-IV or any other classification, but for the official purposes, at the national and international level, the mental health data must be recorded and reported as per ICD-10.

ICD-10 has already incorporated many of the good points of DSM-III, e.g. use of explicit diagnostic criteria, avoidance of terms like neurosis, and acceptance of a multiaxial system. In turn, DSM-IV has incorporated many of the changes introduced in ICD-10. Thus, at present, the differences between the two systems of classifications have been greatly reduced.

In an academic/research department in a developing country, one can use any classification as long as it meets the clinical/teaching and research needs of that department, but it should also be possible to translate that classification into ICD-10 for reporting of national and international data.

ICD-10 at present is probably the best suited classification for the needs of developing countries. It has been developed with the input by experts from many countries in Asia and Africa. It has also been extensively tried in many field centers and found practical and reliable. It has the required flexibility to be useful both at the day-to-day clinical level as well as for the more stringent research purposes. ICD-10 is not *one* but a family of classifications. It offers related but different sets of classifications for clinical psychiatrists, primary care physicians, advanced research workers and for multiaxial use. This flexibility of approach makes it eminently suitable for various types of national needs.

Fabrega [121] highlights the several crucial ways in which culture and social processes limit the establishment of an internationally valid system of diagnosis in psychiatry. Similarly, Stengel [120] and Sartorius [122] reiterated that international classification must not aim to oust or replace regional classifications, which often have valuable functions in the local contexts in which they are devised. No single classificatory system will suffice for all purposes. The correct diagnostic scheme is the one that accomplishes its explicit pragmatic aim by addressing the relevant level of description.

CONCLUSIONS

Mental health professionals in developing countries find themselves in a difficult position in the matter of diagnosis and classification in psychiatry. The psychological concepts and the psychiatric nomenclature of the indigenous traditional systems of medicine, though still popular with the public, are insufficient to accommodate the growing knowledge of psychiatry or the complex needs of modern health services. A total switch over to the American or European classification, however, is equally frustrating. Recognizing the need for an international consensus, psychiatrists in developing countries have generally supported the WHO's efforts to develop international classifications like the current ICD-10.

The research diagnostic criteria of both ICD-10 and DSM-IV need to be widely tested in developing countries. The cultural dimension in psychiatric classification is very important for non-European cultures, i.e. for the countries of Asia, Africa and South America. We have a paradoxical situation that research is least active in cultural settings in which the cultural influence seems to be most important, i.e. in the traditional rural and tribal societies in developing countries.

In the psychiatric classification we have moved forward by adopting empirical criteria for diagnosis. In psychiatric research we will also move a step further if we simplify terms and define them empirically in a neutral way without the load of European philosophical controversies. The language of science should be simple and as far as possible culture-free. The complicated language of psychiatry based on philosophical concepts of nineteenth century Europe makes it very difficult for the non-European to contribute effectively. The rich philosophical heritage of other current world cultures, like the Indian, Islamic or Chinese, is not reflected in the terminology used in psychiatry today. It is true that modern science and psychiatry have a history, which cannot be ignored, and psychiatric language is part of that history. But a simplification of psychiatric terms, reducing their

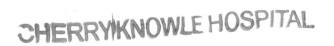

dependency on only one cultural tradition, i.e. European, will make it possible for mental health professionals of other cultures to contribute more effectively to psychiatric research. The overall goal should be the one summarized by Mezzich *et al.* [86]:

> The developments of comprehensive diagnostic modes and regional adaptations of ICD-10 reveal the ebullience of the diagnostic field, especially when appraised from a broad international perspective. It seems likely that the ongoing tension between universality and diversity in diagnostic systems will continue to yield innovative solutions. Emerging proposals are increasingly involving integrated assessments of health status and according pointed attention to the ethical requirements of psychological diagnosis. These proposals must be carefully formulated and thoughtfully and widely evaluated if they are to contribute effectively to the fulfilment of diagnosis as a conceptual and practical tool for clinical care, health promotion and epidemiology.

These are the challenges and opportunities for the future development of psychiatric classification in developing countries.

REFERENCES

1. Martinez C., Marlin H.W. (1966) Folk diseases among urban Mexican-Americans. *JAMA*, **196**: 147–150.
2. Barlett P., Low S. (1980) Nervios in rural Costa Rica. *Med. Anthropology*, **4**: 523–529.
3. Rubel A.J., O'Nell C.W., Collado-Ardon R. (1984) *Susto, a Folk Illness*. University of California Press, Berkeley.
4. Saeed K., Gater R., Hussain A., Mubbashar M. (2000) The prevalence, classification and treatment of mental disorders among attenders of native faith healers in rural Pakistan. *Soc. Psychiatry Psychiatr. Epidemiol.*, **35**: 480–485.
5. Wig N.N. (1990) Indian concepts of mental health and their impact on care of the mentally ill. *Int. J. Ment. Health*, **18**: 71–80.
6. Mora G. (1980) Historical and theoretical trends in psychiatry. In *Comprehensive Textbook of Psychiatry*, 3rd edn (Eds H.I. Kaplan, A.M. Freedman, B.J. Sadock), pp. 4–98. Williams and Wilkins. Philadelphia.
7. Weiss M.G., Desai A., Jadhav S., Gupta L., Channabasavanna S.M., Doongaji D.R., Behere P.B. (1988) Humoral concepts of mental illness in India. *Soc. Sci. Med.*, **27**: 471–477.
8. Dube K.C. (1978) Nosology and therapy of mental illness in Ayurveda. *Comp. Med. East West*, **6**: 209–228.
9. Deb Sikdar B.M. (1961) Glimpses of medico-psychological practices in ancient India. *Ind. J. Psychiatry*, **11**: 250–259.
10. Varma L.P. (1965) Psychiatry in Ayurveda. *Ind. J. Psychiatry*, **7**: 292–312.
11. Narayana Reddy G.N., Ramu M.G., Venkataram B.S. (1987) Concept of manas (psyche) in Ayurveda. *NIMHANS J.*, **5**: 125–131.
12. Balodhi J.P. (1987) Constituting the outlines of a philosophy of Ayurveda— mainly on mental health import. *Ind. J. Psychiatry*, **29**: 127–130.
13. Graziani J.S. (1980) *Arabic Medicine in the Eleventh Century as Represented in the Works of Ibn Jazlah*. Hamdard Academy, Karachi.

14. Lambo T.A. (1965) Psychiatry in the tropics. *Lancet*, **ii**: 1119–1121.
15. Lambo T.A. (1971) The African mind in contemporary conflict. *WHO Chron.*, **25**: 343–353.
16. Ko S.M., Tsoi W.F. (1991) New admissions to psychiatric wards in a general hospital. *Ann. Acad. Med. Singapore*, **20**: 204–207.
17. Tsoi W.F. (1993) First admission schizophrenia: clinical manifestation and subtypes. *Singapore Med. J.*, **34**: 399–402.
18. Erinosho O.A. (1977) Mental health delivery-systems and post treatment performance in Nigeria. *Acta Psychiatr. Scand.*, **55**: 1–9.
19. Binite A. (1981) Psychiatric disorders in a rural practice in the Bendel State of Nigeria. *Acta Psychiatr. Scand.*, **64**: 273–280.
20. Ebigbo P.O. (1982) Development of a culture specific (Nigeria) screening scale of somatic complaints indicating psychiatric disturbances. *Cult. Med. Psychiatry*, **6**: 29–43.
21. Oyarebu K. (1980) Diagnostic and demographic classification of psychiatric patients admission in Bendel state of Nigeria. A review of the University of Benin Teaching Hospital (UBTH) psychiatric inpatients' record of 1980. *Acta Psychiatr. Belg.*, **83**: 501–508.
22. Gureje O., Bamidele R. (1999) Thirteen year outcome among Nigerian outpatients with schizophrenia. *Soc. Psychiatry Psychiatr. Epidemiol.*, **34**: 147–151.
23. Hartog J. (1973) Ninety-six Malay psychiatric patients—characteristics and preliminary epidemiology. *Int. J. Soc. Psychiatry*, **19**: 49–59.
24. Matuja W.P., Ndosi N.K., Collins M. (1995) Nature of referrals to the psychiatric unit at Muhibili Medical Centre, Dar es Salaam. *East Afr. Med. J.*, **72**: 761–765.
25. Avasthi A., Khan M.K.R., Elroey A.M. (1991) Inpatient sociodemographic and diagnostic study from a psychiatric hospital in Libya. *Int. J. Soc. Psychiatry*, **37**: 267–279.
26. Turkson S.N. (1998) Psychiatric diagnosis among referred patients in Ghana. *East Afr. Med. J.*, **75**: 336–338.
27. Johnson F.Y. (1997) Ward Six Psychiatric Unit at the Port Moresby General Hospital: a historical review and admission statistics from 1980 to 1989. *P.N.G. Med. J.*, **40**: 79–88.
28. Saxena S., Nepal M.K., Mohan D. (1988) DSM-III Axis I diagnosis of Indian psychiatric patients with somatic complaints. *Am. J. Psychiatry*, **145**: 1023–1024.
29. Saxena S., Wig N.N. (1983) Psychiatric problems of Afghan refugees in Delhi: a study of 152 outpatients. *Ind. J. Psychiatry*, **25**: 40–45.
30. Saxena S. (1989) Diagnosis of refugees. *Am. J. Psychiatry*, **146**: 410–411.
31. Saxena S., Prasad K.V. (1989) DSM-III sub-classification of dissociative disorders applied to psychiatric outpatients in India. *Am. J. Psychiatry*, **146**: 261–262.
32. Sethi S., Khanna S. (1993) Phenomenology of mania in eastern India. *Psychopathology*, **26**: 274–278.
33. Patel V., Musara T., Butau T., Maramba P., Fuyane S. (1995) Concepts of mental illness and medical pluralism in Harare. *Psychol. Med.*, **25**: 485–493.
34. Keegstra H.J. (1986) Depressive disorders in Ethiopia. A standardised assessment using the SADD schedule. *Acta Psychiatr. Scand.*, **73**: 658–664.
35. Kortmann F. (1988) DSM-III in Ethiopia: a feasibility study. *Eur. Arch. Psychiatry Clin. Neurosci.*, **237**: 101–105.
36. Skodol A.E., Schwartz S., Dohrenwend B.P., Levav I., Shrout P.E. (1994) Minor depression in a cohort of young adults in Israel. *Arch. Gen. Psychiatry*, **51**: 542–551.

37. Mete L., Schnurr P.P., Rosenberg S.D., Oxman T.E., Doganer I., Sorias S. (1993) Language content and schizophrenia in acute phase Turkish patients. *Soc. Psychiatry Psychiatr. Epidemiol.*, **28**: 275–280.
38. Shooka A., al-Haddad M.K., Raees A. (1998) OCD in Bahrain: a phenomenological profile. *Int. J. Soc. Psychiatry*, **44**: 147–154.
39. Okasha A., el Dawla A., Khalil A.H., Saad A. (1993) Presentation of acute psychosis in an Egyptian sample: a transcultural comparison. *Compr. Psychiatry*, 7: 4–9.
40. Inoue S. (1993) Hebephrenia as the most prevalent subtype of schizophrenia in Japan. *Jpn. J. Psychiatry Neurol.*, **47**: 505–514.
41. Singh G., Sachdeva J.S. (1980) A clinical and follow-up study of atypical psychoses. *Ind. J. Psychiatry*, **22**: 167–172.
42. Kapur R.L., Pandurangi A.K. (1979) A comparative study of reactive psychosis and acute psychosis without precipitating stress. *Br. J. Psychiatry*, **135**: 544–550.
43. Pandurangi A.K., Kapur R.L. (1980) Reactive psychosis—a prospective study. *Acta Psychiatr. Scand.*, **61**: 89–95.
44. Kuruvilla K., Sitalaksmi N. (1982) Hysterical psychosis. *Ind. J. Psychiatry*, **24**: 352–359.
45. Indian Council of Medical Research (1983) *Final Report of the Project "The Phenomenology and Natural History of Acute Psychosis"*. Indian Council of Medical Research, New Delhi.
46. Wig N.N., Parhee R. (1988) Acute and transient psychoses: view from developing countries. In *International Classification in Psychiatry—Unity and Diversity* (Eds J.E. Mezzich, M. von Cranach), pp. 115–121. Cambridge University Press, Cambridge.
47. Varma V.K., Wig N.N., Phookun H.R., Misra A.K., Khare C.B., Tripathi B.M., Behere P.B., Yoo E.S., Susser E.S. (1997) First onset schizophrenia in the community: relationship of urbanization with onset, early manifestations and typology. *Acta Psychiatr. Scand.*, **96**: 431–438.
48. Susser E., Wanderling J. (1994) Epidemiology of nonaffective acute remitting psychosis vs schizophrenia: sex and sociocultural setting. *Arch. Gen. Psychiatry*, **51**: 294–301.
49. Jablensky A., Sartorius N., Ernberg G., Anker M., Korten A., Cooper J.E., Day R., Bertelsen A. (1992) Schizophrenia: manifestations, incidence and course in different cultures: a WHO ten country study. *Psychol. Med.*, Suppl. 20.
50. Susser E., Varma V.K., Malhotra S., Conover S., Amador X.F. (1995) Delineation of acute and transient psychotic disorders in a developing country setting. *Br. J. Psychiatry*, **167**: 216–219.
51. Susser E., Varma V.K., Mattoo S.K. (1998) Long-term course of acute brief psychosis in a developing country setting. *Br. J. Psychiatry*, **173**: 226–230.
52. Jablensky A. (1996) Diagnosis and classification. In *Psychiatry for the Developing World* (Eds D. Tantam, L. Appleby, A. Duncan), pp. 27–50. Gaskell, London.
53. Okasha A. (1993) Presentation of acute psychoses in an Egyptian sample: a transcultural comparison. *Compr. Psychiatry*, **34**: 4–9.
54. Kortmann F. (1990) Psychiatric case finding in Ethiopia: shortcomings of the self reporting questionnaire. *Cult. Med. Psychiatry*, **14**: 381–391.
55. Kinzie J.D., Ryals J., Cottington F., McDemott J.F. (1973) Cross-cultural study of depressive symptoms in Hawaii. *Int. J. Soc. Psychiatry*, **19**: 19–24.
56. Giel R., d'Arrigo Busnello E., Climent C.E., Elhakim A.S., Ibrahim H.H., Ladrido-Ignacio L., Wig N.N. (1981) The classification of psychiatric disorder:

a reliability study in the WHO collaborative study on strategies for extending mental health care. *Acta Psychiatr. Scand.*, **63**: 61–74.

57. Jablensky A., Sartorius N., Gulbinat W., Ernberg G. (1981) Characteristics of depressive patients contacting psychiatric services in cultures. A report from the WHO collaborative study on the assessment of depressive disorders. *Acta Psychiatr. Scand.*, **63**: 367–383.

58. Eker D. (1985) Diagnosis of mental disorders among Turkish and American clinicians. *Int. J. Soc. Psychiatry*, **31**: 99–109.

59. Chang W.C. (1985) A cross-cultural study of depressive symptomatology. *Cult. Med. Psychiatry*, **9**: 295–317.

60. Nakane Y., Ohta Y., Uchino J., Takada K., Yan H.Q., Wand X.D., Min S.K., Lee H.Y. (1988) Comparative study of affective disorders in three Asian countries. 1. Differences in diagnostic classification. *Acta Psychiatr. Scand.*, **78**: 698–705.

61. Diefenbacher A., Heim G. (1994) Somatic symptoms in Turkish and German depressed patients. *Psychosom. Med.*, **56**: 551–556.

62. Hsu L.K., Folstein M.F. (1997) Somatoform disorders in Caucasian and Chinese Americans. *J. Nerv. Ment. Dis.*, **185**: 382–387.

63. Alexander P.J., Joseph, S., Das A. (1997) Limited utility of ICD-10 and DSM-IV classification of dissociative and conversion disorders in India. *Acta Psychiatr. Scand.*, **95**: 177–182.

64. Lee S. (1993) Fat phobic and non-fat phobic anorexia nervosa: a comparative study of 70 Chinese patients in Hong Kong. *Psychol. Med.*, **23**: 999–1017.

65. Wig N.N. (1960) Problems of mental health in India. *J. Clin. Soc.*, **17**: 48–52.

66. Singh G. (1985) Dhat syndrome revisited. *Ind. J. Psychiatry*, **27**: 119–122.

67. Behere P.B., Natraj G.S. (1984) Dhat syndrome—the phenomenology of a culture bound sex neurosis of the orient. *Ind. J. Psychiatry*, **26**: 76–78.

68. Chadda R.K. (1995) Dhat syndrome: is it a distinct illness entity?—A study of illness behaviour characteristics. *Acta Psychiatr. Scand.*, **91**: 136–139.

69. Varma V.K. (1971) Classification of psychiatric disorders for use in India (neuroses). *Ind. J. Psychiatry*, **13**: 1–6.

70. Kon Y. (1994) Amok. *Br. J. Psychiatry*, **165**: 685–689.

71. Durust R. (1993) "Brain-fag" syndrome: manifestation of transculturation in an Ethiopian Jewish immigrant. *Israel J. Psychiatry Rel. Sci.*, **30**: 223–232.

72. Loranger A.W., Sartorius N., Andreoli A., Berger P., Buchhein P., Channabasavanna S.M., Coid B., Dahl A., Diekstra R.F., Ferguson B. *et al.* (1994) The International Personality Disorder Examination. The World Health Organization Alcohol, Drug Abuse, and Mental Health Administration international pilot study of personality disorders. *Arch. Gen. Psychiatry*, **51**: 215–224.

73. Moriya N., Miyake Y., Minakawa K., Ikuta N., Nishizono-Maher A. (1993) Diagnosis and clinical features of borderline personality disorders in the east and west: a preliminary report. *Compr. Psychiatry*, **34**: 418–442.

74. Okasha A., Omar A.M., Lotaief F., Ghanem M., Seif el Dawla A., Okasha T. (1996) Comorbidity of axis I and II diagnoses in a sample of Egyptian patients with neurotic disorders. *Compr. Psychiatry*, **37**: 95–101.

75. Reddy Y.C., Girimaji S., Srinath S. (1993) Comparative study of classification of psychosis of childhood and adolescent onset. *Acta Psychiatr. Scand.*, **87**: 188–191.

76. Abiodun O.A. (1992) Emotional illness in a paediatric population in Nigeria. *East Afr. Med. J.*, **69**: 557–559.

77. Bueber M. (1993) Nursing diagnoses for psychiatric patients in China. *Arch. Psychiatr. Nurs.*, **7**: 16–22.
78. Al-Faris E., Al-Subaie A., Khoja T., Al-Ansary L., Abdul-Rehmeem F., Al-Hamdan N., Al-Mazrou Y., Abdul-Moneim H., El Khwsky F. (1997) Training primary health care physicians in Saudi Arabia to recognise psychiatric illness. *Acta Psychiatr. Scand.*, **96**: 439–444.
79. Keshavan K., Sriram T.G., Kaliaperumal V.G., Subramanya K.R. (1991) Mental health knowledge and skills of general hospital nursing staff: an exploratory study. *Int. J. Soc. Psychiatry*, **37**: 280–284.
80. Lee S. (1994) Neurasthenia and Chinese psychiatry in the 1990s. *J. Psychosom. Res.*, **38**: 487–491.
81. Lee S. (1995) The Chinese classification of mental disorders. *Br. J. Psychiatry*, **167**: 216–219.
82. Lee S. (1996) Cultures in psychiatric nosology: the CCMD-2 R and international classification of mental disorders. *Cult. Med. Psychiatry*, **20**: 421–472.
83. Lee S. (1997) A Chinese perspective of somatoform disorders. *J. Psychosom. Res.*, **43**: 115–119.
84. Lee S. (1999) Diagnosis postponed: shenjing shuairuo and the transformation of psychiatry in post-Mao China. *Can. J. Psychiatry*, **44**: 817–881.
85. Zheng Y.P., Lin K.M., Zhao J.P., Zhang M.Y., Yong D. (1994) Comparative study of diagnostic systems: Chinese Classification of Mental Disorders, 2nd edn versus DSM-III-R. *Compr. Psychiatry*, **35**: 441–449.
86. Mezzich J.E., Otero-Ojeda A.A., Lee S. (2000) International psychiatric diagnosis. In *Comprehensive Textbook of Psychiatry*, 7th edn (Eds B.J. Sadock, V.A. Sadock), pp. 839–853. Lippincott, Williams and Wilkins, Philadelphia.
87. al-Issa I. (1990) Culture and mental illness in Algeria. *Int. J. Soc. Psychiatry*, **36**: 230–240.
88. Wig N.N., Singh G. (1967) A proposed classification of psychiatric disorders for use in India. *Ind. J. Psychiatry*, **9**: 158–171.
89. Wig N.N., Narang R.L. (1969) Hysterical psychosis. *Ind. J. Psychiatry*, **11**: 93–100.
90. Sartorius N., Kaelber C.T., Cooper J.E., Roper M.T., Rae D.S., Gulbinat W., Üstün T.B., Regier D.A. (1993) Progress towards achieving a common language in psychiatry. I: Results from the field trial of the clinical guidelines accompanying the WHO classification of mental and behavioural disorders in ICD-10. *Arch. Gen. Psychiatry*, **50**: 115–124.
91. WHO Study Group (1992) ICD-10 field trials in India—a report. *Ind. J. Psychiatry*, **34**: 198–221.
92. Al-Ansazi E.A., Emaza M.M., Mirza I.A., El-Islam M.F. (1989) Schizophrenia in ICD-10: a field trial of suggested diagnostic guidelines. *Compr. Psychiatry*, **30**: 416–419.
93. Okubo Y., Komiyama M., Nakane Y., Takahashi T., Yamashita I., Nishizono M., Takahashi R. (1992) Collaborative multicenter field trial of the draft ICD-10 in Japan—interdiagnostician reliability and disagreement: a report from the WHO project on "Field trials of ICD-10, Chapter V". *Jpn. J. Psychiatry Neurol.*, **46**: 23–35.
94. Okasha A., el Dawla A. (1992) Reliability of ICD-10 research criteria: an Arab perspective. *Acta Psychiatr. Scand.*, **86**: 484–488.
95. Wig N.N. (1983) DSM-III: a perspective from the third world. In: *International Perspectives on DSM-III* (Eds R.L. Spitzer, J.B.W. Williams, A.E. Skodol), pp. 79–89, American Psychiatric Press, Washington.

96. Kala A.K. (1985) Utility of ICD-9 for Indian patients: an opinion survey. *Ind. J. Psychiatry*, **27**: 253–254.
97. Varma V.K., Malhotra S. (1985) Diagnosis and classification of acute psychotic disorders in the developing world. *Ind. J. Soc. Psychiatry*, **1**: 11–21.
98. Kitamura T. (1989) Psychiatric diagnosis in Japan. 2. Reliability of conventional diagnosis and discrepancies with Research Diagnostic Criteria diagnosis. *Psychopathology*, **22**: 250–259.
99. Kitamura T., Shima S., Sakio E., Kato M. (1989) Psychiatric diagnosis in Japan. 1. A study on diagnostic labels used by practitioners. *Psychopathology*, **22**: 239–249.
100. Wig N.N. (1990) Requirement for classification of mental disorders in the world today. In: *Psychiatry: A World Perspective*, vol. 1 (Eds C.N. Stefanis, A.D. Rabavilas, C.R. Soldatos), pp. 26–33. Elsevier, Amsterdam.
101. Wig N.N. (1990) The third-world perspective on psychiatric diagnosis and classification. In *Sources and Traditions of Classification in Psychiatry* (Eds N. Sartorius, A. Jablensky, D.A. Regier, J.D. Burke, Jr., R.M.A. Hirschfeld), pp. 181–210. Hogrefe and Huber, Toronto.
102. Chen H.Y., Luo H.C., Phillips M.R. (1992) Computerised psychiatric diagnoses based on euclidean distances: a Chinese example. *Acta Psychiatr. Scand.*, **85**: 11–14.
103. Khandelwal S.K. (1992) Diagnosis and classification in psychiatry. In *Postgraduate Psychiatry* (Eds J.N. Vyas, N. Ahuja), pp. 316–331. Churchill Livingstone, New Delhi.
104. Daradkeh T.K. (1994) The reliability and validity of the proposed axis V (disabilities) of ICD. *Br. J. Psychiatry*, **165**: 683–685.
105. Joubert P.M., Bodemer W. (1994) Psychiatric classification—an ongoing process. *S. Afr. Med. J.*, **84**: 47–48.
106. Chen E.Y. (1996) Negative symptoms, neurological signs and neuropsychological impairments in 204 Hong Kong Chinese patients with schizophrenia. *Br. J. Psychiatry*, **168**: 227–233.
107. Altshuler L.L. (1998) Who seeks mental health care in China? Diagnoses of Chinese outpatients according to DSM-III criteria and the Chinese classification system. *Am. J. Psychiatry*, **145**: 872–875.
108. Khandelwal S.K. (2000) Classification of mental disorders: need for a common language. In *Mental Health in India (1950–2000)* (Ed. R. Srinivasa Murthy), pp. 60–72. PAMH, Bangalore.
109. Blay S.L., Bickel H, Cooper B. (1991) Mental illness in a cross-national perspective. Results from a Brazilian and a German community survey among the elderly. *Soc. Psychiatry Psychiatr. Epidemiol.*, **26**: 245–251.
110. Hatta S.M. (1996) A Malay cross-cultural world view and forensic review of amok. *Aust. N.Z.J. Psychiatry*, **30**: 505–510.
111. Alarcon R.D. (1999) Clinical relevance of contemporary cultural psychiatry. *J. Nerv. Ment. Dis.*, **187**: 465–472.
112. Lee S. (1997) A Chinese perspective of somatoform disorders. *J. Psychosom. Res.*, **43**: 115–119.
113. Heerlein A., Santander J., Richter P. (1996) Tolerance of ambiguity in endogenous psychoses from the transcultural viewpoint. *Fortschr. Neurol. Psychiatry*, **64**: 358–361.
114. Holloway G. (1994) Susto and the career path of the victim of an industrial accident: a sociological study. *Soc. Sci. Med.*, **38**: 989–997.

115. Guarnaccia P.J., Rogler L.H. (1999) Research on culture bound syndromes: new directions. *Am. J. Psychiatry*, **156**: 1322–1327.
116. Good B.J. (1996) Culture and DSM-IV diagnosis, knowledge and power. *Cult. Med. Psychiatry*, **20**: 127–132.
117. Howard W.T., Loberiza F.R., Pfohl B.M., Thorne P.S., Magpantay R.L., Woolson R.F. (1999) Initial results, reliability and validity of a mental health survey of Mount Pinatubo disaster victims. *J. Nerv. Ment. Dis.*, **187**: 661–672.
118. Pierloot R.A., Ngoma M. (1988) Hysterical manifestations in Africa and Europe. *Br. J. Psychiatry*, **152**: 112–115.
119. Higginbotham N., Connor L. (1989) Professional ideology and the construction of Western psychiatry in South East Asia. *Int. J. Health Serv.*, **19**: 63–78.
120. Stengel E. (1959) Classification of mental disorders. *WHO Bull.*, **21**: 601–663.
121. Fabrega H. (1992) Diagnosis interminable: toward a culturally sensitive DSM-IV. *J. Nerv. Ment. Dis.*, **180**: 5–7.
122. Sartorius N. (1990) Sources and traditions of psychiatric classification: introduction. In *Sources and Traditions of Classification in Psychiatry* (Eds N. Sartorius, A. Jablensky, D.A. Regier, J.D. Burke, Jr., R.M.A. Hirschfeld), pp. 1–6. Hogrefe and Huber, Toronto.

Index

acupuncture 250, 253
acute psychosis
 Determinants of outcome of severe
  mental disorders (DOSMED)
  258
 developing countries 257–9
 Egypt 259
 Indian Council of Medical Research
  (ICMR) 257–9
 non-affective acute remitting
  psychoses (NARP) 258–9
 of uncertain aetiology in India
  266
adaptation of classifications to PC
  needs 228–36
 diagnosis and disability 233–6
 DSM-IV adaptation for use in
  PC 230–3
 other systems 233
 ICD-10 for use in primary care
  (ICD-10-PHC) 228–30
affective disorders 80
 in primary care 223–6
Africa 128, 266
 Manual for North African Practitioners
  266
 Masai 254
 medical traditions 254
 Shona 254
 Unani/Arabic medicine 250
 see also developing countries
Al Razi 253
Alcohol, Drug Abuse, and Mental
  Health Administration
  (ADAMHA) 54, 198
alcohol problems
 in primary care 223–6
 see also substance use disorder
Alcohol Use Disorders Identification
  Test (AUDIT) 241
Alzheimer's disease 6
American Heart Association
  13

American Medical Association (AMA),
  *Standard Classified Nomenclature of
  Diseases* 48–9
American Medico-Psychological
  Association, Committee on
  Statistics 48
American Psychiatric Association
  (APA) 47–77
American Psychiatric Press 184
amok, Cuba 265
amygdaloid subdivision 90
anorexia nervosa, developing
  countries 261
anxiety disorders 26
 in primary care 223–8
APA classification of mental
  disorders 8, 47–77, 79
 collaborative development of DSM-IV
  and ICD-10 55–6
 developmental process for
  DSM-V 63–9
 diagnostic criteria and
  instruments 53–6
 diagnostic instrument development
  and DSM-III 53–4
 DSM system limitations 57–63
 DSM system strengths 56–7
 future directions 69–71
 historical development 48–56
 international classification and
  DSM-III 54–5
 research planning process for
  DSM-V 64–9
apasmara 252
appearance of objects 4, 158
applicability across settings and
  cultures 16
Arabic or Islamic medicine 253–5
 Al-Razi (Rhazes) 253
 Haly Abbas 253
 Ibn Sena (Avicena) 253
 Ibn-Jazleh 253
 Tib-E-Unani (Greek Medicine) 253

Index compiled by Penelope Allport

Acknowledgements

The Editors would like to thank Drs Paola Bucci, Umberto Volpe and Andrea Dell'Acqua, of the Department of Psychiatry of the University of Naples, for their help in the processing of manuscripts.

The publication has been supported by an unrestricted educational grant from Pfizer, which is hereby gratefully acknowledged.